MEMORY, AGING, AND DEMENTIA

Theory, Assessment, and Treatment

Grover C. Gilmore, Ph.D., is an associate professor of psychology and department chair at Case Western Reserve University. He earned his doctorate in experimental psychology from The Johns Hopkins University, where his training emphasized visual perception and human information processing. He has focused his research interests on the perceptual and memory capabilities of healthy elderly adults and Alzheimer's disease patients. He is currently involved with a program of research relating performance on simple cognitive tasks, such as object identification, to basic visual processing capabilities.

Peter J. Whitehouse, M.D., Ph.D., Associate Professor of Neurology and Chief, Division of Behavioral Neurology at Case Western University, is Director of the Alzheimer Center at University Hospitals of Cleveland (UHC AC). He received his M.D. in 1976 and his Ph.D. in psychology in 1977 from The Johns Hopkins University, and he is also trained in neurology, psychiatry, neuropathology, and neuroscience. Dr. Whitehouse established and developed the UHC AC into a program that has gained local and national recognition, including designation by the Ohio Department on Aging, NIMH, and NIA as an Alzheimer Center of Excellence. His research interests lie in the biological and clinical aspects of Alzheimer's disease and related dementias, and in health care delivery; he has published extensively in these areas. His commitment to improving services for the elderly, particularly in long-term care, has led Dr. Whitehouse to become actively involved in such organizations as the National Alzheimer's Association, the Robert Wood Johnson Foundation, and the Health Care Finance Administration as well as chairing the Governor's Task Force on Alzheimer's Disease for the state of Ohio.

May L. Wykle, Ph.D., R.N., F.A.A.N., is the Florence Cellar Professor of Gerontological Nursing and Chairperson of Psychiatric Mental Health and Gerontological Nursing, Frances Payne Bolton School of Nursing, Case Western Reserve University, and Chairperson in Nursing, Hanna Pavilion, University Hospitals, Cleveland, Ohio. She also directs the Case Western Reserve University Center on Aging and Health. A recipient of an NIMH Geriatric Mental Health Academic Award and director of a 5-year Robert Wood Johnson Teaching Nursing Home Project, Dr. Wykle's research area is geriatric mental health, self-care behaviors among aged cohorts, and family caregiving. Her work has been concentrated on enhancing mental health services in long-term care settings.

MEMORY, AGING, AND DEMENTIA
Theory, Assessment, and Treatment

Grover C. Gilmore, Ph.D.
Peter J. Whitehouse, M.D., Ph.D.
May L. Wykle, Ph.D, R.N., F.A.A.N.

Editors

SPRINGER PUBLISHING COMPANY
New York

Springer Publishing Company, Inc.
536 Broadway
New York, NY 10012

89 90 91 92 93 / 5 4 3 2 1

Library of Cataloging-in-Publication Data

Memory, aging, and dementia : theory, assessment, and treatment / Grover C. Gilmore, Peter J. Whitehouse, May L. Wykle, editors.
p. cm.
Grew out of the conference held in Cleveland, Oct. 1987, sponsored by the University Center on Aging and Health of Case Erstern Reserve University and the Alzheimer Center of University Hospitals of Cleveland.
Includes bibliographical references.
ISBN 0-8261-6470-6
1. Memory disorders in the aged—Congresses. 2. Dementia—Congresses. 3. Alzheimer's disease—Congresses. 4. Aging—Psychological aspects—Congresses. I. Gilmore, Grover C. II. Whitehouse, Peter J. III. Wykle, May L.. IV. Case Western Reserve University. Center on Aging and Health. V. University Hospitals of Cleveland (Ohio). Alzheimer Center.
[DNLM: 1. Aging—physiology—congresses. 2. Alzheimer's Disease—congresses. 3. Dementia—congresses. 4. Health Services for the Aged—congresses. 5. Memory Disorders—in old age—congresses. WM 173.7 M5321 1987]
RC394.M46M46 1989
618.97'6831—dc20
DNLM/DLC
for Library of Congress

89-21717
CIP

Printed in the United States of America

Contents

PART II Alzheimer's Disease: From Gene to Mind

PART III Memory, Alzheimer's, and Related Dementias: Intervention and Care

Contributors

Nancy L. Adams, Ph.D., Assistant Professor, Departments of Neurology and Psychiatry, Case Western Reserve University School of Medicine and Cleveland VA Medical Center

Kathleen Coen Buckwalter, Ph.D., R.N., Associate Professor, College of Nursing, University of Iowa

Nelson Butters, Ph.D., Professor, Department of Psychiatry, University of California School of Medicine (San Diego); Chief, Psychology Service, VA Medical Center, San Diego

Cameron J. Camp, Ph.D., Associate Professor, Department of Psychology, University of New Orleans

John Herbert Growdon, M.D., Associate Professor, Harvard Medical School; Neurologist, Massachusetts General Hospital

J. F. Gusella, Ph.D., Neurogenetics Laboratory, Massachusetts General Hospital and Harvard Medical School

Lisa P. Gwyther, M.S.W., Director, Family Support Program, Duke University Aging Center

William C. Heindel, B.S., Psychology Service, San Diego Veterans Administration Medical Center; Neurosciences Department, The University of California School of Medicine at San Diego

Robert L. Kane, M.D., Dean, School of Public Health, University of Minnesota

Donald H. Kausler, Ph.D., Professor, Department of Psychology, University of Missouri-Columbia

James L. Mack, Ph.D., Assistant Professor, Departments of Neurology and Psychiatry, Case Western Reserve University School of Medicine and University Hospitals of Cleveland

Richard Mayeux, M.D., Associate Professor of Clinical Neurology/Psychology, Neurological Institute, Columbia University College of Physicians and Surgeons

D. R. Crapper McLachlan, M.D., F.R.C.P.(C), Departments of Physiology and Medicine, University of Toronto

Marian B. Patterson, Ph.D., Associate Professor, Departments of Neurology and Psychiatry, Case Western Reserve University School of Medicine and University Hospitals of Cleveland

Leonard W. Poon, Ph.D., Director, Gerontology Center; Professor, Department of Psychology, University of Georgia

Kathryn Perez Riley, Ph.D., Assistant Professor, Department of Psychology, Cleveland State University

David P. Salmon, Ph.D., Psychiatry and Neurosciences Departments, The University of California School of Medicine at San Diego

P. H. St. George-Hyslop, M.D., F.R.C.P.(c), Fellow, Neurogenetics Laboratory, Massachusetts General Hospital and Harvard Medical School

Elizabeth A. L. Stine, Ph.D., Senior Research Associate and Adjunct Assistant Professor, Department of Psychology, Brandeis University

Adrian Tomer, M.A., Department of Psychology, University of Florida

Robin Lea West, Ph.D., Assistant Professor, Gerontology Center/Department of Psychology, University of Florida

Peter J. Whitehouse, M.D., Ph.D., Director, Alzheimer Center, University Hospitals of Cleveland and Division of Behavioral Neurology, Case Western Reserve University; Associate Professor, Department of Neurology, Case Western Reserve University School of Medicine

Arthur Wingfield, D. Phil., Professor, Department of Psychology, Brandeis University

Preface

In October, 1987, several hundred people representing the disciplines of medicine, nursing, psychology, and social work met at a conference in Cleveland to discuss memory, aging, and dementia. The conference was cosponsored by the University Center on Aging and Health of Case Western Reserve University and the Alzheimer's Center of University Hospitals of Cleveland. This volume grew out of the presentations and discussions at the conference.

There were several goals for both the conference and this volume. The first was to present contemporary models of memory and relate the concepts and tools of cognitive psychology to an understanding of the memory performance of healthy and impaired elderly adults. A second goal was to demonstrate that interventions can be used to improve the memory performance of both healthy and demented elderly adults. Another goal was to focus on the impact that severe cognitive impairment can have on the family and the caregivers of patients with dementia. Finally, we addressed the medical issues related to Alzheimer's disease by examining the recent evidence on the biological determinants of Alzheimer's disease and addressing the difficulty of clinically diagnosing the disease. The conference and this volume ended with a thoughtful discussion of the ability of our health care delivery systems to deal with the demands of the aging population.

Memory impairment is a focus of the volume, for it represents a major complaint of elderly patients. A person may present relatively mild problems, such as forgetting some items on a grocery list or temporarily misplacing a set of keys. Or there may be evidence of a profound disturbance indicative of dementia. In considering these complaints the psychologist must determine the extent to which the problems may be attributed to a competence or a performance deficit. That is, are the problems related to a true loss of ability, or does the person have difficulty because of an intervening variable, such as depression? If the latter case holds, then the intervention strategy may be to treat the intervening variable (depression). However, if there is a loss of competence, then the intervention will focus on the enhancement of performance through the maintenance and effective strategic use of remaining abilities. The effective assessment of the nature of the memory problem and the design of the memory intervention requires an understanding of the multiple facets of memory. This volume will sensitize the reader to these assessment issues in the context of contemporary theory of memory function.

While there is some controversy surrounding care and treatment issues of persons suffering from dementia, it is agreed upon by all disciplines that care planning for these individuals is a major concern for the professional. Treatment varies from interventions to help recover memory to techniques for reducing environmental stimuli that may cause catastrophic reactions in the Alzheimer patient. Other care and treatment issues surround the ability of the patient and family to manage health care delivery service costs. Since dementia is a disorder that has an impact on the entire society as well as the individual patient and family, attention to the impact of the health care policies on quality care is critical. An interdisciplinary approach is needed to examine assessment, care, treatment, and cost needs of dementia patients.

Alzheimer's disease is the most common cause of dementia in the elderly. Although dementia is defined by the presence of impairment in a number of spheres of cognitive activity, memory problems are often the earliest and most dysfunctional intellectual deficits. Considerable advances are being made in AD to understand the neurobiological basis of the memory impairment. More drugs, as well as behavioral strategies, are being developed to ameliorate the effects of the disease. Yet despite these advances, the burden of the disease on the patient, family, and entire society is becoming increasingly apparent. Moreover, because of the growing number of people who will be affected in the future, AD is a lead issue in promoting reform in our health care delivery system.

To assist the reader, the volume is divided into three parts. The first presents contemporary memory theory and illustrates the assessment of memory abilities in both healthy and impaired elderly adults. The second section examines the medical issues of the etiology and diagnosis of Alzheimer's disease. The last section illustrates how professionals from three disciplines—nursing, psychology, and social work—address the problems of both the demented patient and the caregivers and provides a challenging discussion of the reforms needed in our health care delivery systems.

We wish to recognize the following persons for their help in the preparation of the manuscripts: Greg Knapik, Rose Bouch, Nandita Verma, Doug Lanska, Cheryl Cowan, and Tsui Chan. Work was supported in part by NIMH Center Grant MH-43-4401, Ohio Department of Aging Alzheimer's Disease Research

Center Grant No. ADR-2, NIA Alzheimer's Disease Research Center Grant, and the David S. Ingalls Neurological Center for the Study of Dementia.

We also wish to thank Diane Ferris for her dedication in producing both the conference and this volume. Without her tireless effort and professionalism, neither project would have succeeded.

GROVER C. GILMORE
PETER J. WHITEHOUSE
MAY L. WYKLE

PART I
Memory and Aging: Theory and Assessment

Memory complaints are common among older adults, but severe memory disturbance is the hallmark of Alzheimer's disease. To understand the specific nature of memory disturbances and to properly differentiate the problems experienced by healthy elderly adults from those experienced by sufferers of dementia, it is important to grasp the multidimensional character of memory. Great strides have been made recently in uncovering the intricate nature of a variety of memory processes. This section provides an introduction to current conceptualizations of memory and illustrates the application of theory in the memory assessment of both healthy and cognitively impaired individuals.

The first two chapters provide an overview of current memory theory as it relates to the cognitive changes associated with aging. The major concepts and terms employed in memory research are introduced in the context of research methodologies. In the first chapter, Arthur Wingfield and Elizabeth Stine note that successful memory is dependent in large part on the uniqueness or distinctiveness of the initial encoding of the stimulus information. The elderly adult may exhibit poor memory because of limitations on encoding, such as sensory deficits and processing speed. However, Wingfield and Stine emphasize that such limitations may be overcome when the individual uses his or her rich knowledge base to supplement the initially available information. This point is clearly illustrated by their research on the processing of spoken language. Elderly listeners have difficulty recalling random strings of words but yield excellent recall performance when presented with normal sentences. The final message here is a very important one. While aging is associated with diminished processing abilities, it also brings experience and knowledge that may compensate for the decline and yield good cognitive performance.

Donald Kausler introduces the concept of age-associated memory impairment (AAMI) and explores several competing hypotheses of its cause. In a well-balanced presentation, he examines the evidence in support of each alternative. Kausler illustrates that AAMI is present in varying degrees in the different forms of memory. There is little impairment in the ability to retrieve information from generic or semantic memory, but the recall of episodic information is difficult, particularly when the information must be retained for a relatively long period of time. Because of the multiple forms of memory and the different types of impairment, Kausler emphasizes that the assessment of an individual's memory must involve a number of different memory tasks. This theme is further developed in later chapters that examine clinical memory assessment.

The memory complaints of healthy elderly adults are addressed by Robin West and Adrian Tomer, who suggest intervention strategies to improve memory performance. The authors stress that the specific needs and abilities of the participants must be considered in order to maximize the effectiveness of a memory training program. In reviewing the value and effectiveness of a number of intervention strategies, they note that there is not a single best approach. Indeed, West and Tomer suggest that memory training programs should teach elderly adults to evaluate their memory goals and to apply the best memory strategy to attain those goals. Such flexible training will take into account the abilities and needs of the client and may lead to generalization of the training effects.

A significant obstacle for memory investigators is the problem of translating research findings obtained in a laboratory into practical clinical applications. Leonard Poon argues in Chapter 4 that the challenge is to take the researcher's knowledge "from lab to life." A major problem is that laboratory investigations are designed to understand the memory processes exhibited by a group of people, while a clinician desires a test that will predict memory performance for individuals. Sounding a common theme of this volume, Poon suggests that performance be evaluated on a wide range of tests. He demonstrates the effectiveness of this approach by evaluating the capabilities of healthy, demented, and depressed elderly adults on tests that tap skills from attention to semantic processing. The cognitive speed profiles that emerge from this analysis capture the strengths and weaknesses of the individuals. Poon suggests that such a profile analysis may be a useful clinical diagnostic tool.

The specific cognitive deficits that underlie the poor memory performance associated with various forms of dementia and amnesia are addressed by William Heindel, David Salmon, and Nelson Butters in Chapter 5. In a careful review of a broad set of studies in cognitive neuropsychology, the authors demonstrate that tasks and concepts developed in cognitive psychology laboratories can be useful diagnostic tools. The authors stress that patients with dementias of different etiologies can be differentiated from each other and from patients with amnesia.

Their chapter illustrates the benefits of bringing the "lab to life" through an interaction between experimental and clinical approaches to clinical psychology.

The application of memory concepts and tests in the clinical setting is discussed by James Mack, Marian Patterson, and Nancy Adams. They challenge clinicians to consider the advances of contemporary cognitive psychology in seeking assessment techniques to distinguish the multiple aspects of memory function. Drawing on an extensive review of the clinical literature and their own broad clinical assessment experience, the authors provide a thoughtful consideration of the issues in cognitive assessment and discuss the relevance of a variety of assessment tools. A very valuable portion of the chapter is the presentation of case histories that illustrate the authors' approach to assessment and diagnosis.

Taken together, these chapters provide an excellent review of contemporary concepts and theory relevant to memory and aging. The authors stress the multidimensional nature of memory function, which requires the use of assessment tools that tap the separate dimensions. A clear message is that the advances of cognitive psychology provide useful tools for the diagnosis of memory problems and the design of intervention strategies. Psychologists in the lab and the clinic are sharing their skills and knowledge to yield conceptually rich, theory-based assessment tools that help the investigator understand and predict the memory performance of the elderly adult.

GROVER C. GILMORE

1

Modeling Memory Processes: Research and Theory on Memory and Aging

Arthur Wingfield and Elizabeth A. L. Stine

Our goal in this chapter is to paint, with a fairly broad brush, the recent revolution of modern memory theory. In so doing, we hope first to introduce many of the concepts, terms, and research methodologies that will appear throughout the remainder of this volume. Second, we hope to offer a broad theoretical base on which to understand age-related memory deficits, whether it be the benign forgetfulness of normal aging or the debilitating memory losses associated with the tragedy of Alzheimer's disease. We will, wherever possible, refer the reader to other chapters in this volume in which each of these issues is discussed in detail.

WHY A THEORY OF MEMORY?

In memory research, it is surprisingly easy to gather a lot of facts. Research efficiency, on the other hand, depends on the availability of theory, which guides us to the most productive or interesting places to look for our facts and helps

The preparation of this chapter was facilitated by PHS Grant AGO4517 from the National Institute on Aging.

us to interpret the facts that we find. This need for theory stands, whether the need is to understand the biological basis of memory, to develop sensitive clinical tests for memory assessment, or to devise techniques to improve memory using various memory aids.

It is our contention that people *always* have a theory. There has *never* been a neutral science of psychology, or neurobiology, or education—it is only a question of whether there is an open, clearly articulated, explicit theory or simply an implicit theory that remains unarticulated. Thus it is not a question of whether to have a theory, but a question of developing the best, most *practical* theory.

While this latter point may sound like a conflict in terms, F. C. Bartlett, one of the pioneers of early memory research, was among those who felt strongly that there is nothing quite so practical as a good theory (Bartlett, 1932). Bartlett held the view that many of the best theories are constructed while trying to solve practical problems. A good theory should be practical. It should help us to understand why we forget, and how we can prevent (or at least retard) this process. We would also like to know how memories are maintained, and how they support the knowledge that allows us to answer questions and to solve problems. The most fundamental question of memory, then, is a practical one (Wingfield & Byrnes, 1981).

SHORT-TERM MEMORY AND LINEAR-STAGE MODELING

Invariably, when most of us think of memory, we think first of why we cannot remember more than we do. Most of us wish, in short, that there were some way we could improve our memory.

In fact, history shows no shortage of ideas, some more fanciful than others, for improving "weak" memory. Poor memory has often been seen as a problem to be fixed, or "cured," with remediation. We have referred to this as the "pink pill" approach to memory—that is, a remedy that would operate in all situations and require as little personal effort as possible: a metaphorical "pink pill" as an all-purpose cure-all for forgetting (Wingfield, 1979). The seventeenth century was an especially rich time in this regard, with a variety of cures offered for poor memory. Among the more exotic were herbal treatments (cinnamon being a favorite), the advice to wear a cap made of beaver skin, and instructions to anoint the head and spine monthly with drops of castor oil (Hunter, 1964).

An early memory aid that survives today is the use of *mnemonics*, specially designed sets of associations or plans for organizing to-be-remembered materials (e.g., the use of imagery, associations, or mediators to which otherwise difficult-to-organize learning materials can be attached). Named after *Mnemosyne*, the Greek goddess of memory, mnemonics were considered in medieval times to be so powerful that they were classed among the "magic arts." What magic there is, however, lies solely in the fact that mnemonics work best when they mimic the natural organizing schemata ordinarily associated with meaningful material.

Can we "enlarge" memory by practice at memorizing? Martin and Fernberger (1929) had undergraduate volunteers spend up to 50 days in repeated memorization of random-digit lists. Their two-part question was whether one could increase digit spans beyond the usual 7 or 8 digits, and, if so, whether this might increase memory capacity in general. The answer to the first part of the question was yes: one volunteer increased his digit span recall to 15 digits without error. (He reported treating the lists as if they were composed of three groups of 5 digits each.) The answer to the second part was no: general principles of learning—concentration, grouping, and so forth—may be learned, but there were no other positive effects on memory span in general. Other attempts at improving memory span by practice seem to reinforce these early findings. Memory is not so much a "muscle" exercised by practice as it is a skill. Like other skills, memory performances can be improved by practice and the discovery of techniques that work for the user. Like improving other skills, however, generalization across different tasks cannot be taken for granted. (A broader discussion of cognitive training and plasticity across the life span can be found in Baltes, 1987.)

In spite of these efforts, the modern history of memory theory ironically shows an opposite search. For most theorists, an ideal memory system should *not* retain everything. Indeed, life would be a nightmare if all memories were retained. Imagine, for example, doing math exercises and remembering at the end of the day all of the numbers you punched into your calculator keyboard, or imagine remembering all the names of *everyone* you have ever met—every store clerk and every bus driver with a name tag—or every telephone number you ever dialed. From the beginning, modern theorists looked at places and mechanisms where memory could be protected from the overload and confusions that would surely result from storing too much information.

Memory Processes versus Memory Structures

There are many ways to divide memory as a heuristic for understanding. One of these has been to contrast memory *processes* and memory *structures*.

Memory processes are those mental activities we perform in order to analyze information, to store the results of these analyses, and to perform those activities necessary to make later use of this information. The literature usually distinguishes between three memory processes, any of which could be the locus for a memory failure. The first process, *acquisition*, refers to the registration and analysis of the experienced stimulus and the preliminary formation of a suitable memory code in the nervous system. A failure to remember could be the result of inattention during the orginal experience or a misunderstanding or misperception of the experience. The second process is *retention*, the storage and maintenance in store of the acquired information. It is this trace that will serve as the basis for the final process: the act of remembering, or *retrieval* of the information. Often fleshed out by other knowledge and creative inference, this recall can take the form of an overt response, or an internal activation of the trace for such activity as solving a mental problem.

For these distinctions to have utility, however, it must be recognized that such processes are interdependent elements of a complex cognitive act of remembering. For example, effective retrieval depends first on an adequate, or "distinctive," encoding of the stimulus, and second, on a compatibility between the features used in original encoding and the features used in attempted retrieval (Fisher & Craik, 1977; Tulving & Thomson, 1973; Watkins & Tulving, 1975; Wingfield, 1980).

Questions about memory *structure* have to do with the nature of memory storage itself: how this information is represented, how long the representations last, and how memories are organized. One early hope was that by understanding the structure of memory, one could also understand its process.

Limiting the Input

Figure 1.1 shows the general form structural models of memory took throughout the 1960s and early 1970s. It represents a good starting point for our discussion of the development of modern memory theory.

Note that a major distinction is made between what is labeled in the diagram as *short-term memory* (STM), a transient, "buffer" memory for the temporary holding of recent information, and the more permanent store of *long-term memory* (LTM). Short-term memory was presumed to have a limited capacity, a rapid loss without rehearsal, and to be easily erased if disrupted by almost any sort of interference. The contents of short-term memory could be kept alive by rehearsal. With sufficient rehearsal, the material could be passed on to long-term memory.

It became obvious, however, that if STM were to be viewed as a temporary, limited-capacity "buffer," then there would have to be some way to filter the sensory input to prevent too much information from overloading this STM system. One of the earliest solutions was to propose that all information might be held in an even briefer *sensory memory*. This brief "echo" of the sensory stimulus could hold, for a fraction of a second, far more than could ever be processed for meaning and awareness. The visual sensory store was referred to as *iconic* memory, and its auditory counterpart as *echoic* memory (Neisser, 1967).

For example, if several people were speaking at once, sensory memory would receive and hold, for a few seconds or fractions of a second, a transient trace of all of the conversations in an unanalyzed form. To keep the higher level systems from overload, only one of the conversations (a single "channel" of information), could be passed through the attentional filter at one time. The other channels would be filtered or blocked from input.

According to this theory, a person could attend to one conversation while eavesdropping on others (something we often do) by rapidly switching between the

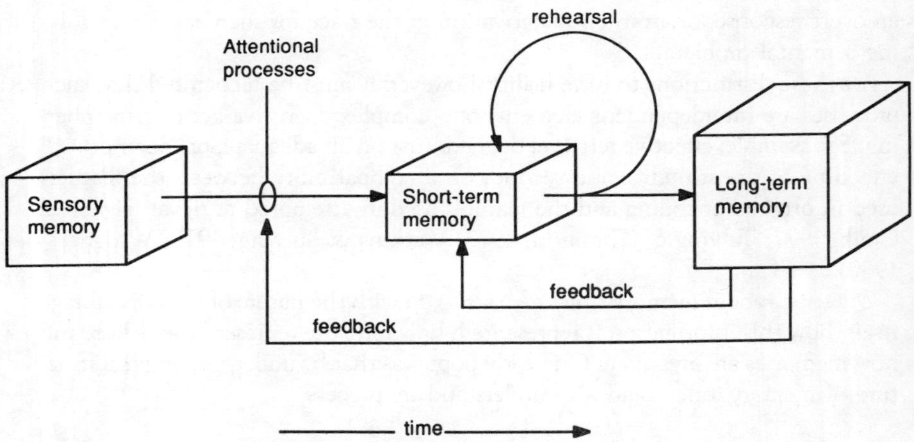

FIGURE 1.1 A linear-stage model of memory showing the flow of information over time, from the moment of stimulus receipt to eventual storage in long-term memory. Later theories have shifted the focus from discrete stages to more dynamic process models that empahsize levels of analysis and working memory capacity.

decaying sensory traces of the conversations, the way several TV programs can be followed by rapidly switching the channel selector from one channel to another. If we sample frequently enough, and if the programs (i.e., conversations) have enough redundancy, we can easily piece together those small elements we have missed (Broadbent, 1971).

Models of the sort shown in Figure 1.1 are sometimes called "information processing," or "linear stage," models, because they attempted to represent the flow of information from one stage to the next over the course of time (in this case, over the first few seconds after a stimulus has been received). The nature of the memory code is also presumed to change across the stages, with each stage representing progressively more abstract coding of the stimulus, from its raw sensory form in sensory memory to a semantic representation in LTM. As indicated by the directional arrows in the diagram, although information moves from one stage of processing to the next, some feedback occurs to allow monitoring and control of processing operations.

The diagram in Figure 1.1 is intended to be a generic one, but it owes much to the linear stage modeling of, for example, Broadbent (1958, 1971) and Atkinson and Shiffrin (1968; see also Waugh & Norman, 1965). All of this effort, we should emphasize, was a result of the recognition that information processing must be conducted within a limited-capacity system (Welford, 1968).

The idea of STM as an ecologically advantageous "buffer" memory with limited capacity is usually attributed to Donald Broadbent (1958), while George Miller (1956) can be credited with defining its capacity as 7 ± 2 items, or "chunks," of information. (Trying to remember a seven-digit telephone number is a good example of a short-term store with a limited number of "slots" and that is subject to rapid decay without rehearsal.) These early theories, incidentally, tended to emphasize verbal rehearsal. For example, even when visually presented, there is a tendency for digits and letters to be named, and then for the names to be given verbal maintenance rehearsal. Recall errors for visually presented letters of the alphabet often show the result of this verbal rehearsal in the form of acoustic errors (e.g., *P* for *B*, or *Q* for U), rather than visually similar errors (e.g., *P* for *F*, or *O* for *Q*) (Baddeley, 1976; Conrad, 1972; Wickelgren, 1965).

The function of this verbal short-term store as a phonological buffer, or "rehearsal loop," would thus be influenced by such factors as the time it takes to articulate each of the letters (or digits, or words) as part of the rehearsal process. The longer it takes to articulate the words in rehearsal, the fewer items one is able to recall. This is so because such a list gets less rehearsal than a list that can be articulated through the rehearsal loop at a faster rate (Baddeley, Thomson, & Buchanan, 1975).

Maintaining Material in Short-Term Memory

William James (1890) made a distinction between what he called Primary Memory (PM) and Secondary Memory (SM), and many writers have preferred to use these terms rather than STM and LTM. James described PM as representing the psychological present: those events, thoughts, or perceptions that are part of one's immediate awareness at any given moment. Recent, short-term memory would, of course, be in this category, but so, too, would other kinds of memories. James used SM to refer to knowledge acquired in the past, that is not ordinarily part of current conscious experience.

Although immediate memory processing does contain some elements of STM as we have described it, the development of memory theory over the past decade has found fault with the concept of STM as a distinct memory structure, and the term itself no longer carries its earlier implications. Like most authors, we will use short- and long-term memory in the remainder of this chapter as only descriptive terms rather than to imply specific memory structures. The reasons for this will soon become apparent.

In contrast to memory of meaningful or easily organized materials, however, remembering sets of unrelated stimuli such as digit and word lists is a very difficult task requiring considerable conscious effort. If such materials are not rehearsed, or if some distraction occurs, this information, or at least access to it, will become quickly lost (Peterson & Peterson, 1959). Figure 1.2 comes from an experiment by Wingfield and Byrnes (1972) that shows how sharply limited memory can be when rehearsal is prevented and attention must be shared between two potential inputs.

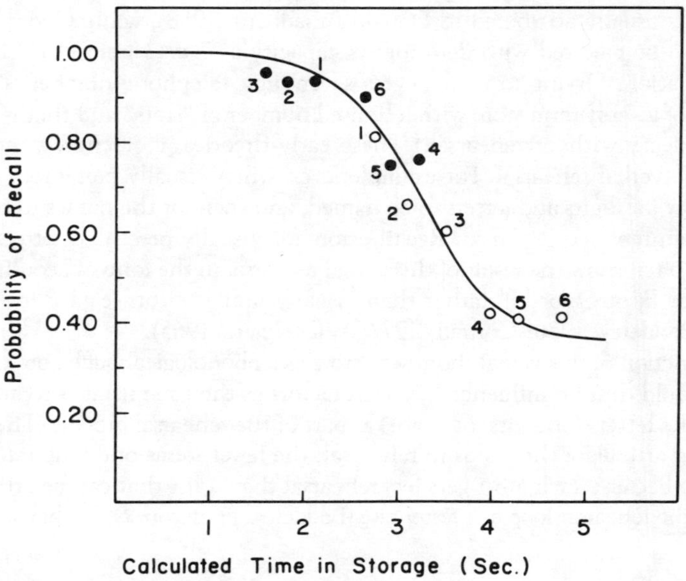

FIGURE 1.2 Probability of recall for simultaneous digit lists recalled either pair-by-pair (O) or list-by-list (•) as a function of calculated time in storage. Numbers along the curve art the orders of recall specified by the two recall conditions. (From Fig. 2 of Wingfield & Byrnes, 1972, p.691.)

In this experiment, subjects heard three pairs of digits spoken simultaneously by two different speakers (i.e., two simultaneous lists of three digits each). The task was to recall the six digits either pair-by-pair (the open circles in Fig. 1.2), or first the three digits spoken by one speaker, then the three digits spoken by the other speaker (filled circles). As we had been able to show previously, these two different orders of report will reliably produce very different temporal output patterns of the responses.

Figure 1.2 shows the probability that each of the six digits of the two lists would be recalled, plotted as a function of the mean time in seconds from the instant a digit was heard to the instant it was recalled aloud by the subject. (The small numbers along the curve indicate the specified orders of recall of the six digits as required by the two recall conditions.) As we can see, after only 4 seconds, item recall probability under these conditions has dropped to only .40.

Note that we do not specify whether this rapid loss is due just to the passage of time or whether it is due to the interference that may go on during that interval. Discussions of this question can be found in Crowder (1976), or Wingfield and Byrnes (1981, pp 258–271). Rather, our point here is that unrelated materials (in this case, digit strings) represent a form of stimuli for which the nervous system is hardly best suited. Contrast the rapid loss shown in Figure 1.2, for example, with our ability to remember long sentences or prose passages after only one hearing or reading. It is precisely for this reason that memory training techniques tend to focus not only on concentration and rehearsal, but also on the importance of organizing the materials and using mnemonic techniques such as linking items to images. (See Chapters 2, 3, and 10.)

There are, of course, no end of "boxes" one could postulate (e.g., primary, secondary, tertiary memory, or short, intermediate, long-term memory). It is because memory is so complex that theorists attempted to simplify the problem by parsing memory into its presumed elements, structures, or processes. The fact is that stimulus acquisition is based less on a sequence of stages than on a rapid, probably parallel, spread of activation across extraordinarily complex neural networks (McClelland & Rumelhart, 1985; McClelland, Rumelhart, & the PDP Research Group, 1986; Rumelhart, McClelland, & the PDP Research Group, 1986).

The idea that there are components of memory, however, is a powerful one, especially as it has led investigators to attempt to specify with greater precision where memory deficits associated with adult aging might lie. In this connection, we would like to quote one of our elderly volunteers who was being recorded as she attempted to recall word strings presented at a very fast rate. As we noted earlier, we all have theories, and this particular experimental subject had a theory about the locus of memory difficulty with age.

> "I really can't remember; that part of my brain must be getting weak."
>
> (We must have looked at her a bit quizzically, because she went on.)
>
> . . . "You see, you really have three parts to your brain: the part you [use to] remember [what happened] just now, the part back a bit, and the part back farther. Yes, that's why some people in my age range can remember everything that happened years ago, but [they] can't remember what happened five minutes ago . . . Three parts to the brain, and they're all working differently."

BEYOND LINEAR STAGE MODELING

Declarative Knowledge and the Neural Basis of Memory

One goal of modern neuroscience is to understand memory on the cellular or molecular level by asking such questions as how synapses and synaptic circuits change as memories are formed (Kandel & Schwartz, 1985). A second approach is that of examining behavioral consequences of accident- or disease-induced lesions to specific areas of brain. This latter approach has led to our further understanding of the structure of human (and animal) memory.

As this work has progressed, it has led to evidence in support of some aspects of a distinction between short- and long-term memory functions, and to at least hint at their neural loci. This evidence also supports a necessary differentiation between memory for at least two kinds of knowledge: *declarative knowledge* and *procedural knowledge*.

Based on the selectivity of memory deficits observed following brain damage, Squire (1986) has pointed to a biological distinction between long-term and short-term memory functions. Specifically, it would appear that the consolidation of temporary short-term memories into a more enduring long-term form involves the important participation of the medial aspects of the temporal lobe and especially the hippocampus, a twisted band of fibers underlying the temporal lobes (and so named because its peculiar shape reminded early anatomists of a sea horse). Also important is the midline diencephalic region, especially the mediodorsal thalamic nucleus and the mammillary nuclei, which have strong anatomic connections to the medial temporal region. The hippocampus, it should be noted, is especially rich in afferent and efferent pathways, giving extensive (if sometimes indirect) communication to the many areas of the cortex responsible for information processing, a point to which we will return later.

As is discussed in detail in Chapter 5, patients with damage to these areas are referred to as amnesics; although they can recall early memories quite well, their ability to remember new information is poor, often dramatically so. Because amnesic patients can recall early memories quite well, it seems unlikely that the mediotemporal region is a permanent storage site for long-term memory. Rather, this area seems to be important for the consolidation of memories, or for the transfer of short-term memories to long-term memory (Squire, 1986).

An important principle of memory is that information that has been processed to a semantic or "deep" level (i.e., information that has received the most extensive perceptual and semantic analysis) will be retained best; far better, for example, than material that we try to retain through rote rehearsal. Memory might thus be, at least in part, a representation or record of the perceptual operations that the nervous system undertook when the stimulus was first presented (Craik & Lockhart, 1972). It is not unreasonable, then, to suppose that the neural representations of these memories may be stored in the same neural systems (roughly, brain regions) that were involved in the initial perception and analysis of the information when it was learned.

The literature already suggests that the cortical areas that subserve higher-order visual processing may also serve as the site of storage of the visual memories that resulted from that processing (Squire, 1986). That is, while the integrity of the temporal and diencephalic regions may be necessary for long-term traces to develop, both temporary short-term storage and permanent long-term storage may reside in those cortical regions associated with the cortical processing of stimuli drawn from that particular domain (Monsell, 1984; Squire, 1986). This biological data is important to the question of domain-specific memory in working memory theory, a topic we will address in a later section. (See Squire [1987] for further coverage of these issues and Sherry & Schacter [1987] for an interesting discussion of multiple memories from an adaptive cross-species perspective.)

As is discussed in detail in Chapter 5, the memory impairments of amnesic patients support a major distinction between memory for two general kinds of knowledge. The first, *declarative knowledge*, refers to our ordinary memories of the facts and events of everyday life, knowledge that is accessible to conscious awareness and that can be articulated to others. Declarative knowledge includes *episodic memory*, those memories for the experiences and events of our lives, and some elements of *semantic memory*, those context-free, long-held areas of knowledge, such as knowledge of the syntactic rules of our language or how to add two numbers (Tulving, 1983).

As we have indicated, declarative knowledge is explicit in the sense that it is accessible to conscious awareness and that we can describe, or declare, this knowledge to others. Declarative memory acquisition seems uniquely vulnerable in the amnesias we have been describing.

By contrast, *procedural knowledge*, or memories for procedures such as motor skills, seems relatively spared in these patients. These are implicit memories in the sense that they are accessible only through performance, as when one actually engages in the skill, or when the effects of the knowledge are seen in some other behavior (Squire, 1986). Chapter 5 will have more to say on this issue, and on its implications for the importance of different brain regions in memory representation.

It Takes Attention to Pay Attention

The filtering of unwanted, or potentially overloading, input has as its basis what one might call *attentional resources*. Recall that Broadbent offered a very reasonable way of explaining the limits on attention using the metaphor of a mechanical "filter" or switch, which would have to be tuned either to one input channel or another in a rapid, time-sharing fashion. There are other ways to conceptualize our limits on attention. One of these has been to postulate that individuals have a limited pool of "attentional" or "processing" resources at their command at any one time.

Imagine, for example, a small computer with an upper limit on the amount of information it can accommodate at any one time. The more complex the instructional program giving the operations to be performed on the data, the less space there will be for storing the data itself. Conversely, the more data the computer must store, the less space will be available for storing the operating routines and for carrying them out. By analogy, we can view sensory input and the operations that must be performed on it as competing for a limited pool, or "capacity," of available resources. For example, if a stimulus input is of poor quality or is degraded in some way, more capacity will have to be allocated for its perceptual analysis. As a result, less capacity is available for other operations one might wish to perform on the results of this analysis. Similarly, if complex cognitive operations have to be performed on stimuli already received, little spare capacity is available for the analysis of new, incoming stimuli (Moray, 1969).

In principle, parallel processing, or the ability to do two things at one time, is possible, provided the total capacity is not exceeded by the combined demands of the task requirements and the analysis of the sensory input. Thus our inability to follow two conversations at once could be a result of the unavailability of sufficient processing resources to allow both to be analyzed to a complete semantic level. Both inputs might receive simultaneous processing, but not to a level necessary for awareness of content or for recall of what was heard.

Although the idea of a limited pool of attentional resources appeared very early in the psychological literature (Titchener, 1908), a true capacity model of attention was first articulated in a complete form by Kahneman (1973). Specifically, Kahneman argued that there is flexibility in how one can choose to allocate one's resources, or effort, among several possible activities (e.g., processing stimulus inputs, holding their analyses in memory, and organizing a complex response). Most processing resources could be allocated to one of these activities at the expense of the others, or the same limited resources could be divided more evenly across all of these activities. This second strategy would allow some success at several simultaneous activities, but no one activity would have sufficient resources for more than low-level performance. (Kahneman also inserted an interesting caveat: while processing resources may be limited, they need not be fixed. That is, a highly motivated subject could give more effort to a task and hence make more resources available for its performance than a less motivated subject.)

Kahneman, incidentally, was very careful to note the possibility that not *all* mental activities might have to draw on the same pool of resources. This, as the literature was to show, was a wise caution. Now, however, we will introduce two important notions. The first is that deep encoding and memory maintenance require effort, and there are upper limits to the amount of attentional or processing resources available at any one time (*resource capacity*). The second notion is that there is some flexibility in the amount of resources that can be allocated to any one particular task or mental activity. For example, we do not always encode information as completely as possible. Rather, we often encode stimuli just to the level necessary for distinctions that are meaningful or important to us.

One implication of this argument is that mere exposure, even massively repeated exposure, to stimuli will not be sufficient to produce deep, discriminative learning as long as adequate resources are not allocated for their analysis. A case in point is illustrated by Figure 1.3, taken from Nickerson and Adams (1979). All of these U.S. "pennies" are plausible, but which penny is the correct one is not easy for most people to say. (Only one of them is correct. All of the others have specific features omitted, mislocated, or added.) You can see how difficult a task this is, even though you have experienced pennies countless times. We should note that the difficulty is not simply a confusion of seeing all these variations

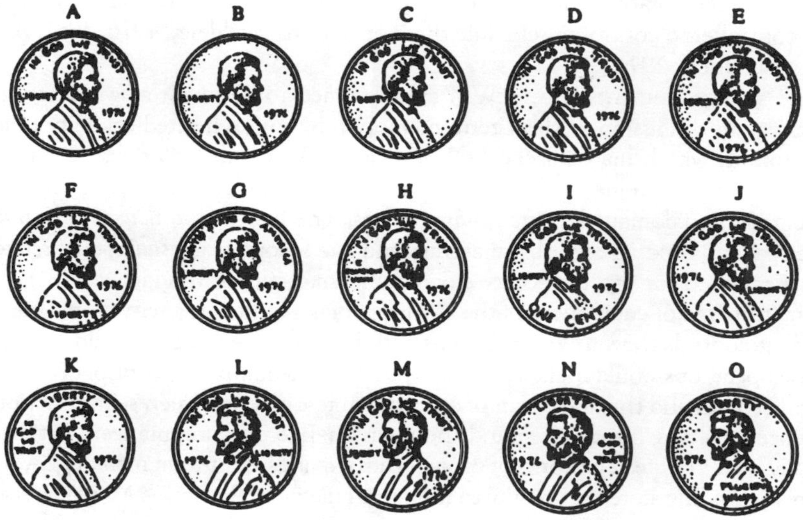

FIGURE 1.3 Fifteen drawings of the head of a U.S. penny used in recognition study. The task is to determine which of these pennies is correct. (From Nickerson and Adams, 1979.)

together. Nickerson and Adams also recorded poor performance when subjects were asked to draw or describe a penny from memory or when they were shown a single example and asked to say if it was correct, and if not, why not.

The concept of resource limitations, although first proposed in the context of divided attention (Johnston & Heinz, 1978; Kahneman, 1973; Norman & Bobrow, 1975), has had an important impact on memory theory. Most notable in this regard has been the development of working memory theory and the role played within the theory by the concept of resource limitations.

RESOURCE LIMITATIONS AND WORK MEMORY

We have seen that the temporary holding of unrelated elements such as digit strings and word lists is one capability of our memory system. One hint that we have to look farther, however, is that, at least within broad limits, digit spans do not correlate well with many other cognitive task performances (Daneman & Carpenter, 1980), nor do they appear to be especially age-sensitive (Craik & Rabinowitz, 1984).

The memory function that enables the maintenance of such materials through rehearsal is now seen as but one function of a more complex memory and processing system collectively referred to as *working memory* (WM). The most common conceptualization of WM is that of a limited-capacity system which contains components of temporary holding, components to process what is held, and an executive controller to control or schedule these operations (Baddeley, 1976, 1981; Baddeley & Hitch, 1974).

The storage elements within WM are presumed to be much as we described them in our discussion of short-term memory function: a limited-capacity holding store in which material can be lost as a result of time, interference, or the displacement of old material by new. As currently formulated, however, the WM system has two domain-specific holding stores. The first is an *articulatory loop* for rehearsal and holding of verbal material, and the second is a *visual-spatial scratch pad* specialized for the temporary storage of visual stimuli (Baddeley, 1981).

The third major component of the WM system is a limited capacity *central executive* that controls the various operations performed on the materials held in store. These operations would include, for example, the scheduling and control of rehearsal procedures and the allocation of attentional resources between such functions as processing new information and the maintenance or manipulation of stimuli already held in store. The concept of WM thus expands short-term memory beyond simply a holding store on the way to long-term memory. Rather, WM is now seen as a kind of scratch pad, or computational space, in which information can be manipulated and considered and where interim results of these manipulations can be held for further computation.

To get a feeling for the role of shared resources within a limited-capacity WM system, imagine being asked to read or listen to a set of five unrelated sentences and (to make sure you are paying attention) to say after each sentence whether the statement was true or false (e.g., "Albany and Springfield are both state capitals"). In addition, you are also told that after hearing all five sentences, you will be asked to recall the final word of each of the five sentences. (From this example, the word to be retained would be "capitals.")

The difference between simple recall of a five-item word list and this task illustrates the difference between a simple holding store and current conceptions of working memory. That is, WM differs from older notions of STM in its emphasis on the manipulation of information rather than on simple storage or maintenance capacity.

Daneman and Carpenter (1980) have used this kind of task to study the impact of WM limitations on text memory among young adults. In so doing, they attempted to examine the "operational capacity" reflected by their subjects' performance levels (see also Salthouse, in press). The notion they wished to convey was that capacity must subsume both storage capacity and processing power.

Reference to WM as a limited-capacity system implies that the more processing resources that are required for one WM task, the fewer processing resources that will be available for the performance of other tasks. By contrast, "automatic" tasks, or tasks demanding minimal processing resources, leave the WM system relatively free for other activities (Hasher & Zacks, 1979; Shiffrin & Schneider, 1977). In short, current models of WM show a number of elements ordinarily associated with more general capacity models of attention and resource allocation within a limited resource pool (Baddeley, 1981; Craik & Simon, 1980; Kahneman, 1973; Norman & Bobrow, 1975; Wingfield & Sandoval, 1980).

Currently, most authors use STM or PM to refer to the temporary holding of stimulus materials in a relatively untransformed fashion, and WM to refer to situations where materials in memory have to be manipulated, transformed, or recombined. In fact, most memory tasks reflect varying degrees of all of these elements (Craik & Rabinowitz, 1984; Wingfield et al., 1988). One reason simple digit spans are such poor predictors of subjects' abilities on other tasks may be that such span tests rely on simple storage capacity, and require little WM involvement. Thus, as Daneman and Carpenter (1980) have suggested, it may be that our interest should be in processing capacity, not storage capacity, as a predictor of general performance.

Modularity of Function and Domain Specificity

One question theorists have begun to ask is whether WM should be viewed as a single, if complex, memory system, or as a generic term for a variety of autonomous, domain-specific, processing subsystems (Monsell, 1984).

Let us consider for a moment the arguments for this position and its implications for memory theory. Perhaps the first step is to recall Squire's (1986) position that memories arising from different neural processing subsystems (e.g., complex visual processing) may be represented in memory in those brain regions primarily involved in their original encoding. Note also that current conceptions of working memory already include the notion of both articulatory and visual-spatial stores. There is certainly good evidence for temporary storage uniquely associated with visual memory, or a visual-spatial representation (Baddeley & Lieberman, 1980; Kosslyn, 1980; Sherry & Schacter, 1987). It is thus a small step to propose that there may be numerous cognitive operations, with each such operation requiring its own domain-specific memory store.

Although the term *modularity* has come into wide use with numerous meanings, its most strict usage refers to cognitive modules as autonomous, probably hard-wired, and impenetrable processing subsystems (Fodor, 1983). By autonomous and impenetrable we mean that stimuli within a particular cognitive domain (e.g., speech or music) are processed independently of each other, and that processing within a module is uninfluenced by other cognitive operations. According to this proposal, processing operations within such modules are inaccessible to conscious awareness and are neither facilitated nor impaired by information or events external to that module (Swinney, 1979). There are, for example, claims that verbal rehearsal and visual-spatial memory tasks can be accomplished simultaneously without significant interference (Peterson, Rawlings, & Cohen, 1977).

Modularity is by no means currently well defined, nor is there complete understanding of what might even constitute a domain. For example, a processing domain might be as general as language or as specific as certain aspects of lexical or syntactic processing (Grodzinsky & Shapiro, 1988). Thus one of our questions must be how numerous and how specific the memory stores within a WM system might be. The second and equally fundamental question is whether such putative subsystems are controlled and regulated by a single central executive with its presumed pool of limited resources. While most authors currently assume the central processing notion of WM, still other writers, such as Monsell (1984), make clear that the issue is still in doubt.

The concept of central processing resources has had considerable descriptive utility for many years, especially in the cognitive aging literature (Craik & Simon, 1980). We must thus leave this issue simply with the caution that memory processing may be modular: certain memory operations may be distributed over linked, but autonomous, subsystems (Monsell, 1984, p. 330). If this is the case, its implications are clear: since autonomous processors might reasonably have different processing rates, the full system would also need further buffer stores between processors. The picture that emerges is thus one of considerably greater complexity than that of several domain-specific holding stores controlled by a central processor drawing resources from a single undifferentiated resource pool.

Even with this critique of working memory theory, the distinction between memory storage and manipulative operations performed on that store remains a useful one. We believe that this will remain so, even if, as Monsell suggests, working memory may come to denote an aggregate of numerous specific capacities and operations.

Working Memory and Age: An Experimental Demonstration

It is within this context that we must view the traditional question of where to place the primary source of memory declines in later adulthood. There is now general agreement that while immediate memory processes remain relatively unscathed in normal aging (Burke & Light, 1981; Craik, 1977), significant age differences begin to appear with increased involvement of WM (Craik & Rabinowitz, 1984).

Figure 1.4 illustrates these points with data taken from one of our own studies (Wingfield et al., 1988). Our elderly subjects were 34 community-dwelling men and women (mean age, 70 years; SD = 6.3). All of our subjects were active, in excellent health for their ages, and had good scores on standard tests of verbal ability. (This information is important, since these are the characteristics of elderly adults known to show the smallest memory deficits with age.) Our young group included 34 university undergraduates with verbal ability scores comparable to those of the elderly group.

The two vertical bars to the left in Figure 1.4 show the mean forward digit spans for the two subject groups. These were measured simply by requiring immediate recall of progressively longer sets of spoken digits and plotting the average number

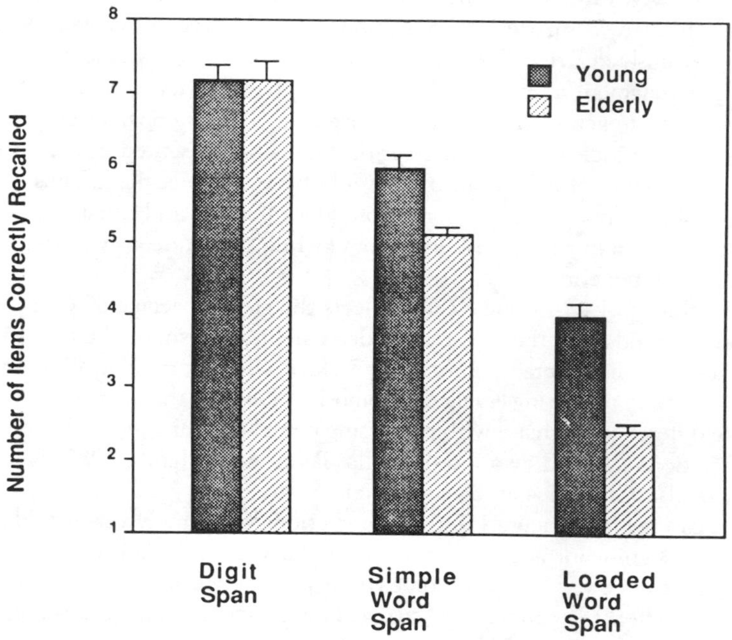

FIGURE 1.4 Mean number of items correctly recalled by young and elderly adults using three span measures representing increasing involvement of working memory capacity. (From Fig 1 of Wingfield, Stine, Lahar, and Aberdeen, 1988.)

of digits reported correctly. Digits represent a small, well-defined set and require very little processing except storage. As such, digit spans represent a fairly pure test of short-term, or primary, memory. As expected, the elderly subjects performed no worse than the young (mean digit spans were 7.2 for both groups). The identity of these values also confirms that hearing acuity for speech was adequate to the task for both groups.

The next set of vertical bars shows the mean simple word spans for the two subject groups; the mean number of unrelated words (in this case, nouns) subjects could recall as progressively longer word strings were presented for immediate recall. Although traditionally also seen as a test of short-term or primary memory, the larger potential ensemble of words could require more extensive identification operations than digits. If so, this would represent some increase in processing involvement in addition to simply holding the items in immediate memory. As we look at the data in Figure 1.4, we see that there is indeed a small but significant age effect ($p < 0.001$). Note, however, that the difference in real terms is a very small one.

The final pair of vertical bars on the right in Figure 1.4 represents our attempt to increase WM involvement in a major way. This task, which we refer to as a loaded word span, was patterned after Daneman and Carpenter's (1980) WM span test as previously described. Subjects listened to a series of statements and made a true/false judgment after each. At the end of the set, they were to try to recall the last word of each of the statements heard in that set. Spans were measured by progressively increasing the number of statements presented in each set, and hence the number of final words that would have to be recalled. Thus the task required subjects not only to perform word identification and storage operations, but also to maintain these words in memory while simultaneously processing the subsequent statements.

Of the three tasks, this one clearly reflects the greatest degree of WM involvement and should show the greatest age decrement. This should be true whether one takes the specific prediction that the elderly have particular difficulty with working memory processing (Craik & Rabinowitz, 1984), or the more general notion that age differences increase with processing complexity or the number of cognitive operations required by a task (Cerella, Poon, & Williams, 1980; Salthouse, 1982; see also Chapter 4 in this volume).

As we can see from Figure 1.4, these predictions were amply verified. Not only was there a significant age difference on the loaded word span test ($p < 0.001$), but this difference was clearly an order of magnitude greater than the age difference observed on the simple word spans. This visual appearance was confirmed by an analysis of variance (ANOVA) conducted on the simple and loaded word span tests. The ANOVA showed not only a significant effect of age and of task, but also a significant age × task interaction ($p < 0.001$).

The issue of age-related reductions in WM capacity remains an intriguing one, especially as it relates to attempts to use these measures to predict other cognitive performances (Hartley, 1986; Light & Anderson, 1985; Stine & Wingfield, 1987). One of our questions must be whether WM limitations, when they occur, play a larger or a smaller role in different tasks and at different stages of processing within a task (Stine & Wingfield, 1987).

LONG-TERM MEMORY AND ENCODING SPECIFICITY

To this point we have focused on short-term, or working memory, processes. As we move to a brief discussion of long-term memory, we will see that the principles of processing resources and resource limitations continue to have strong implications. The literature has for some time contained claims that age-sensitive memory deficits in long-term as well as short-term recall may be attributable to diminished resources with age (Craik & Simon, 1980).

The principle of *levels of processing* as articulated by Craik and Lockhart (1972) began with the information processing sequence as sketched in Figure 1.1, but emphasized the continuous nature of stimulus transformations. In this formulation, information is processed to varying "depths," or levels, which begin with the sensory analysis of the physical stimulus and end with a completed semantic analysis. A semantic analysis typically includes detecting the relationship between this stimulus and other aspects of knowledge. "Deep" processing implies semantic analysis, and "shallow" processing implies an analysis limited to the physical or superficial features of a stimulus.

The claim that deep processing results in better memory than intentional rote rehearsal came from incidental learning experiments in which subjects performed various orienting tasks at the time of stimulus presentation. These tasks were intended to encourage different levels of processing, either "shallow" or "deep." When followed by a surprise test, recall is invariably better for stimuli that have been given deeper processing. Indeed, deeply processed stimuli followed by surprise testing can sometimes be remembered as well as stimuli actively rehearsed for intentional memory (Craik & Lockhart, 1972).

It became apparent that depth of processing *per se* was not the only determinant of good recall. There could be an enrichment of the memory code at almost any level of processing, even at a relatively shallow one. Such elaboration or "spread" of processing at a given level could include encoding features of the context or in some other way produce a more unique, specifiable memory code for the stimulus (Craik & Tulving, 1975).

Thus, while it is usually the case that deeper processing produces more unique or distinctive codes, it is the *distinctiveness* of the code and not its depth that best predicts recall performance (Lockhart, Craik, & Jacoby, 1976; Stein, 1978). In other words, depth and spread of encoding produce their effects by increasing the distinctiveness of the memory trace, which in turn makes it easier to discriminate that trace from others at the time of recall. (Note that we made a similar point when we described Nickerson and Adams' [1979] study of recognition memory for pennies, Figure 1.3.)

This emphasis on encoding operations for success at later retrieval also implies that retrieval cues will be useful only to the extent that they are compatible with the specific encoding processes that occurred during the initial encoding (Morris, Bransford, & Franks, 1977; Nelson, Walling, & McEvoy, 1979). In general then, initial encoding will determine to a very large extent how, and how well, memories will later be retrieved (Tulving & Thomson, 1973; Watkins & Tulving, 1975). (To facilitate our subsequent discussion, we will use the term "deep processing" as a generic term to include its ordinary consequence of distinctive encoding.)

Resource Allocation and Encoding Specificity

As we saw in our earlier discussion of capacity models and working memory, the availability of attentional resources was presumed to regulate both the amount and the kind of processing a stimulus could receive. The relationship between depth (distinctiveness) of processing and resource allocation reflects the same principles. Deep processing, especially if the demands of the task are complicated and the stimuli are unfamiliar, will ordinarily require a great deal of processing capacity. On the other hand, complex shallow processing (e.g., detecting consecutive letters of the alphabet in a written text) might also require considerable resources. Little processing capacity might be required for deep processing when the task demands are simple or when the stimulus is a highly familiar one (e.g., detecting your own name).

The most direct way of studying expended processing capacity during encoding is to use a dual-task, or divided-attention, experiment (Wingfield & Sandoval, 1980). In one such study, Eysenck and Eysenck (1979) asked subjects questions about presented words in order to encourage either deep or shallow processing. At the same time, subjects also received a concurrent secondary task in which reaction times were measured to detecting the occurrence of a sound or light signal. If we take the reaction time to the signal as an index of capacity allocation on the primary task (Johnston & Heinz, 1978), then Eysenck and Eysenck's results showed that more capacity was being expended when deep processing was required. Their results were consistent with the proposition that deeper processing consumed more capacity on the primary task, such that less capacity was available for performance of the simple reaction time task. A dual-task procedure has also been used by Craik and McDowd (1987) to show that memory deficits in later adulthood are due to, or at least correlate with, limitations in processing resources. While the elderly were found to show particular memory deficits in cued recall relative to recognition, they were also especially slower in responding on a concurrent choice reaction time task.

One consequence of an age-related reduction in processing resources would be an inefficiency or slowing of semantic processing of to-be-remembered stimuli. This in turn would reduce the likelihood of distinctive encoding. The importance of this encoding specificity, or elaboration, is that such memories will be tagged in a way to make them unique, and hence discriminable, from other memories, at the time of recall (Craik & Simon, 1980; Eysenck, 1974).

Consider, for example, a subject who has been asked to memorize a word list that includes the word "cloud" as one of the items. If on a later recall test our subject left out the word, it would not be that "cloud" was "forgotten." Our subject still knows what a cloud is; it remains in his or her semantic memory. Rather, we would argue, our subject is uncertain *when* he or she heard the word. Was the word "cloud" heard a minute ago as part of the experimental list, or was it heard or read several hours ago, perhaps in the course of an everyday conversation or reading? Indeed, if we use common words in our experiments (as most investigators do), they are that much more likely to have been encountered recently. (See Wingfield & Byrnes, 1981, pp. 262–263, for a discussion of temporal discrimination in traditional short-term recall tasks.)

It would be reasonable to assume that whenever a stimulus or an event occurs, there is some activation or reactivation of the trace in memory. Thus the level of activation of a neural trace would give direct information about the recency of encountering that stimulus or event. Common (i.e., frequently encountered) words and events would have high levels of activation and hence be difficult to discriminate in time from the even more recently experienced experimental stimuli. Thus, memory failures for such common events may result from a lack of sufficient temporal discrimination.

In a typical memory experiment, such temporal confusions should not be especially likely. On the one hand, repeated rehearsal of a list of words would make their traces discriminably fresh. Both recency and frequency would be operating conjointly to raise the trace's level of activation. It would be unlikely in this case for the subject to mistake an "old" item for a new one, or vice versa. Also, if the stimuli can be given deep or elaborative processing, or some linking associations created, the subject would not have to rely on temporal discrimination at all. That is, temporal discrimination would be a discriminator of last resort, when no other distinguishing feature of the memory trace can be found. As we shall see, however, this can be the case for many routine daily activities.

When Uniqueness Fails: A Temporal Tagging Hypothesis

A recent report by Cohen and Faulkner (1989) makes the important point that many memories are for things that never happened. Cohen and Faulkner's major concern, especially in the case of the elderly, is that of distinguishing between intended and actual memories: a confusion of the memory of an action performed with the memory of an action planned. In one of their examples, they cite a person's uncertainty about whether he or she has added salt to a bowl of soup, or whether what is remembered is the intention of doing so. As Cohen and Faulkner note, the direction of the confusion will affect the type of error that is made. A plan misidentified as an action will cause the action to be omitted. An action misidentified as a plan may be repeated. Such confusion could be serious if the misidentifications related to whether one had turned off the stove or had taken one's medication.

To the extent that an elderly adult's memory for an actual event is fuzzy (i.e., less distinctive), so the likelihood of confusion between intention and actuality may be greater. This is an area we expect to see attract considerable attention in cognitive aging research. The topic is of both theoretical and practical interest (Cohen & Faulkner, 1989).

It would follow from our earlier discussion of temporal discrimination that what might appear as a failure of reality monitoring could in fact sometimes be a result of temporal uncertainty. This would be especially so for activities that are performed frequently and without much thought (e.g., locking your car or brushing your teeth). For example, if you try to remember whether you locked your door when you left home this morning, you might say that you had done so. You have a clear memory image of yourself turning the key in the lock. A temporal tagging confusion, however, could result in your memory of having done so yesterday being mistaken for having done so today. It is not a question of whether the event did occur and is in memory. It is a question of how recently it last occurred. The more frequently such routine tasks are performed, the more likely this temporal confusion is.

Our failure in such cases is most probably a failure to attend to the distinctive features of the task when it was performed. By this we mean a failure to find some contextual elaboration at the time of task performance that might be encoded with the task to make this performance somehow unique. Even when the resources for creating a more distinct code are available, they may not necessarily be utilized. A question for future research is whether elderly adults may be less likely to encode these events with clarity and hence tend to rely more frequently on temporal tagging, the most fallible of memory distinctions.

USING MEMORY

Memory is more than an abstraction or a biochemical change. It is an ability—some would say a skill—of practical significance. Memory is something we use. Thus if our understanding of memory theory is to be of value, it should tell us not only how to characterize the aspects of memory that seem most vulnerable to the aging process, but should also tell us how those abilities that are still intact could potentially compensate for areas of weakness.

As we have already seen, limitations in working memory resources have been frequently cited in relation to age-related performance declines in a variety of cognitive domains (Craik & Rabinowitz, 1984; Stine & Wingfield, 1987). Because some upper limit on resource capacity is part of the presumed nature of working memory, changes caused by resource limitations would be expected to be a matter of degree rather than a reflection of a fundamental change in the way a task is performed. A good rule in cognitive aging is that those tasks that are difficult or complex for the young will be even more so for the elderly (Cerella, Poon, & Williams, 1980; Salthouse, 1982). It is for this reason that qualitative differences in task performances, when they appear, are of special interest.

Along with resource limitations, the literature also holds suggestions that performance declines in normal aging may result from a general slowing of behavior or reduction in processing speed (Birren, Woods, & Williams, 1980; Salthouse, 1980; Wingfield et al., 1985). Although we should not presume a direct correlation between time and depth of processing (Craik & Tulving, 1975), perceptual processing and stimulus encoding do take time. A slowing of processing speed could thus leave shallow traces vulnerable to loss enroute to more complete processing (Salthouse, 1980; Waugh & Barr, 1980; Wingfield, 1980).

We should say at the outset that the relationship between slowing, resource limitations and processing efficiency is a complex one. We suffer in part from inadequate definitions of some of these underlying concepts and in part from an inability to determine directions of causality. For example, in the above illustration, we showed how slowing could cause inefficient processing and hence, poor recall. It is also the case, however, that apparent slowing could be a consequence of an inefficient, or resource-limited, system: an inefficient system would require more time to complete any given activity. To fully exhaust the argument, we must also record that both slowing and resource limitations could co-occur in normal aging, and each could contribute to observed performance declines. There seems no question that elderly adults have more difficulty than young adults in rapidly and/or spontaneously organizing to-be-remembered materials, or rapidly seeing connections between stimulus elements (Rankin, Karol, & Tuten, 1984; Smith, 1980). One final element in this mix is our as yet rudimentary understanding of how acquired experience, or "expertise," may operate within a declining biological system to produce what may, on an output level, be quite excellent levels of performance.

In order to pursue these questions, one could pick almost any domain of stimulus processing and memory performance (e.g., visual scene perception and visual memory or reading skill and text recall). The domain we have chosen to explore these questions is that of the perceptual processing and immediate recall of spoken language. It might be instructive to say why.

One notable feature of ordinary spoken language is its very rapid rate. Ordinary conversation typically proceeds at rates of between 140 to 180 words per minute (wpm), while a radio or TV news reader working from a prepared script can easily exceed 210 wpm. Further, unlike reading, where we can control our input rate and backtrack for review, speech processing must follow the rate of the speaker. What cannot be accomplished *on-line* (i.e., as the speech is being heard), must at least be accomplished within the span of memory for what has just been heard. In principle, then, spoken language processing should put a high demand on both working memory and processing speed.

There is a second set of reasons for choosing speech. Although we do not wish to underrate the importance of memory for written text, by far our greatest communicative interaction with the world comes through speech. We get news of family and friends from spoken conversation. When lonely, we do not want to read a book, we want to talk to a friend or neighbor. For news of the world around us, we now know that newspapers have been supplanted by TV and radio. This is so even though the visual "aids" (the films, pictures, maps) that accompany TV news and weather reports are of dubious value for either comprehension or memory of program content (Waagenar, Varey, & Hudson, 1984).

At the same time, most of us are aware that hearing impairment of one form or another can be a serious problem among the elderly. Hearing impairment is, in fact, the third most prevalent problem in the community-dwelling elderly population, after arthritis and hypertensive disease. The incidence of hearing impairment rises from just over 1% for people under 17, to 12% for people between 45 and 64, 24% for those between 65 to 74, and 39% for those 75 and older (U.S. Congress, Office of Technology Assessment, 1986).

The issue of hearing impairment associated with aging (*presbycusis*) is a complex one, and good introductory reviews are available for the interested reader in addition to the congressional report just cited (e.g., Corso, 1984; Stine, Wingfield, & Poon, 1989). It is important to note, however, that many elderly adults do not have a clinically significant hearing loss, and that many of those who do still retain adequate hearing for good interaction with the world. It remains equally clear that an understanding of auditory processing by the elderly, especially as it relates to speech, should be high on our list of priorities.

Processing Demands for Spoken Language

We can often make a formal distinction between comprehension and memory: one can memorize nonsense syllables or words without knowing their meaning, and one can comprehend a message when hearing it but later remember very little of its content. In general, however, when a person recalls sentences or narratives, comprehension is an inherent part of the memory task (Bartlett, 1932; Clark & Clark, 1977). For example, incorrectly recalled passages are invariably consistent with the meanings of the utterances, whether the errors are of omission or commission (for examples and a review, see Wingfield, 1975; Wingfield & Byrnes, 1981, pp. 93–107). It is for this reason that although our focus is on memory, we must, as part of our analysis, be aware that memory for natural language will always involve syntactic and semantic processing as part of the task.

One reason speech can be recognized so rapidly is the role played by context in on-line language processing. For example, words in context can be recognized, on average, within 200 milliseconds (ms) of their onset, or when less than half of their full acoustic signal has been heard (Grosjean, 1980; Marslen-Wilson & Welsh, 1978; Wingfield & Wayland, 1988). This is true even though many words in ordinary speech are so poorly articulated that they would be totally unintelligible if they were spliced out and presented in isolation (Hunnicutt, 1985).

Current conceptions of on-line language processing postulate an interactive system in which listeners continually analyze the speech input for structural information such as the detection of main clauses and the completion of functional relationships within these clauses. These would have to be predictive hypotheses that would either be confirmed or modified as further speech input is received. Although these operations would be conducted primarily on-line, as the speech is being heard, we would also have to postulate a necessary memory component. That is, as the speech is being heard, either the individual words (or their analytic representations) would have to be saved and integrated with both past and subsequent speech elements to determine the full structure, and hence meaning, of the utterances. Although most theorists have stressed on-line operations (Marslen-Wilson & Welsh, 1978) or on-line operations with memory constraints (Wingfield & Butterworth, 1984; Wingfield & Nolan, 1980), not all processes can be conducted on-line. Just one example is the fact that the recognition of some words requires the use of linguistic context that follows the word (Grosjean, 1985). This would have to require *post hoc*, or memory-dependent, processing.

Such *post hoc* processes, those which must be retrospectively accomplished after the speech signal has gone by, are called off-line processes. Extreme cases involve "garden path" sentences, such as, "The old man the boats." These are apparently anomalous sentences that, on reflection, do have meaning. For successful comprehension, such utterances must be held in memory while the listener re-analyzes their linguistic elements to discover the initial encoding mistake. (In this case, we would have to recode "old" as a noun, and "man" as a verb.) Other notable memory-dependent analyses include working out anaphoric reference, such as connecting pronouns (it, he, she, they, them) with their specific referents.

It thus seems to be that some transient memory storage is necessary for language processing and comprehension, and there have been suggestions that up to two sentences at a time may be held in memory during speech processing (Glanzer, Fischer, & Dorfman, 1984). There is general agreement, however, that whatever the nature of the interim memory component in natural language processing, it is not the kind of short-term passive store maintained by a simple rehearsal loop as was envisaged by the early memory theorists. The nature of the transient memory representations in rapid language processing remains of interest to investigators (Clark & Clark, 1977; Monsell, 1984; Wingfield & Butterworth, 1984).

Speed of Processing in Normal Aging

Along with the evidence for resource limitations and reductions in working memory capacity (Craik & Rabinowitz, 1984), a major source of performance deficits observed in elderly adults may be a general slowing of behavior (Birren, Woods, & Williams, 1980). In our previous discussion of processing depth, we made the argument that slowed processing could retard effective stimulus encoding and hence have a negative impact on memory performance (Salthouse, 1980; Waugh & Barr, 1980; Wingfield, 1980). If this were the case, one would expect to see especially great age effects on memory for speech because of the very high speech rates of normal conversation and the complexity of processing demands.

We examined this question by constructing speech materials in which we increased the processing demands placed on the listener by systematically varying the speech rate of the speech recordings (Stine, Wingfield, & Poon, 1986, experiment 1). We did not want to increase speech rate by varying the speed on a tape recorder, as this would distort the pitch and sound quality. Rather, we made use of the so-called *sampling method* of time-compression on a dedicated computer designed for this purpose. Our method of time-compression was to remove 20-ms segments at regular intervals from the speech signal and then to abut the remaining segments in time. When played back at normal speed, the result is speech reproduced in less than its normal time but without the distortions in pitch or quality that would, for example, accompany tape-recorder playback at a faster speed (Foulke, 1971). The degree of time compression is controlled by the frequency with which the tape segments are deleted.

Studies have shown that young adults can follow time-compressed speech quite well, often to the point of handling speech rates of as much as twice the normal speech rates (Foulke, 1971; Wingfield, 1975). Beyond some point (depending on features such as content complexity and redundancy), however, recall performance will decline with increasing speech rates. Although removal of any of the speech signal is bound to eliminate some richness of the signal, these declines are thought to be due, at least within limits, more to the loss of ordinarily available processing time than to degrading of the speech signal per se (Aaronson, Markowitz, & Shapiro, 1971; Chodorow, 1979).

As in the previous experiment, our elderly subjects were active, community-dwelling men and women with good education and good scores in general verbal ability. Our young subjects were again a matched group of university undergraduates. The subjects heard prerecorded sentences through earphones at rates varying from 200 to 400 wpm. The particular sentences heard at each speech rate were counterbalanced across the experiment. The subjects' task was to listen to each sentence as it was presented, and when the sentence had finished, to recall as much of it as possible, as accurately as possible.

Figure 1.5 shows data taken from this experiment, in which we have plotted the percentage of propositions, or "idea units," recalled by both young and elderly subjects as a function of speech rate in terms of propositions per second (Kintsch & Keenan, 1973). For both groups, recall performance shows an approximately linear decline with increasing speech rate, but the rate of this decline is much steeper for the elderly subjects than for the young. The elderly subjects do show a measureable processing deficit for rapid speech. Note, however, that at our slowest input rate on the left side of the graph (a rate that is in fact much higher than one would ordinarily encounter), our elderly subjects performed almost as well as the young.

Linguistic Structure and Compensation for Loss

It is clear that we can demonstrate age-related decrements in processing speed, just as we previously demonstrated age differences in tests of working memory

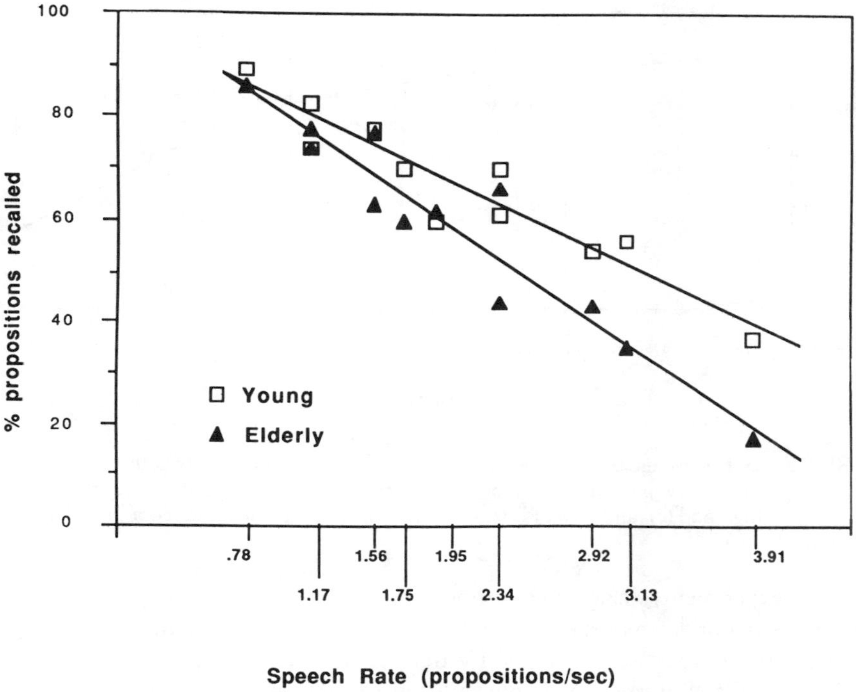

FIGURE 1.5 Percentage of propositions recalled by young and elderly adults as a function of speech input rate (propositions/sec).

capacity. In spite of these losses, however, most elderly adults, like those who took part in our experiment, do handle spoken language well. Indeed, it was only when our subjects were put under especially heavy processing loads that the age differences began to appear.

Our answer to this apparent paradox is that natural language processing is not just a highly practiced skill. Normal language contains highly structured internal organization that is as well appreciated by the elderly as by the young (Wingfield & Stine, 1986). While elderly adults may lose some degree of processing speed, they do not lose knowledge of the rules or the structure of their language. It would seem likely that these subjects were using this knowledge to compensate for what would otherwise be very real processing deficits.

Figure 1.6 shows the results of another experiment in which we looked more closely at the question of processing deficits, linguistic structure, and recall performance (Wingfield et al., 1985). In this experiment, young and elderly adults heard three different kinds of sentence-length sets of verbal materials. As in the

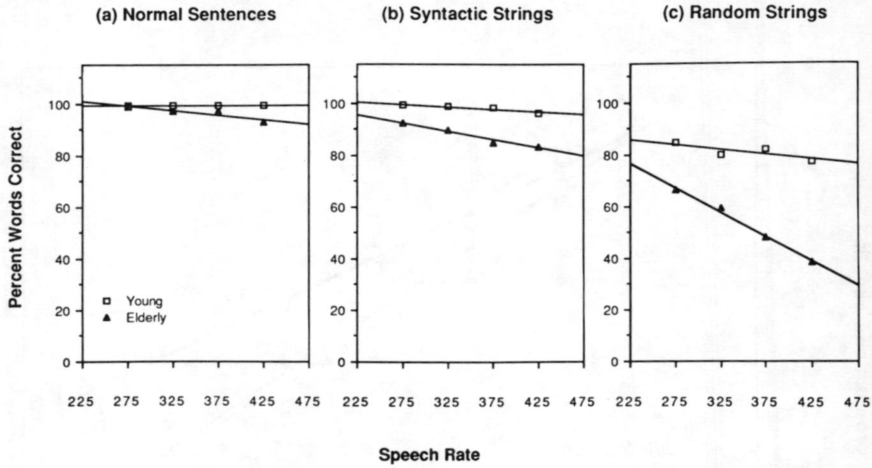

FIGURE 1.6 Percentage of words recalled correctly by young and elderly adults as a function of speech rate (wpm) for three types of speech meterials: (a) normal sentences, (b) syntactic strings, and (c) random word strings. (Data taken from Wingfield, Poon, Lombardi, & Lowe, 1985.)

previous experiment, we again used time-compression to vary speech rate. In this case we used four different speech rates (275, 325, 375, and 425 wpm), all of which were faster than the fastest radio or TV news reader one could possibly imagine! The subjects' task was again simply to listen to each speech passage, and then to recall, as accurately as possible, as much as they could remember.

Figure 1.6 (*c*) shows our best attempt to examine "pure" processing ability by measuring recall performance for what we have called "random strings." These were five- and eight-word strings of unrelated words spoken in a monotone. (The curves shown here are the average of the two string lengths.) We can see that the elderly adults' recall is poorer at all speech rates and that the slope of performance against increasing speech input rate is again notably greater for the elderly than for the young subjects. An ANOVA verified the significant overall effects of speech rate ($p < 0.001$), and age ($p < 0.001$), and also a significant speech rate × age interaction ($p < 0.001$).

Figure 1.6 (*b*) shows performance for the same subjects listening to verbal materials of the same lengths and same speech rates. Suddenly, however, the processing deficit seems to have been reduced! We have called these passages "syntactic strings": word sequences without meaning, but which follow the general constraints of normal English grammar. That is, the nouns, verbs, adjectives, and grammatical endings are all there, but the "sentences" themselves do not make sense. These materials, a very old favorite in psycholinguistics research, take the form of strings like, "Colorless green ideas sleep furiously," or "Frisky water drank clear dogs."

As we can see, the elderly subjects do show poorer overall performance than the young, and also a steeper slope decline. An ANOVA confirmed both main effects of speech rate and of age ($p < 0.001$) and also a significant speech rate × age interaction ($p < 0.01$). Note, however, that in absolute terms the age gap has been dramatically reduced. This is true both in terms of the general levels of performance for young and elderly subjects, but also in terms of the slopes of the speech rate functions.

Figure 1.6(a), shows the full effect of contextual and linguistic constraints on performance. These curves show recall performance for fully normal, ordinary sentences of the same lengths, and heard at the same speech rates as those in (b) and (c). In this case, the age deficits have been virtually eliminated.

The performance of the two age groups were not equal, and an ANOVA showed significant effects of speech rate ($p < 0.005$), of age ($p < 0.005$), and a speech rate × age interaction ($p < 0.005$). As we can also see, however, in absolute terms these differences were very small indeed. That is, at the slowest speech rate we used (still a very rapid 275 wpm), the young and the elderly are essentially equivalent in their level of performance. They are both virtually at a "ceiling" of 100% accuracy. Further, even at the fastest speech rate we tested (425 wpm), the age difference remains small in absolute terms. In fact, had we tested only normal sentences, we would have come to the erroneous conclusion that the elderly subjects had virtually no processing deficit for speech.

In subsequent work we have also looked more specifically at the role of *prosody* (i.e., intonation contour, temporal patterning, word stress, etc.) as an important source of linguistic information (Stine & Wingfield, 1987; Lahar, Wingfield, & Stine, 1987). In these studies we were able to show that elderly adults make good use of prosody in speech processing, often to a higher degree than do the young (Cohen & Faulkner, 1986; Wingfield, Lombardi, & Sokol, 1984). Our main point, however, is that one cannot treat the processing deficits associated with aging as independent of the compensatory mechanisms that may be used by the subjects as part of their on-line processing operations.

Compensation and Knowledge-Task Interactions

Some of the possibilities of interactions between loss and compensation are represented in Figure 1.7, taken from Rybash, Hoyer, and Roodin (1986, p. 85). This is a graph of idealized performance curves for three hypothetical tasks, each of which involves a different degree of experience-based skill.

The top solid curve in the graph is intended to represent the gradual build-up of knowledge and experience that can accumulate over a lifetime. As a general rule, practice and experience at a task produces the sort of curve of *diminishing returns* shown here: the build-up of experience brings improvement, but each gain from one period to the next is smaller than the change that occurred in the previous

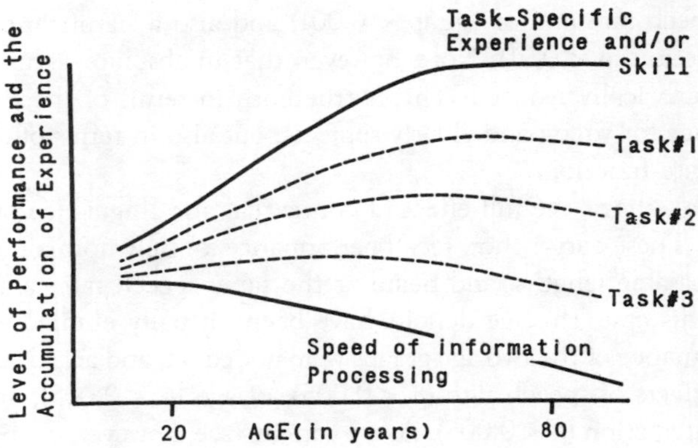

FIGURE 1.7 Hypothetical performance curves for three tasks representing different ratios of task-related experience or skill (which increase with age) to processing speed or efficiency (which decrease with age). (From Fig. 5.3 of Rybash, Hoyer, & Roodin, 1986, p. 86.)

period. While the curve does asymptote at a certain point, however, this point may occur very late in a lifetime of acquiring knowledge and experience. For example, not only does vocabulary tend to continue to increase well into late adulthood, but so do many procedural skills (Wingfield, 1979, pp. 143–166). This is the good news.

The lowest, solid line curve, is the bad news. As we have seen, with age comes a diminution of what we have called *processing power*, whether we characterize this loss in terms of reduced processing resources or, as indicated in Figure 1.7, as a gradual loss of processing speed. Just as the rate and duration of knowledge and skill acquisition will vary from person to person over their lifetimes, so too does the rate of biological aging show wide variations, not only from individual to individual but also from one system to another within a single individual. Thus the lowest curve in Figure 1.7 ("speed of information processing"), is intended to represent a general decline, rather than to depict a specific rate or shape of such a decline across the late life span (Berg, 1985).

The three dotted line curves lying between these two solid line curves show age-related changes in performance levels on three hypothetical tasks representing different proportional combinations of experience or skill versus declining processing power or speed (Rybash, Hoyer, & Roodin, 1986, pp. 85–86). Task #1 is an idealized representation of a performance curve for a highly practiced skill based on a lifetime of accumulated knowledge or experience. The argument here is that the greater the involvement of experience or highly practiced skill, the more this skill or experience can be used to compensate for age-related processing declines and hence, the less likely it will be to see performance declines with advancing years (Denney, 1984). In this connection, Rybash, Hoyer, and Roodin cite a report by Salthouse (1984), who compared typing speed for young and older typists. As implied by the curve for Task #1, he found that the older typists were able to maintain good typing speed in spite of very real declines in general sensorimotor performance.

The curve labeled Task #2 shows a hypothetical age-performance curve for a more balanced skill-processing power mix, and the curve labeled Task #3 represents performance on an unfamiliar, perhaps speeded, task, where past experience or practiced skills cannot easily be brought to bear.

Where then is language in this mix? The answer, of course, is that "language" is not a single task, and the mix of experience versus processing power will vary as a function of the skill of the listener, the nature of the materials to be processed, and the characteristics of the processing demands. For example, as we have seen, the same person who shows significant age-sensitive speeded processing declines for recall of random-word lists may well show excellent recall for meaningful speech, virtually equivalent to that of the younger adult. Indeed, to the extent that mental operations may be modular within rather narrow domains (Fodor, 1983; Monsell, 1984), so the potential for experience- or "top-down"-based compensation will vary. One of our questions must be to determine those elements of perceptual processing and memory that are autonomous versus those interactive components that function through integration of the products of multiple sources.

CONCLUSIONS

Over the years of modern gerontological research, there has been a continuing focus on deficits in memory and cognitive function related to age, and where the loci of these deficits may reside. This work has, quite correctly, followed the trends and paradigms of cognitive psychology and memory research, with its traditional focus on tight control of the experimental procedures and stimuli. To the criticism that the focus of many of these studies seems far from everyday memory, we must argue that this is legitimate when their purpose is to test theory rather than to represent everyday cognitive behavior.

Indeed, this approach has a long and respected history in the experimental psychology of memory, beginning with Ebbinghaus' (1913) goal of "simplifying the stimulus and isolating the response." His way of meeting this dual challenge was to model "pure" memory by using nonsense syllables learned by rote repetition. In the words of one of Ebbinghaus' severest critics: "He [Ebbinghaus] realized that if we use continuous passages of prose or verse as our material to be remembered, we cannot be certain that any two subjects will begin on a level. Such material sets up endless streams of cross-association which may differ significantly from person to person." (Bartlett, 1932, p. 3).

As Bartlett went on to argue, however, if one attempts too much simplification or artificiality (he speaks specifically in this case of using rote retention of very well rehearsed nonsense syllables as one's window on memory), "the remedy is at least as bad as the disease."

While our own view sides very much with Bartlett, there was, of course, merit to both sides of this debate. It is the case that a good test of theory can rest on stimuli and taks as unrepresentative of everyday memory as repetition-memory for word lists or paired-associate learning. Much of the basic work reported in this chapter did in fact derive from such studies. Bartlett's point, however, was that we should be careful of "throwing out the baby with the bathwater": in the case of natural language, with its "endless streams of cross-associations," in its complexity lies its essence.

It is in this spirit that we have offered illustrations drawn from the most natural of daily activities: the processing of spoken language. Listening to, comprehending, and recalling radio and TV news and conversations with neighbors and friends are, in fact, our primary sources of communicative contact with the world and our primary means of acquiring new information. Our reason for studying speech processing in aging is not only because of its dominance in everyday activity and because of the concern we have for auditory processing deficits in the elderly, but also because language processing can stand as the severest test of many of our theories of memory and cognitive decline with age. It can serve as a model for the study of those processes that remain labile with age and those that do not, and how the two can interact to produce the final behavior we see.

Our research goal should thus not only be to enumerate and try to understand the losses that accompany old age; our goal should also be to show how the capacities that do remain can interact with acquired knowledge and experience and produce the full potential of cognitive behavior we might hope to see.

REFERENCES

Aaronson, D., Markowitz, N., & Shapiro, H. (1971). Perception and immediate recall of normal and "compressed" auditory sequences. *Perception & Psychophysics*, 9(4):338–344.

Atkinson, R. C., & Shiffrin, R. M. (1968). Human memory: A proposed system and its control processes. In K. W. Spence, & J. T. Spence (eds.), *The Psychology of Learning and Motivation*, vol. 2. New York: Academic Press.

Baddeley, A. D. (1976). *The Psychology of Memory*. New York: Basic Books.

Baddeley, A. D. (1981) The concept of working memory: A view of its current state and probable future development. *Cognition*, 10:17–23.

Baddeley, A. D., & Hitch, G. J. (1974). Working memory. In G. A. Bower (ed.), *The Psychology of Learning and Motivation*, vol. 8. New York: Academic Press.

Baddeley, A. D., Lieberman, K. (1980). Spatial working memory. In R. S. Nickerson (ed.), *Attention and Performance*, vol. VIII. Hillsdale, NJ: Erlbaum Associates, pp. 521–540.

Baddeley, A. D., Thomson, N., & Buchanan, M. (1975). Word length and the structure of short-term memory. *Journal of Verbal Learning and Verbal Behavior*, 14(6):575–589.

Baltes, P. B. (1987). Theoretical propositions of life-span developmental psychology: On the dynamics between growth and decline, *Developmental Psychology*, 23(5):611–626.

Bartlett, F. C. (1932). *Remembering. A study in experimental and social psychology*. Cambridge: Cambridge University Press.

Berg, S. (1985, July). *Intelligence and terminal decline*. Paper presented at the Thirteenth International Congress of Gerontology, New York.

Birren, J. E., Woods, A. M., & Williams, M. V. (1980). Behavioral slowing with age: Causes, organization, and consequences. In L. W. Poon (ed.), *Aging in the 1980s: Psychological issues*. Washington, DC: American Psychological Association.

Broadbent, D. E. (1958). *Perception and Communication*. New York: Pergamon Press.

Broadbent, D. E. (1971). *Decision and Stress*. New York: Academic Press.

Burke, D. M., & Light, L. L. (1981). Memory and aging: The role of retrieval processes. *Psychological Bulletin*, 90(3):513–546.

Cerella, J., Poon, L. W., & Williams, D. M. (1980). Age and the complexity hypothesis. In L. W. Poon (ed.), *Aging in the 1980s: Psychological issues*. Washington, D.C.: American Psychological Association.

Chodorow, M. S. (1979). Time-compressed speech and the study of lexical and syntactic processing. In W. E. Cooper, & E. C. T. Walker (eds.), *Sentence processing: Psycholinguistic Studies Presented to Merrill Garrett* (pp. 87–102). Hillsdale, NJ: Erlbaum Associates.

Clark, H. H., & Clark, E. V. (1977). *The Psychology of Language*. New York: Harcourt Brace Jovanovich.

Cohen, G., & Faulkner, D. (1986). Does 'elderspeak' work? The effect of intonation and stress on comprehension and recall of spoken discourse in old age. *Language and Communication*, 6:91–98.

Cohen, G., & Faulkner, D. (1989). The effects of aging on perceived and generated memories. In L. W. Poon, D. C. Rubin, & B. A. Wilson (eds.), *Everyday Cognition in Adulthood and Late Life*. Cambridge: Cambridge University Press.

Conrad, R. (1972). Short-term processing in the deaf: A test for speech coding. *British Journal of Psychology*, 63:173–180.

Corso, J. F. (1984). Auditory processes and aging: Significant problems for research. *Experimental Aging Research*, 10:171–174.

Craik, F. I. M. (1977). Age differences in human memory. In J. E. Birren & K. W. Schaie, (eds.), *Handbook of the Psychology of Aging*. New York: Van Nostrand Reinhold.

Craik, F. I. M., & Lockhart, R. S. (1972). Levels of processing: A framework for memory research. *Journal of Verbal Learning and Verbal Behavior*, 11:671–684.

Craik, F. I. M., & McDowd, J. M. (1987). Age differences in recall and recognition. *Journal of Experimental Psychology: Learning, Memory, and Cognition*, 13(3):474–479.

Craik, F. I. M., & Rabinowitz, J. C. (1984). Age differences in the acquisition and use of verbal information. In H. Bouma, & D. G. Bouwhuis (eds.), *Attention and Performance X*, (pp. 471–499). Hillsdale, NJ: Erlbaum Associates.

Craik, F. I. M., & Simon, E. (1980). Age differences in memory: The roles of attention and depth of processing. In L. W. Poon, J. L. Fozard, L. S. Cermak, D. Arenberg, & L. W. Thompson (eds.), *New directions in memory and aging: Proceedings of the George A. Talland Memorial Conference*, (pp. 95–112). Hillsdale, NJ: Erlbaum Associates.

Craik, F. I. M., & Tulving, E. (1975). Depth of processing and the retention of words in episodic memory. *Journal of Experimental Psychology: General*, 104:268–294.

Crowder, R. G. (1976). *Principles of Learning and Memory*. Hillsdale, NJ: Erlbaum Associates.

Daneman, M., & Carpenter, P. A. (1980). Individual differences in working memory and reading. *Journal of Verbal Learning and Verbal Behavior*, 19(4):450–466.

Denney, N. W. (1984). A model of cognitive development across the life span. *Developmental Review*, 4:171–191.

Ebbinghaus, H. (1913). *Memory: A contribution to experimental psychology*. Translated by H. A. Ruger & C. E. Bussenius. New York: Teachers College, Columbia University. (Originally published Leipzig: Altenberg, 1885).

Eysenck, M. W. (1974). Age differences in incidental learning. *Developmental Psychology*, 10(6):936–941.

Eysenck, M. W., & Eysenck, M. C. (1979). Processing depth, elaboration of encoding, memory stores, and expended processing capacity. *Journal of Experimental Psychology: Human Learning and Memory*, 5(5):472–484.

Fisher, R. P., & Craik, F. I. M. (1977). Interaction between encoding and retrieval operations in cued recall. *Journal of Experimental Psychology: Human Learning and Memory*, 3(6):701–711.

Fodor, J. A. (1983). *The Modularity of Mind*. Cambridge, MA: MIT Press.

Foulke, E. (1971). The perception of time-compressed speech. In D. L. Horton & J. J. Jenkins (eds.), *The Perception of Language*. Columbus, OH: Merrill.

Glanzer, M., Fischer, B., & Dorfman, D. (1984). Short-term storage in reading. *Journal of Verbal Learning and Verbal Behavior*, 23(4):467–486.

Grodzinsky, Y., & Shapiro, L. P. (1988). Two perspectives on the modularity of language. *Aphasiology*, 2: 295–298.

Grosjean, F. (1980). Spoken word recognition processes and the gating paradigm. *Perception & Psychophysics*, 28(4):267–283.

Grosjean, F. (1985). The recognition of words after their acoustic offset: Evidence and implications. *Perception & Psychophysics*, 38(4):299–310.

Hartley, J. T. (1986). Reader and text variables as determinants of discourse memory in adulthood. *Psychology and Aging*, 1:150–158.

Hasher, L., & Zacks, R. T. (1979). Automatic and effortful processes in memory. *Journal of Experimental Psychology: General*, 108(3):356–388.

Hunnicutt, S. (1985). Intelligibility versus redundancy—conditions of dependency. *Language and Speech*, 28:47–56.

Hunter, I. M. L. (1964). *Memory*. Baltimore: Penguin Books.

James, W. (1890). *Principles of Psychology*, vol. 1. New York: Holt.

Johnston, W. A., & Heinz, S. P. (1978). Flexibility and capacity demands of attention. *Journal of Experimental Psychology: General*, 107(4):420–435.

Kahneman, D. (1973). *Attention and Effort*. Englewood Cliffs, NJ: Prentice-Hall.

Kandel, E. R, & Schwartz, J. H. (1985). *Principles of Neural Science* (2nd ed.). New York: Elsevier.

Kintsch, W., & Keenan, J. (1973). Reading rate and retention as a function of the number of propositions in the base structure of sentences. *Cognitive Psychology*, 5(3):257–274.

Kosslyn, S. M. (1980). *Image and Mind*. Cambridge, MA: Harvard University Press.

Lahar, C. J., Wingfield, A., & Stine, E. L. (1987, August). *Effects of prosody and age on running memory for speech*. Paper presented at the Annual Meeting of the American Psychological Association, New York.

Light, L. L., & Anderson, P. A. (1985). Working-memory capacity, age, and memory for discourse. *Journal of Gerontology*, 40(6):737–747.

Lockhart, R. S., Craik, F. I. M., & Jacoby, L. (1976). Depth of processing, recognition, and recall. In J. Brown (ed.) *Recall and Recognition* (pp. 75–102). New York: Wiley.

Marslen-Wilson, W. D., & Welsh, A. (1978). Processing interactions and lexical access during word recognition in continuous speech. *Cognitive Psychology*, 10(1):29–63.

Martin, P. R., & Fernberger, S. W. (1929). Improvements in memory span. *American Journal of Psychology*, 41:91–94.

McClelland, J. L., & Rumelhart, D. E. (1985). Distributed memory and the representation of general and specific information. *Journal of Experimental Psychology: General*, 114(2):159–188.

McClelland, J. L., Rumelhart, D. E., & the PDP Research Group. (1986). *Parallel distributed processing: Explorations in the microstructure of cognition. Volume 2: Psychological and biological models*. Cambridge, MA: Bradford Books/MIT Press.

Miller, G. A. (1956). The magical number seven, plus or minus two: Some limits on our capacity for processing information. *Psychological Review*, 63(2):81–96.

Monsell, S. (1984). Components of working memory underlying verbal skills: A "distributed capacities" view. In H. Bouma & D. G. Bouwhuis (eds.), *Attention and Performance*, X. Hillsdale, NJ: Erlbaum Associates.

Moray, N. (1969). *Listening and Attention*. Baltimore: Penguin Books.

Morris, C. D., Bransford, J. D., & Franks, J. J. (1977). Levels of processing versus transfer appropriate processing. *Journal of Verbal Learning and Verbal Behavior*, 16(5):519–533.

Neisser, U. (1967). *Cognitive Psychology*. New York: Appleton-Century-Crofts.

Nelson, D. L., Walling, J. R., & McEvoy, C. I. (1979). Doubts about depth. *Journal of Experimental Psychology: Human Learning and Memory*, 5:24–44.

Nickerson, R. S., & Adams, M. J. (1979). Long-term memory for a common object. *Cognitive Psychology* 11(3):287–307.

Norman, D. A., & Bobrow, D. G. (1975). On data-limited and resource-limited processes. *Cognitive Psychology* 7(1):44–64.

Peterson, L. R., & Peterson, M. J. (1959). Short-term retention of individual verbal items. *Journal of Experimental Psychology* 58(3):193–198.

Peterson, L. R., Rawlings, L., & Cohen, C. (1977). The internal construction of spatial patterns. In G. H. Bower (ed.), *The Psychology of Learning and Motivation*, vol. 11. New York: Academic Press.

Rankin, J. L., Karol, R., & Tuten, C. (1984). Strategy use, recall, and recall organization in young, middle-aged, and elderly adults. *Experimental Aging Research* 10:193–196.

Rumelhart, J. L., McClelland, J. L., & the PDP Research Group. (1986). *Parallel Distributed Processing: Explorations in the Microstructure of Cognition. Volume 1: Foundations*. Cambridge, MA: Bradford Books/MIT Press.

Rybash, J. M., Hoyer, W. J., & Roodin, P. A. (1986). *Adult Cognition and Aging. Developmental Changes in Processing, Knowing and Thinking.* New York: Pergamon Press.

Salthouse, T. A. (1980). Age and memory: Strategies for localizing the loss. In L. W. Poon, J. L. Fozard, L. S. Cermak, D. Arenberg, & L. W. Thompson (eds.), *New Directions in Memory and Aging: Proceedings of the George A. Talland Memorial Conference* (pp. 47–66). Hillsdale, NJ: Erlbaum Associates.

Salthouse, T. A. (1982). *Adult Cognition*. New York: Springer-Verlag.

Salthouse, T. A. (1984). Effects of age and skill in typing. *Journal of Experimental Psychology: General* 113(3):345–371.

Salthouse, T. A. (in press). The role of processing resources in cognitive aging. In M. L. Howe & C. J. Brainerd (eds.), *Cognitive Development in Adulthood*. New York: Springer-Verlag.

Sherry, D. F., & Schacter, D. L. (1987). The evolution of multiple memory systems. *Psychological Review*, 94:439–454.

Shiffrin, R. M., & Schneider, W. (1977). Controlled and automatic human information processing: II. Perceptual learning, automatic attending, and a general theory. *Psychological Review*, 84(2):127–190.

Smith, A. D. (1980). Age differences in encoding, storage, and retrieval. In L. W. Poon, J. L. Fozard, L. S. Cermak, D. Arenberg, & L. W. Thompson (eds.), *New directions in Memory and Aging: Proceedings of the George A. Talland Memorial Conference*. Hillsdale, NJ: Erlbaum Associates.

Squire, L. R. (1986). Mechanisms of memory. *Science*, 232:1612–1619.

Squire, L. R. (1987). *Memory and Brain*. New York: Oxford University Press.

Stein, B. S. (1978). Depth of processing reexamined: The effects of the precision of encoding and test appropriateness. *Journal of Verbal Learning and Verbal Behavior*, 17(2):165–174.

Stine, E. L., & Wingfield, A. (1987). Process and strategy in memory for speech among younger and older adults. *Psychology and Aging*, 2:272–279.

Stine, E. L., & Wingfield, A., & Poon, L. W. (1986). How much and how fast: Rapid processing of spoken language in later adulthood. *Psychology and Aging*, 1:303–311.

Stine, E. L., Wingfield, A., & Poon, L. W. (in press). Speech comprehension and memory through adulthood: The roles of time and strategy. In L. W. Poon, D. C. Rubin, & B. A. Wilson (eds.), *Everyday Cognition in Adulthood and Later Life*. New York: Cambridge University Press.

Swinney, D. A. (1979). Lexical access during sentence comprehension: (Re)consideration of context effects. *Journal of Verbal Learning and Verbal Behavior*, 18(6):645–659.

Titchener, E. B. (1908). *Lectures on the Elementary Psychology of Feeling and Attention*. New York: Macmillan.

Tulving, E. (1983). *Elements of Episodic Memory*. New York: Oxford University Press.

Tulving, E., & Thomson, D. M. (1973). Encoding specificity and retrieval processes in episodic memory. *Psychological Review*, 80(5):352–373.

U.S. Congress, Office of Technology Assessment (1986, May). *Hearing impairment and elderly people—A background paper.* (OTA-BP-BA-30). Washington, DC: U.S. Government Printing Office.

Waagenar, W. A., Varey, C. A., & Hudson, P. T. W. (1984). Do audiovisuals aid? A study of bisensory presentation on the recall of information. In H. Bouma & D. G. Bouwhuis (eds.), *Attention and Performance, X*. New York: Academic Press.

Wales, R., & Toner, H. (1979). Intonation and ambiguity. In W. E. Cooper & E. C. T. Walker (eds.), *Sentence Processing: Psycholinguistic Studies Presented to Merrill Garrett*. Hillsdale, NJ: Erlbaum Associates.

Watkins, M. J., & Tulving, E. (1975). Episodic memory: When recognition fails. *Journal of Experimental Psychology: General* 1:5–29.

Waugh, N. C., & Barr, R. A. (1980). Memory and mental tempo. In L. W. Poon, J. L. Fozard, L. S. Cermak, D. Arenberg, & L. W. Thompson (eds.), *New Directions in Memory and Aging: Proceedings of the George A. Talland Memorial Conference* (pp. 251–260). Hillsdale, NJ: Erlbaum Associates.

Waugh, N. C., & Norman, D. A. (1965). Primary memory. *Psychological Review*, 72(2):89–104.

Welford, A. T. (1968). *Fundamentals of Skill*. London: Methuen.

Wickelgren, W. A. (1965). Acoustic similarity and intrusion errors in short-term memory. *Journal of Experimental Psychology*, 70(1):102–108.

Wingfield, A. (1975). Acoustic redundancy and the perception of time-compressed speech. *Journal of Speech and Hearing Research*, 18:96–104.

Wingfield, A. (1979). *Human Learning and Memory: An Introduction*. New York: Harper and Row.

Wingfield, A. (1980). Attention, levels of processing, and state-dependent recall. In L. W. Poon, J. L. Fozard, L. S. Cermak, D. Arenberg, & L. W. Thompson (eds.), *New Directions in Memory and Aging: Proceedings of the George A. Talland Memorial Conference* (pp. 135–142). Hillsdale, NJ: Erlbaum Associates.

Wingfield, A., & Butterworth, B. (1984). Running memory for sentences and parts of sentences: Syntactic parsing as a control function in working memory. In H. Bouma & D. G. Bouwhuis (eds.), *Attention and Performance, X* (pp. 351-364). New York: Academic Press.

Wingfield, A., & Byrnes, D. L. (1972). Decay of information in short-term memory. *Science*, 176:690–692.

Wingfield, A., & Byrnes, D. L. (1981). *The Psychology of Human Memory*. New York: Academic Press.

Wingfield, A., Lombardi, L., & Sokol, S. (1984). Prosodic features and the intelligibility of accelerated speech: Syntactic versus periodic segmentation. *Journal of Speech and Hearing Research*, 27:128–134.

Wingfield, A., & Nolan, K. A. (1980). Spontaneous segmentation in normal and in time-compressed speech. *Perception & Psychophysics*, 28(2):97–102.

Wingfield, A., Poon, L. W., Lombardi, L. & Lowe, D. (1985). Speed of processing in normal aging: Effects of speech rate, linguistic structure and processing time. *Journal of Gerontology* 40(5):579–585.

Wingfield, A., & Sandoval, A. W. (1980). Perceptual processing for meaning. In L. W. Poon, J. L. Fozard, L. S. Cermak, D. Arenberg, & L. W. Thompson (eds.), *New Directions in Memory and Aging: Proceedings of the George A. Talland Memorial Conference* (pp. 205-238). Hillsdale, NJ: Erlbaum Associates.

Wingfield, A., & Stine, E. L. (1986). Organizational strategies in immediate recall of rapid speech by young and elderly adults. *Experimental Aging Research*, 12:79–83.
Wingfield, A., Stine, E. L., Lahar, C. J., & Aberdeen, J. (1988). Does the capacity of working memory change with age? *Experimental Aging Research*, 14(2): 103–107.
Wingfield, A., & Wayland, S. (1988). Object-naming in aphasia: Word-initial phonology and response activation. *Aphasiology*, 2: 423–425.

2

Impairment in Normal Memory Aging: Implications of Laboratory Evidence

Donald H. Kausler

"Reagan Memory Loss Astonishing, Muskie Says" (*Columbia Daily Tribune*, March 2, 1987). Mr. Muskie appeared to be referring to what once was labeled *benign senescent forgetfulness* (Kral, 1962). The current popular term is *age-associated memory impairment* (AAMI), (Crook et al., 1986). Alas, if Mr. Muskie is correct, even the former President of the United States is not immune to the ravages of time and the occurrence of AAMI.

How extensive is memory impairment with normal aging? An answer to this question is not easy to obtain. There are at least four important issues to be considered. The first is the fact that the human memory system is imperfect at all ages. Consequently, the extent of impairment in late adulthood on any memory task must be evaluated relative to the performance of younger adults on the same task. Laboratory studies of aging's effects on memory are therefore necessarily studies of adult age differences, and they require comparisons between older and younger adults.

The second issue rests in the possibility that age differences in memory proficiency may be attributable to factors other than aging per se, particularly age differences in generational membership. A popular favorite in recent years has been to place the responsibility for age-related deficits in many cognitive tasks on the wide generational span separating young and elderly adults. That is, age differences in performances may be the consequence of a cohort effect rather than a true aging effect. I feel that as far as memory is concerned, this is an unlikely possibility (see Kausler, 1982, for an elaboration). However, there are other factors that frequently covary with age. They merit more serious attention and will be discussed later in this chapter.

The third issue concerns the degree to which age differences in memory proficiency found in the laboratory generalize to age differences found in the everyday world. A common criticism of laboratory research is that it employs tasks that are artificial and often seemingly unrelated to memory's everyday operations. Conceivably, age differences favoring younger adults are exaggerated by performances under laboratory conditions. However, it may be argued that it is *memory processes*, not the tasks they mediate, that are at stake in laboratory research, and these processes are comparable to those mediating everyday memory performances. Nevertheless, it is true that we need to encourage more research that demonstrates the covariation between performances on laboratory tasks and everyday memory tasks (Kausler, 1985; Kausler, in press).

The final issue, and to me the most important, stems from the complexity of the human memory system. Recent years have seen a remarkable change in our conceptualization of human memory. Instead of one memory system, we now consider memory to be composed of several interacting but somewhat independently functioning components, or subsystems. The postulation of different forms of memory greatly complicates our understanding of age-related impairment. Some components may be impaired modestly, if at all, while other components may be severely impaired. My coverage will be restricted to what I consider to be the three major components: *generic* (or *semantic*) memory, *episodic* memory, and *metamemory* (in so doing, I will touch upon another component, implicit memory). Still another component, procedural memory, has been postulated, but thus far it has had little impact on gerontological research. A brief overview of the three primary components is in order before we begin our discussion of age-related memory impairment.

THE HUMAN MEMORY SYSTEM: AN OVERVIEW

Generic (or semantic) memory (Tulving, 1972) is the subsystem involved in the storage and retrieval of permanent knowledge. A basic component of generic memory is the internal lexicon, a store presumed to contain the representations of the thousands of words we know and use in language comprehension and production as well as the concepts those words represent. Note how rapidly and smoothly you gain access to the lexicon as you comprehend the stream of words presently reaching your eyes. Generic memory also contains our knowledge of the universe: for example, our knowledge that Columbus is the capital of Ohio, 12 is the square root of 144, and so on. Knowledge in generic memory is stored without reference to context, that is, information pertaining to when and where that knowledge was acquired. Do you remember when and where you learned that Columbus is the capital of Ohio?

By contrast, episodic memory is the repository for personally experienced episodes or events. Will you remember next week what food you ate tonight? Will you remember a year from now the name of the author of the chapter you are now reading? Information in episodic memory is stored in reference not only to the content of the experienced event, but also to when and where it was experienced. In addition, the episodic subsystem is assumed to mediate both short-term and long-term memory of experienced events, and it is assumed to be governed by both effortful (or rehearsal-dependent) and automatic (or rehearsal-independent) processes. I will have more to say about these distinctions shortly.

Metamemory is essentially an individual's knowledge of his/her own memory system and the regulation of that system. Given a set of new material to memorize, how would you go about doing it? How would you rehearse it? How much time and effort would you allow for the memorization? How would you know when you have the material fully memorized? These are the kinds of processes that collectively make up metamemory. Understanding potential age differences in metamemorial processes is quite important to the understanding of age differences in performances on episodic memory tasks. It is possible that some impairment with aging in episodic memory proficiency may be the consequence of age-related deficits in metamemory proficiency.

Generic Memory: Age Differences

Our discussion of generic memory will focus on the internal lexicon, simply because most laboratory research on adult age differences in generic memory proficiency has been concerned with it. Shown in Figure 2.1 is a popular model of the lexicon's associative network. Note that the concept of "Health practitioner" has stored with it the word "Doctor" and information about the sound and the orthography of that word. Also stored with the word are associative pathways leading to such related words as "Nurse" and "Bill." Activation of "doctor" by hearing or seeing that word spreads automatically, (that is, without the expenditure of attentional resources) to these related words, resulting in their indirect activation. However, the probability of activating "nurse" is greater than the probability of activating "bill," simply because the distance separating "doctor" from each is greater for the latter. There is now convincing evidence to indicate that this automatic spreading of activation operates as proficiently for elderly adults as for young adults (Balota & Duchek, 1989; Burke, White, & Diaz, 1987). One of the tasks demonstrating this comparability requires subjects simply to pronounce a word as soon as it is

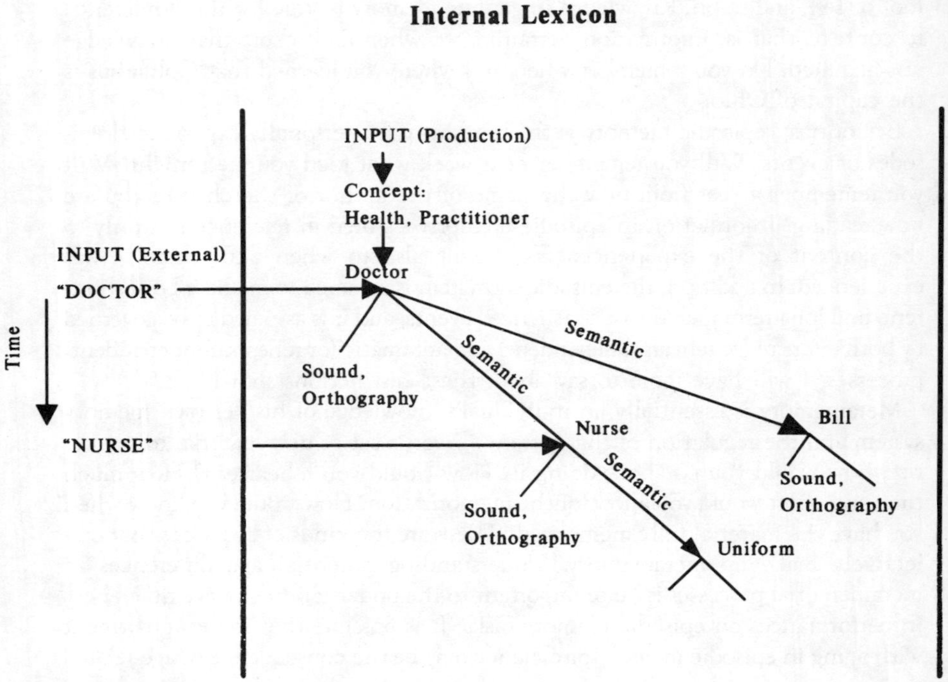

FIGURE 2.1 Model of the internal lexicon's associative network.

exposed on a computer screen. For example, the word "nurse" is one of the to-be-pronounced words in a lengthy series of words, and it is preceded in the series by either the related word "doctor" or the unrelated word "grass." The latency in pronouncing "nurse" is less when preceded by "doctor" than when preceded by "grass," provided there is sufficient time separating the successively exposed words. Most important, the facilitation attributable to relatedness (i.e., latency for unrelated word minus latency for related word) is as pronounced for old as for young subjects. This may be seen in the results obtained by Balota and Duchek (1989) (Fig. 2.2); relatedness/unrelatedness was varied in their study by the use of category names and exemplars or nonexemplars of those categories. Activation of words in the network doesn't always proceed automatically, of course. There are many occasions when self-directed, or attentional, processes are demanded in order to gain access to a word. Even these attention processes seem to be relatively unimpaired in normal aging (Burke, White, & Diaz, 1987). By contrast, it is attentional processes that seem to be markedly impaired in patients with Alzheimer's disease (Nebes & Madden, 1988).

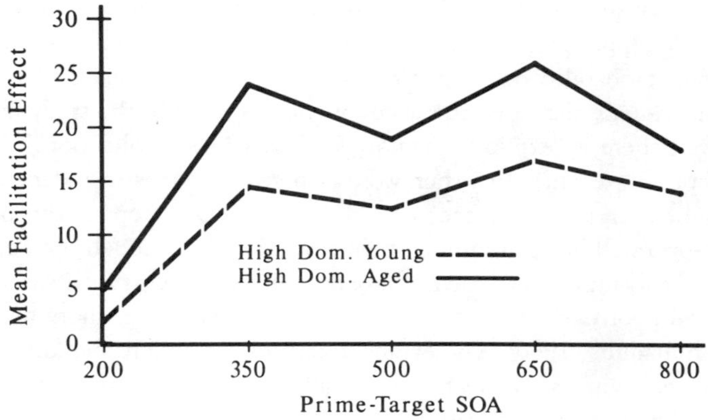

FIGURE 2.2 Facilitation from spreading activation for target words (high dominance exemplars) preceded by category names as primes. (Adapted from Figure 2 in Balota & Duchek, 1989.)

Moreover, there is also good reason to believe that the basic structure of the associative network is relatively unaltered over the course of the adult life span. This may be seen from various studies comparing the word associations of young and elderly individuals (Burke & Peters, 1986). The basic attributes of associations are roughly comparable regardless of age.

The tendency to conclude that generic memory is remarkably spared from impairment with normal aging is tempered, however, by recent evidence indicating that some components of its operations diminish in proficiency during late adulthood (see Light & Burke, in press, for further coverage). For example, Balota and Duchek (1989) recently demonstrated that lexical access time is greater for older than for younger individuals. In addition, elderly adults appear to be less proficient than young adults in movement within the network from concept to word—for example, from "Health practitioner" to "Doctor" (see Fig. 2.1). This is evident from the fact that elderly adults have greater difficulty than young adults in finding words that match definitions of those words (Bowles & Poon, 1985) and also the fact that elderly adults have more "tip of the tongue" experiences (i.e., word-finding difficulties in spontaneous speech) than do younger adults (Burke, Worthley, & Martin, 1987).

There is a phenomenon known as implicit memory that may be closely related to the operations of semantic memory. The phenomenon is attracting considerable attention these days because of its potential diagnostic value in distinguishing between individuals with organic-based amnesia, individuals with Alzheimer's disease, and individuals with AAMI. A popular task for demonstrating implicit memory is to have individuals study a lengthy list of words in preparation for a subsequent recognition or recall memory test. The subjects also receive a series of word fragments, such as "sha—," and they are asked to complete the word. If the word "shade" appeared in a prior study list, then implicit memory is demonstrated by a high probability of completing the word with the letters "de," whether or not the individuals identified the word "shade" as being in the study list (i.e., whether or not there is "explicit" memory, or "conscious recollection," for the underlying episodic event). In other words, there is stochastic independence between implicit and explicit memory (Tulving, 1985). Apparently, organic amnesics perform well on such implicit memory tasks, even though their explicit memory is markedly impaired (Cohen, 1984). By contrast, patients with Alzheimer's disease perform poorly on the implicit as well as the explicit memory test (Butters, 1987; Shimamura, 1986). The evidence regarding implicit memory impairment with normal aging is less clear. Conceivably, implicit memory is a phenomenon closely related to the activation of concepts in the internal lexicon, an activation that persists sufficiently over time to make those concepts highly salient at the time of the implicit memory test. If generic memory functions are largely immune to normal aging impairments, then we would expect little in the way of an age difference between young and older individuals in their implicit memory performances. Some support for this position comes from studies by Light, Singh, and Capps (1986) and Light and Singh (1987). On the other hand, a rather substantial difference favoring young adults was reported by Chiarello and Hoyer (1988). We can expect to find a number of similar studies conducted in the near future. Hopefully, they will resolve the currently conflicting evidence.

Rehearsal-Dependent Episodic Memory

Nature

A model of the operations underlying what I prefer to call rehearsal-dependent episodic memory is shown in Figure 2.3. By rehearsal dependency I mean that some form of rehearsal is needed either to assure proficient transmission to a long-term store for later long-term memory or to maintain information in working memory for short-term memory. In general, the better the quality of the rehearsal or the greater the amount of the rehearsal, the greater the amount of transmission to the long-term store. Proficient rehearsal is assured by the activation of a rehearsal strategy store in metamemory, usually initiated by an individual's intent to encode episodic events and to commit them to long-term storage. That is, intentionality is usually a precursor to long-term rehearsal-dependent memory. Information in the to-be-remembered events (e.g., words in a lengthy series of words) is matched initially with the representations of those events in generic memory. These representations are then transmitted to working memory where they are

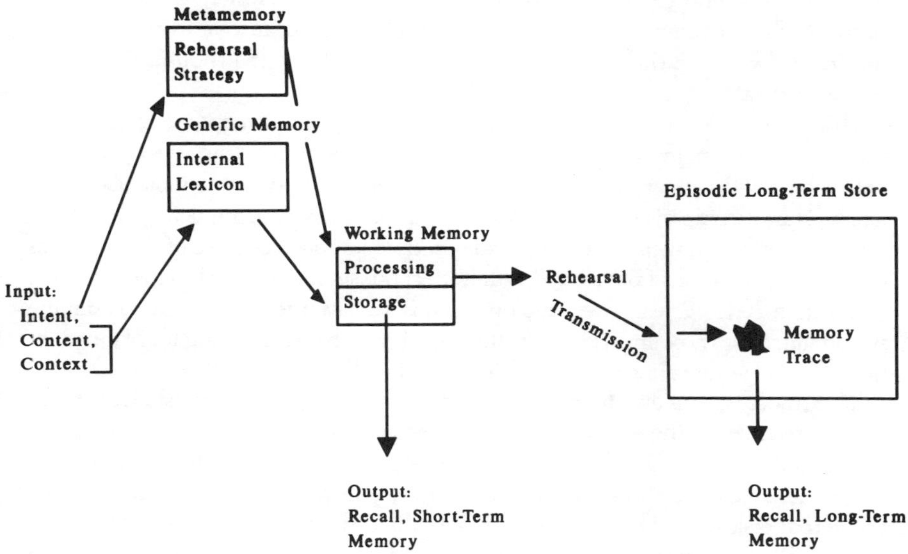

FIGURE 2.3 Model of the episodic memory system.

stored briefly, encoded (or processed), and rehearsed. Rehearsal results in the transmission of this encoded information as memory traces to the long-term store. In the laboratory, long-term rehearsal-dependent memory is studied by giving subjects such tasks as a lengthy list of paired-associates to "learn." That is, subjects receive a list containing pairs of unrelated words, such as *table-apple*, to practice until they are able to recall each second word in the pair when the first word is presented alone. In the real world, this form of memory is involved when we try to learn what name goes with what face when we are introduced to a number of people at a party. By contrast, short-term rehearsal-dependent memory is studied by giving subjects a short list of rapidly presented items (e.g., digits, letters, or words) and asking for recall of those items immediately or shortly after their presentation. An everyday counterpart occurs when we try to recall a telephone number someone just gave us to dial.

Adult Age Differences in Proficiency

Research on rehearsal-dependent episodic memory, both short-term and long-term, has dominated the activities of cognitive aging researchers for a number of years. The evidence gathered from numerous studies employing many different specific forms of memory tasks has been quite consistent. Age-related deficits on short-term tasks tend to be modest to moderate, while age-related deficits on long-term memory tasks tend to be moderate to pronounced (see Kausler, 1982, and Salthouse, 1982, for summaries). I will not attempt to be exhaustive in my coverage, but instead will cite the outcome of a single recent study (Salthouse, Kausler, & Saults, 1988a).

This study is unique in three important respects. First, the same subjects performed both short-term memory tasks and a long-term memory task (they also performed both rehearsal-dependent and rehearsal-independent memory tasks—more about this later). Thus a comparison of the differential magnitudes of aging deficits for short-term and long-term memory can be made on the same subjects, free of the problems of sampling variations from study to study. Second, several hundred subjects ranging in age from 20 to 79 years were employed. Thus we have the opportunity to examine performance for those individuals in the vast terrain between young and late adulthood, as well as for young and elderly individuals. Third, none of these subjects were college students, thus avoiding the common confounding of age with student status.

For convenience, the subjects across the age range were placed in three age groups: young adults (20–39), middle-aged adults (40–59), and elderly adults (60–79). Each subject received two short-term memory tasks, one verbal, the other spatial. For the verbal task seven letters were made visually distinctive within a matrix of 25 letters (5× 5 array; three-second exposure), with subjects recalling which letters were the distinctive ones. A subject's score consisted of the average number of letters correctly recalled across four trials. For the spatial task, seven boxes were made visually distinctive within a matrix of 25 boxes (5 × 5 array; three-second exposure). Here a subject's score consisted of the average number of target positions correctly recalled across four trials. The results are shown in Figure 2.4. Note that there is only a modest decline in performance from young adulthood to middle age, and another modest decline from middle age to late adulthood. Alzheimer's patients are characterized by a moderately greater deficit in short-term memory proficiency, and the magnitude of their deficit appears to increase as the severity of the disease increases (see Kaszniak, Poon, & Riege, 1986; and Storandt, Botwinick, & Danziger, 1986, for reviews).

Our long-term task consisted of two trials on a paired-associate list composed of eight pairs of unrelated nouns (two-second exposure). Our interest will be only on the percentage of pairs on the second trial in which the second word of a pair was correctly recalled, given the first word of the pair as a cue. The results are shown in Figure 2.5. Note the rather substantial decline in proficiency of recall from young adulthood to middle age, with a more moderate further decline from middle age to late adulthood. This pattern is, of course, quite different from that found for our short-term memory tasks. In addition, the pattern is quite different from that found with Alzheimer's patients. Their paired-associate learning proficiency is well below the level of matched aged controls, as is their proficiency on other rehearsal-dependent long-term memory tasks (see Kaszniak, Poon, & Riege, 1986, for a review).

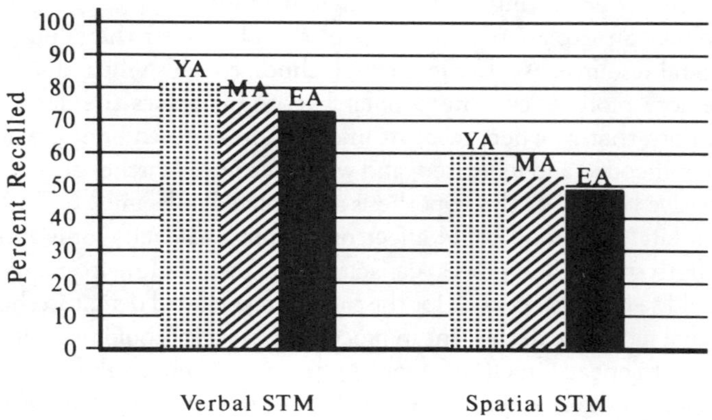

FIGURE 2.4 Differences in verbal and spatial short-term memory proficiency for young (Y), middle-aged (MA), and elderly (E) adults. (Adapted from data in Salthouse, Kausler, & Saults, 1988a.)

Why AAMI?

The reasons underlying age-related deficits in rehearsal-dependent memory, whether moderate or pronounced, have been investigated intensively in recent years. In effect, there has been a major shift away from research simply identifying and describing adult age differences in memory to explanatory research. The objective,

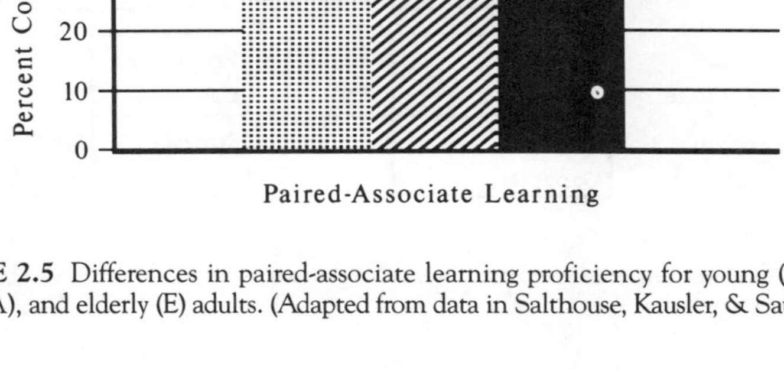

FIGURE 2.5 Differences in paired-associate learning proficiency for young (Y), middle-aged (MA), and elderly (E) adults. (Adapted from data in Salthouse, Kausler, & Saults, 1988b.)

of course, is to identify the causes of AAMI. For our purposes, explanatory research may be regarded as consisting of three different kinds.

The first seeks an explanation in terms of a decline over the adult life span in some general resource. As that resource declines, so does rehearsal-dependent episodic memory proficiency. One popular hypothesis places the decrement in working memory, that is, where relevant information is stored briefly, where that information is encoded and rehearsed, and where retrieval searches are conducted. Three alternative versions of this hypothesis are depicted in Figure 2.6. The decline from early to late adulthood could affect only storage capacity, only processing capacity, or both storage and process capacity. A modest decline in storage capacity alone would seemingly account for the modest age-related deficit in short-term memory. Even a moderate decrement in processing capacity could make it difficult for older adults to engage in effortful forms of encoding/rehearsal and in effortful searches of traces in the long-term store (Craik & Byrd, 1982). Alternatively, others, particularly Salthouse (1985), have argued that the general resource that diminishes with normal aging is the rate at which information is processed. That is, there is a "slowing down" in processing rate from early to late adulthood, with an accompanying decline in memory proficiency.

One means of testing the validity of any general resource hypothesis is to assess subjects on one or more "markers" of the suspected resource and then determine the relationship between scores on these markers and scores on an episodic memory task. For the working memory hypothesis (whatever its specific form), a favorite

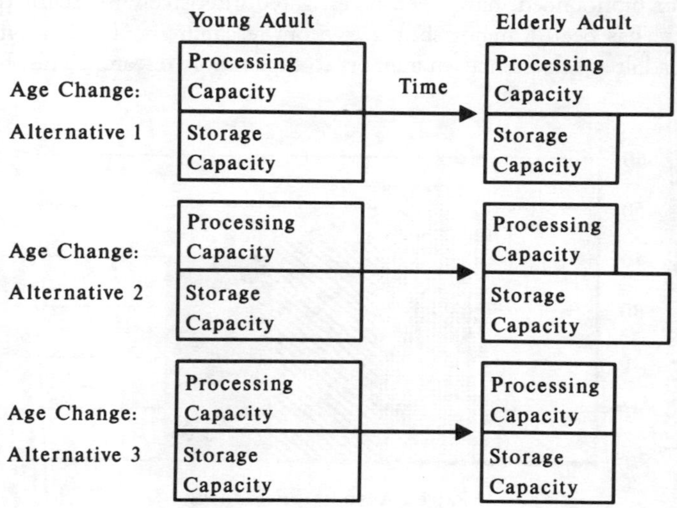

FIGURE 2.6 Alternative conceptualizations of an age-related decrement in working memory's capacity.

marker has been a subject's reading span score (Daneman & Carpenter, 1980). Subjects read several related sentences with the intent both to comprehend those sentences and to remember the last word in each sentence. The more sentences that can be spanned without error in "last word" memory, the greater the reading span—and, presumably, the greater the capacity of working memory. Both Light and Anderson (1985) and Hartley (1986) failed to find a significant correlation between span scores and recall scores for discourse material. Moreover, Hartley even found comparability in span scores between young and elderly subjects—an anomaly, indeed, if we believe both that span scores assess working memory's capacity and that this capacity declines with normal aging. On the other hand, evidence supporting the hypothesis was reported recently by Stine and Wingfield (1987). They substituted a "listening span" measure for reading span. Subjects heard several sentences and had to recall the last word in each sentence (score = number of sentences spanned without error in recall). Span scores were substantially correlated with recall scores of sentences presented aurally, in support of the capacity decrement hypothesis. The difference in outcomes for different sensory modalities is an intriguing one that clearly merits further investigation. Perhaps the most discouraging evidence for any general resource hypothesis comes from Salthouse, Kausler, and Saults' (1988b) follow-up analysis of their data collected on multiple tasks. A path analysis failed to support either the working memory hypothesis (scores on the verbal and spatial short-term memory tasks served as markers) or the slowing-down hypothesis (scores on several speeded tests, such as a digit symbol test, served as markers).

There is another means of testing the validity of the capacity hypothesis, one that may prove in the long run to be more effective than the correlational method. It calls for having subjects perform under dual-task conditions—that is, perform two tasks simultaneously. The primary task requires the performance of a designated memory operation, such as recalling the words from a just-studied list; the secondary task requires performance on a task independent of the primary task, such as detecting the presence of a targeted sensory signal (Craik & McDowd, 1987; Macht & Buschke, 1983). The study by Craik and McDowd is especially informative. Their secondary task was performed while their subjects attempted either to recall or to recognize previously studied words. It was also performed in the absence of the primary task (i.e., a baseline condition). The difference between dual-task and baseline reaction times on the secondary task was much greater for elderly than for young subjects when recall provided the primary task. The difference between age groups, however, was considerably less when recognition served as the primary task. Craik and McDowd concluded, " . . . that recall tasks demand more processing than do recognition tasks and that because older people have a smaller pool of processing resources at their disposal, they are disproportionately penalized" (1987, p. 478). The "smaller pool of processing resources" presumably refers to a diminished capacity of working memory. The implication is that the search for traces in the long-term episodic store for their retrieval in recall is a cognitively effortful process, and it therefore draws upon a limited processing capacity that, in turn, decreases with increasing age.

What about encoding/rehearsal processes? Are they too cognitively effortful and therefore similarly affected by normal aging? That is, is the locus of the age-related deficit in rehearsal-dependent memory proficiency only in the retrieval of stored information, or is it also in the encoding and transmission of that information? The traditional method of answering this question has not been very satisfactory. The rationale for its application is simple enough. It is the searching component of retrieval that is presumed to be effortful and therefore age sensitive. Searching enters into recall, but not into recognition. Consequently, if an age-related deficit is found for recall, but not for recognition, then it may be concluded that only retrieval processes are age sensitive. By contrast, if an age-related deficit occurs for recognition as well as for recall, then it may be concluded that the encoding/rehearsal stage of rehearsal-dependent episodic memory is also age sensitive.

Unfortunately, recall versus recognition comparisons have only served to confuse the issue. Some investigators have found slight, if any, age differences in recognition, but pronounced age deficits in the recall of the same materials (Craik & McDowd, 1987; Schonfield & Robertson, 1966). However, others have found large age differences for recognition as well as for recall (although the latter is likely to be greater; Erber, 1974). The recall versus recognition issue is complicated further by the argument made by some researchers (Howe, 1988) that recognition, like recall, requires an effortful search process. If true, then an age-related deficit in recognition may be the consequence of a retrieval deficit rather than an encoding deficit. A further complication is the possibility that the retrieval problem resulted from poor encoding of the to-be-remembered events in the first place. That is, because of impoverished encoding, the separate traces may lack distinctiveness and are therefore difficult to retrieve. What is needed to tease apart the encoding/retrieval confusion regarding the source of age-related deficits in rehearsal-dependent memory are studies that employ the dual-task procedure factorially—that is, during study only, during retrieval only, during both study and retrieval, and during neither study nor retrieval. We are likely to discover a flood of such studies in the future. Until evidence is gathered from these future studies, the locus issue (i.e., encoding/rehearsal versus retrieval as *the* stage or the stages of age sensitivity) will remain in limbo.

Many hypotheses have been offered over the years as to what encoding processes are effortful and therefore susceptible to age-related declines in proficiency. From my perspective, the distinction between rehearsal-dependent and rehearsal-independent forms of episodic memory rests only in the encoding stage. My assumption is that there is a single long-term episodic store and that retrieval from that store is an effortful process regardless of the nature of the earlier encoding processes. That is, retrieval is as likely to be effortful for rehearsal-independent memory as for rehearsal-dependent memory. What distinguishes the two forms of episodic memory is the degree of effort required to encode events. Examples of so-called effortful encoding processes include the generation of images of to-be-remembered items (Hulicka & Grossman, 1967), the elaboration of those items (Craik, 1977), the encoding of specific attributes of items (as opposed to the encoding of more general attributes; Craik & Simon, 1980), the encoding of contextual information (Burke & Light, 1981), and the utilization of organizational processes (Smith, 1980). In general, there is some support from laboratory studies for the age sensitivity of each of these processes. However, for reasons to be discussed later, the extent to which such effortful processes contribute to age-related deficits in everyday memory performances is uncertain.

The second kind of explanatory research examines causation in terms of a defective memory process, with the fault resting outside of the encoding/retrieval processes of episodic memory per se. Specifically, metamemorial processes are suspected of being a major contributor, if not the sole contributor, to age-related deficits in rehearsal-dependent memory. From this perspective, older adults are viewed as being as capable as younger adults in the processing of information for episodic long-term storage. The problem is in translating that competence into actual performance. For example, older adults may simply terminate their rehearsal too soon, ending it before sufficient information has been transmitted to the store to assure later retrievability. An interesting demonstration of this possibility, at least for some kinds of material, was provided recently by Murphy et al. (1987). Their subjects received a series of drawings of common objects that were to be recalled in the order of their presentation. Young adults, relative to old adults, studied the list for a longer period of time, rehearsed the items more, and tested themselves more often before they attempted overt recall of the items—and, as a result, they recalled more items correctly. However, as may be seen in Figure 2.7, the age-related deficit disappeared when old subjects were required either to monitor their readiness for recall or to rehearse for as long as young subjects do. I suspect, nevertheless, that relatively little of the elderly adult's impairment on most long-term episodic memory tasks can be attributed to age differences in metamemorial processes.

The final kind of explanatory research searches for causation from nonaging factors that covary with age. Educational level is one of these factors. It is a fact that younger adults average more years of formal adult education than do older adults. This may be a fact, but it is unlikely to be an artifact in most aging studies on memory. Usually, young and old groups are carefully matched on years of formal education—and AAMI is still apparent. Nor did the age differences reported by Salthouse, Kausler, and Saults (1988a) disappear when years of formal education served as an adjustment variable.

There is another nonaging factor that relates somewhat to educational level: namely, current student status. In most aging studies on memory, the young subjects are currently college students, while the elderly subjects with whom they are being compared are years removed from active student status. Somehow, argue

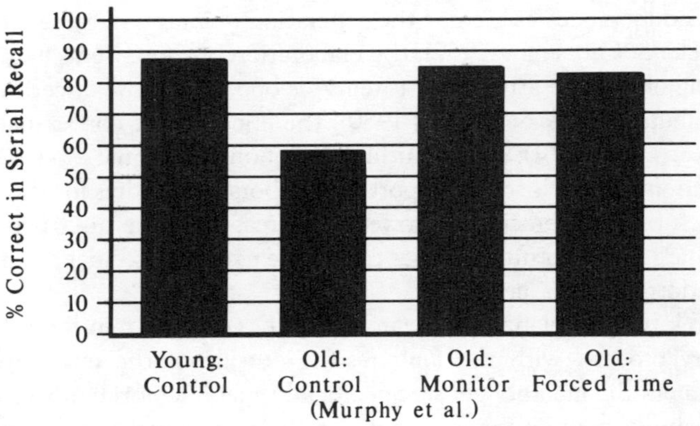

FIGURE 2.7 Adult age differences in serial recall as affected by variations in practice conditions. (Adapted from Table 1 in Murphy et al., 1987.)

some gerontologists, being a student keeps the memory mechanism "lubricated" and running smoothly. After years away from the mental challenges of academia, the mechanism becomes "rusty" and "sluggish." Return the individual to student status, and the "rust" wears off. This is an old argument in gerontology (Thorndike et al., 1928) that resurfaced dramatically following the publication of a study by Zivian and Darjes (1983). They compared young college students (18–26 years of age), middle-aged college students (35–44 years of age), middle-aged nonstudents (36–49 years of age), and elderly nonstudents (60–86 years of age) in performance on a rehearsal-dependent memory task (free recall of a taxonomically categorizable word list). Young and middle-aged students were roughly comparable in their performance, with both being clearly superior to middle-aged and elderly nonstudents. Missing, of course, was a group of elderly students. Would they also have approximated the memory proficiency of young college students? Probably not, at least according to the results obtained by both Hartley (1986) and Parks, Mitchell, and Perlmutter (1986). In each study, elderly college students performed no more proficiently than elderly nonstudents on a rehearsal-dependent memory task (memory for connected discourse in the Hartley study [1986]; paired-associate learning in the Parks, Mitchell, and Perlmutter study [1986]).

Remember, too, that Salthouse, Kausler, and Saults (1988a) found an age-related deficit for nonstudent elderly subjects, relative to nonstudent young subjects, that approximated the deficit commonly found when the young comparison group consists of college students. This point is important in that it could be argued that the use of only young college students in aging memory research leads to an exaggeration of the extent of AAMI. That it may lead to a moderate exaggeration for some kinds of memory tasks was demonstrated by Ratner et al. (1987) for discourse memory. The deficit in memory proficiency was greater when elderly nonstudents were contrasted with young students than when contrasted with young nonstudents.

Activity level is yet another nonaging factor suspected by some of being a major culprit in determining adult age difference in rehearsal-dependent memory proficiency. Younger adults are presumed to be more active than older adults, both physically and mentally, and this difference somehow affects performance on memory tasks. Some suggestive evidence for this position was reported by Craik, Byrd, and Swanson (1987). Elderly residents of a retirement community that provided them with a physically and cognitively active and enriched environment scored considerably higher on several memory tasks than did elderly individuals living a seemingly more passive existence. In fact, the "active" elderly subjects scored as high on these tasks as did young college students! Craik, Byrd, and Swanson (1987) were quick to point out, however, that a hidden variable in their study may have been the healthy status of their subjects. That is, physically and cognitively active elderly individuals may maintain a high level of activity (relative to more sedentary elderly individuals) simply because their superior health permits it. Interestingly, Milligan et al. (1984) did find that elderly individuals who reported their health to be poor performed less proficiently on a rehearsal-dependent memory task (serial learning) than did elderly individuals who reported their health to be good or superior. Of course, the health issue is seemingly avoided in most memory studies by employing only subjects who report their health to be "good" or better—and AAMI is still found. However, "good" health for an older individual may mean only "for someone my age." If it were to mean instead "as good as when I was 20 years old," would AAMI disappear? The answer is unclear. However, age-related deficits reported for the current generation of elderly adults really aren't much different from the deficits reported 30 or more years ago (Kausler, 1982). Surely the health status of today's elderly population is superior to that of 30 years ago.

Training on Rehearsal-Dependent Memory Tasks

A by-product of this emphasis on nonaging factors as the source of AAMI is the belief that age-related deficits in memory may be alleviated, if not eliminated, by appropriate training on to-be-remembered materials. This belief is fostered by evidence indicating that elderly individuals benefit considerably in their acquisition rate for paired-associate lists following mnemonic training (Yesavage, Rose, & Bower, 1983). However, it is uncertain how effectively these trained individuals will retain these newly acquired skills and how extensively they will actually employ them in their everyday memory performances. Moreover, it is unlikely that mnemonic training will result in any major reduction in the magnitude of age differences in performances. Young adults equally trained in the use of mnemonics also show dramatic improvements in rate of acquisition (Bugelski, Kidd, & Segman,

1968). Young versus old performance differences are likely to be as great for trained subjects as for untrained subjects. Of interest here is the fact that Salthouse and Somberg (1982) found that elderly subjects profit considerably from extended practice on a memory scanning task—but so do young subjects. The net effect is essentially no change in the magnitude of the advantage of young over old.

Forgetting

Even when episodic events are stored as effectively by older as by younger individuals, there remains the possibility of age differences in the rate of forgetting those events. Elderly adults are often viewed as being more "interference prone" than younger adults (Kausler, 1970, 1987). Interference refers to other events acquired either before (proactive interference) or after (retroactive interference) the to-be-retained events in question. It is these other events that are commonly assumed to cause forgetting, and not the passage of time per se. Equality over the adult life span in the acquisition of new material would be relatively meaningless if older adults forget that material more quickly because of their greater susceptibility to the effects of interference. Tests of adult age differences in rate of forgetting are complicated greatly by a fact of life that must be faced by any researcher working in this area: the primary factor determining rate of forgetting is how well the material was acquired in the first place. Poorly mastered material is likely to be forgotten more rapidly than thoroughly mastered material. Therein lies the problem for tests of age differences in rate of forgetting. Assurance is needed that young and old subjects are matched in the amount of original acquisition. Without such assurance we have no way of knowing whether an age difference in rate of forgetting is simply an artifact produced by an age difference in amount acquired.

Of interest to us are potential age differences in forgetting for both short-term and long-term episodic memory. For short-term memory, forgetting concerns the loss of information from working memory over a retention interval (measured in seconds) when that information is not sustained by deliberate rehearsal. There are several methods available for assuring equality of the amount of information stored in working memory by young and elderly subjects at the beginning of the retention interval. Recent studies applying these methods have demonstrated that forgetting over brief retention intervals (e.g., 15 seconds) occurs no more rapidly for elderly than for young adults (Parkinson, Inman, & Dannenbaum, 1985; Puckett & Stockburger, 1988). Puckett and Stockburger's study is especially informative. They employed the Brown-Peterson procedure (Brown, 1958; Peterson & Peterson, 1959), in which strings of words were to be remembered in the order of their presentation over a retention interval that varied from 0 to 15 seconds. Equality of acquisition was assured by having string length set by a subject's word span (which turned out to be five words for young subjects, four words for elderly subjects). Thus each subject received to-be-retained information that consumed all working memory storage capacity, regardless of the subject's age. Deliberate rehearsal of the word strings during the retention interval was prevented by having subjects perform a decision task involving either words or nonwords. In addition, various procedures were used to identify and eliminate those subjects who did engage in rehearsal of the word strings, despite the instructions not to do so. When interference was moderate during the retention interval (the interpolated nonword decision task), the rate of forgetting of the word strings was moderate for both young and old subjects. When a greater degree of interference was present (the interpolated word decision task), forgetting was much greater—but equally so for young and old subjects. For short-term memory at least, there is no reason to believe that interference proneness increases over the adult life span.

For long-term memory, the issue of age differences in rate of forgetting has received less attention than it deserves, probably because of the "assurance of equality of acquisition" problem. Several studies in the 1960s approached the issue by assessing the long-term (e.g., 1 week) retention of either a single paired-associate list learned alone in the laboratory or a paired-associate list that was followed by the acquisition of a second list (i.e., a retroactive interference paradigm) (see Kausler, 1982, for a detailed review). The results of these studies are difficult to interpret, given their inadequate consideration of equality of initial acquisition over the age groups. Two recent studies, however, by Park et al. (1988) and Rybarczyk, Hart, and Harkins (1987) did provide adequate assurance of equal acquisition. In each study, subjects received a lengthy series of pictures: line drawings of complex scenes in Park et al.'s study, and line drawings of familiar objects in Rybarczyk, Hart, and Harkins' study. Subjects were tested for recognition memory on different subsets of the pictures after varying intervals (immediately after study, and again after 48 hours, 1 week, 2 weeks, and 4 weeks in Park et al.'s study; 10 minutes after study, and again after 2 hours and 48 hours in Rybarczyk, Hart, and Harkins' study). The results obtained in these studies are given in Figure 2.8. Note the striking agreement in outcomes for the 48-hour retention interval common to the two studies. There is no age difference—young and old alike show the same precipitous drop in retention after only 48 hours. After that, Park et al.'s elderly subjects appear to manifest a greater further drop as the retention interval increases. However, after 4 weeks, the age groups appear to be converging on the same modest level of retention. In my opinion, we have no more reason to believe that elderly adults are more interference prone than young adults for long-term episodic memory than they are for short-term episodic memory.

Our focus thus far has been on the forgetting of the same material that is acquired when one is either young or old. There is another facet of forgetting that also deserves our attention. What happens to the material we acquired years

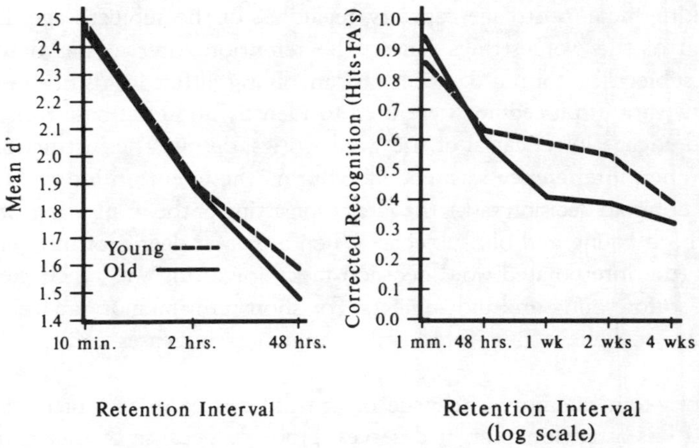

FIGURE 2.8 Adult age differences in rate of forgetting pictures as list items. (Left panel: from Table 1 in Rybarczyk, Hart, & Harkins, 1987; right panel: from Figure 1 in Park et al., 1988.)

ago—the names of our schoolteachers, the names of old television shows, the Spanish vocabulary learned in high school, the names of popular songs from long ago, and so on? Thanks to a series of remarkable studies by Bahrick (Bahrick, 1979, 1984; Bahrick, Bahrick, & Wittlinger, 1975), we now have a reasonably clear picture of the fates of these old memories. The typical outcome is illustrated in Figure 2.9. Forgetting is quite rapid for the first few years after initial acquisition. After that it levels off, and retention remains fairly stable for the rest of one's lifetime, with 20–40% of the original material being retained. The material that remains recallable resides in what Bahrick calls a permastore, presumably because it was that portion of the original material that was highly overlearned at the time of acquisition. You can probably be assured that people 20 years younger than you remember no more names of television shows aired 10 years ago than you remember.

Rehearsal-Independent Episodic Memory

Nature

Even a cursory examination of your everyday memory experiences should reveal to you that most of your memories of episodic events occur without intentionality and without active rehearsal. Do you remember brushing your teeth this morning? Showering? Do you remember the content of the headline in this morning's

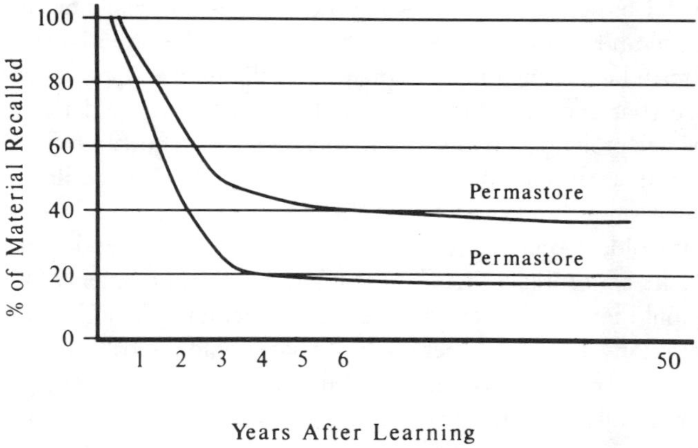

FIGURE 2.9 Rate of forgetting of material learned early in adulthood, with 20–40% remaining in permanent storage. The curves indicate the upper and lower limits of permanent storage.

newspaper? The gist of the conversation you had with your spouse this morning before leaving for work? How many times you saw commericals for a light beer on television last night? You probably do, but not necessarily. Did you intend to remember these events? Did you rehearse them? Probably not—but memory frequently persists anyway. For such activities as showering, simply planning them and performing them seems to be sufficient to assure transmission of a trace to the long-term store. For remembering the gist of a conversation, the comprehension of its content provides similar assurance. Such memories are representative of what I call rehearsal-independent memory—that is, memory without intentional rehearsal. It seems to be the kind of memory Mr. Muskie had in mind in his reference to the President.

Until the past 10 years or so, memory research concentrated nearly exclusively on rehearsal-dependent forms of long-term episodic memory. This isn't hard to understand in that the typical subject population in these studies is that of college students. Rehearsal-dependent memory is surely more involved in the daily living of college students than it is in the daily living of elderly people. What is surprising has been the comparable focus of gerontological research on rehearsal-dependent forms of memory. The frequent complaints of elderly people about their memory problems (Gilewski & Zelinski, 1986) commonly include many examples of impairment in rehearsal-independent memory (e.g., "I thought I turned off the stove, but it turns out that I didn't"). The situation has changed greatly, however, since the appearance of the influential article by Hasher and Zacks (1979). Their emphasis on basic differences between "effortful" and "automatic" forms of episodic memory has resulted in considerable interest in rehearsal-independent memory, both for basic and gerontological memory researchers. The distinction between effortful and automatic refers to the nature of the underlying encoding operations. Effortful encoding processes draw upon the limited capacity of working memory. Since that capacity diminishes with normal aging, elderly adults are expected to be less proficient than younger adults on such effortful tasks as paired-associate learning, as they are indeed. By contrast, automatic encoding processes bypass working memory, and they should therefore be rehearsal-independent and as proficient for older adults as for younger adults. Rehearsal-independence in Hasher and Zack's conceptual scheme means that incidental memory of the events in question should be as proficient as intentional memory of those same events. That is, intentionally activated rehearsal processes should contribute little, if anything, to the enhancement of the memorability of those events. Age insensitivity is expected because variation in working memory's capacity is not a factor in determining variation in memorability.

My preference is to refer to this kind of memory as being rehearsal-independent rather than automatic. Long-term episodic memory requires processing of some kind, and even under incidental memory conditions, such processing would surely involve working memory. For example, in a frequency judgment task the events that vary in their frequencies of occurrence are "studied" in some way, even though the subject is unaware of an impending memory test of those frequencies. What is critical under incidental memory conditions is the absence of deliberate rehearsal of those events. Rehearsal-independency implies that such rehearsal is unnecessary to promote subsequent memorability. Most important, there is no a priori reason to expect immunity to age-related deficits.

Rehearsal-independency and age insensitivity, from the perspective of automaticity, has been postulated to be characteristic of memory both for certain noncontent attributes of episodic events and for certain kinds of content. The primary noncontent attributes postulated to be rehearsal-independent have been the frequency of occurrence of episodic events and the temporal sequencing of episodic events (Hasher & Zacks, 1979, 1984; Zacks et al., 1984). Memory for frequency of occurrence, in fact, has been the prototypal task for testing the basic tenets of Hasher and Zacks's position regarding automaticity. Research on content has been more limited, concentrating largely on memory for continuous activities and discrete actions performed in the laboratory.

Noncontent Attributes

The standard procedure for research on frequency-of-occurrence memory is to present a series of episodic events (usually words or activities performed in the laboratory) in which the individual events vary in the number of times they occur in the series (e.g., 0, 1, 3, and 5). Young and old subjects perform under both incidental and intentional memory conditions. Following the completion of the series, they are asked to judge the frequency with which each event appeared in the series. The results obtained with this procedure have been somewhat conflicting. Most studies have found incidental memory to be as proficient as intentional memory (Attig & Hasher, 1980; Kausler, Lichty, & Hakami, 1984; Kausler & Puckett, 1980), but there have been exceptions (Greene, 1986). Similarly, some investigators have reported a null effect for age variation (Attig & Hasher, 1980; Kausler & Puckett, 1980), while others have found a modest advantage favoring young adults in terms of accuracy of frequency judgments (Kausler, Lichty, & Hakami, 1984; Kausler, Salthouse, & Saults, 1987). A frequency judgment task was one of the many tasks included in our large-scale normative study (Kausler, Salthouse, & Saults, 1987; Salthouse, Kausler, & Saults, 1988a). The results for young, middle-aged, and elderly subjects are shown in Figure 2.10. Note the modest difference, but nevertheless sufficient to attain statistical significance. A comparable outcome was reported by Kausler, Lichty, and Freund (1985) for judging the frequency with which each laboratory activity was performed in a series of activities. I suspect that there is a slight decline in the proficiency of frequency-of-occurrence memory over the adult life span, but so slight that it is likely to be detected in some studies, but not in other studies, contingent on the extent of sampling error. Interestingly, Alzheimer's patients seem to be very poor at giving accurate frequency estimations (Strauss, Weingartner, & Thompson, 1985). The possibility of employing a frequency judgment task in the early detection of Alzheimer's disease should be given serious consideration by those investigators searching for improved diagnostic tests.

The procedure for research on temporal memory calls for presenting a series of episodic events (usually words or activities performed in the laboratory, with each event occurring only once). At the end of the series, temporal memory is assessed by asking subjects either to judge the temporal placement of each event in the series (e.g., first fourth, second fourth, and so on) or to reconstruct the order in which the event occurred. In general, the rehearsal-independent nature of temporal memory is supported by the usual finding of a null effect for instructional variation (i.e., incidental memory equals intentional memory; Kausler, Lichty, & Davis, 1985; McCormack, 1981; Toglia & Kimble, 1976). On the other hand, evidence from our laboratory in Missouri clearly indicates that temporal memory is highly age sensitive, whether the events consist of words or performed activities. A word temporal memory task was part of the battery in Salthouse, Kausler, and Saults' study (1988a; Kausler, Salthouse, & Saults, 1988). Sixteen words were presented in the series, and their order was then reconstructed. The correlation coefficient between true order and reconstructed order constituted each subject's word temporal memory score. As may be seen in Figure 2.10, the magnitude of the age-related deficit was considerably more pronounced than that found for frequency-of-occurrence memory. Another form of temporal memory was also assessed in this study. After completing a number of tasks in the battery, subjects were unexpectedly asked to reconstruct the order in which those tasks had been

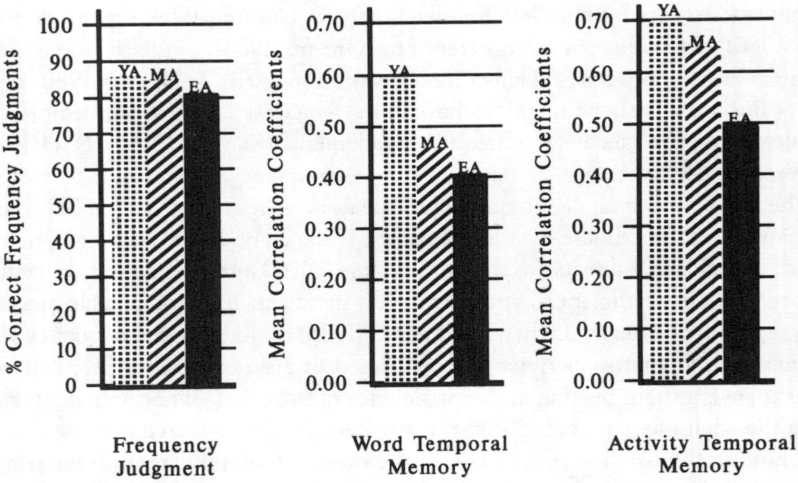

FIGURE 2.10 Adult age differences in memory for three noncontent attributes. (Adapted from data in Salthouse, Kausler, & Saults, 1988a.)

performed. The correlation between true and reconstructed order of performance defined each subject's activity temporal memory score. Note in Figure 2.10 that a pronounced age-related deficit was also apparent for this form of temporal memory (a deficit comparable to that found in one of our earlier studies; Kausler, Lichty, & Davis, 1985). However, the pattern of decline differs from that found for word temporal memory. That is, for activity temporal memory the greatest decline occurs between middle age and late adulthood, whereas for word temporal memory the greatest decline is from young adulthood to middle age.

Memory for a number of other noncontent attributes has been tested in terms of the presence or absence of age-related deficits. These include memory for the spatial location of episodic events (e.g., buildings on a map; Light & Zelinski, 1983; Zelinski & Light, 1988), memory for the modality in which events are presented (i.e., visual or auditory; Lehman & Mellinger, 1984, 1986), memory for the sex of voice (male or female) in which words as events are presented (Kausler & Puckett, 1981), and memory for source of information (McIntyre & Craik, 1987). Age-related deficits are manifested for each of these attributes.

Content

Hasher and Zacks (1979) reasoned that memory for such noncontent attributes as frequency of occurrence is essential for effective adaptation to the environment, and for this reason, its automaticity may be genetically assured. An even stronger case for "natural" automaticity, at least in terms of rehearsal-independency, can be made for certain forms of content memory. Why do we remember having balanced our checkbooks? Surely not because we rehearsed it. Memory for the content of our own activities seems to me to be an everyday example of rehearsal independent memory. Accordingly, several years ago, my students and I began a series of laboratory studies on memory for the content of activities. Our objectives were to confirm its rehearsal-independent nature and to demonstrate its probable immunity to age-related deficits in proficiency, assuming the validity of Hasher and Zacks's position on the age insensitivity of automatic forms of memory.

Our procedure called for subjects, young and old, to perform for several minutes on each of a series of tasks (e.g., connecting dots, solving arithmetic problems), with half of the subjects at each age level performing under incidental memory conditions, the others under intentional memory conditions. After the series was completed, subjects were instructed to recall, in whatever order that came to mind, as many of the just-performed activities as possible. Our results have been quite consistent over a number of studies employing this basic procedure (Kausler & Hakami, 1983; Kausler, Lichty, & Davis, 1985; Kausler et al., 1986; Lichty, Kausler, & Martinez, 1986; see also Kausler & Lichty, in press, for a detailed review). Intent to memorize what activities are being performed has little effect on subsequent memorability, regardless of age, nature of the activities (i.e., motor or cognitive; Lichty, Kausler, & Martinez, 1986), and duration of performing the activities (Kausler et al., 1986), thus offering strong support for the rehearsal independency of activity memory. By contrast, our results clearly indicate that there is an age-related deficit in the recall of activities. Elderly adults recall about 15% fewer activities than do young adults (Fig. 2.11).

Other investigators have approached the same topic, but they have had their subjects perform discrete brief actions (e.g., "snap your fingers," "touch your nose"), rather than prolonged continuous activities (Backman & Nilsson, 1984, 1985; Cohen, 1983; Cohen, Sandler, & Schroeder, 1987; Lichty, 1986). Despite the difference in task requirements, the outcome is much the same as that found in our activity memory studies. That is, action memory is also rehearsal-independent (Cohen, 1983), but age sensitive, at least as measured by recall (Cohen, Sandler, & Schroeder, 1987; Lichty, 1986) (see Fig. 2.11). I am convinced that activity memory and action memory are essentially minor variants of the same basic phenomenon (see Kausler & Lichty, 1988, for elaboration). The potential diagnostic value of activity/action memory assessments for the early detection of Alzheimer's disease is an important topic for future research. Alzheimer's patients are likely to be very deficient in their recall of both continuous activities and discrete actions.

There remains the haunting question, however, of whether or not the age-related deficit in activity/action memory is truly an encoding deficit. Conceivably, memory traces of performed activities/actions are indeed transmitted automatically (i.e.,

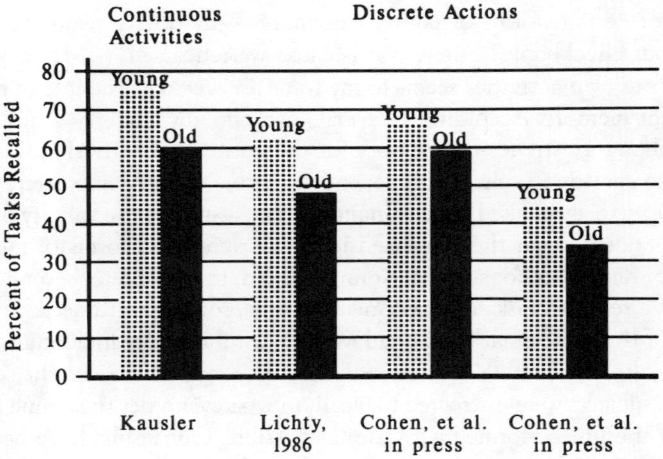

FIGURE 2.11 Adult age differences in recall of continuous activities (Kausler, averaged from several studies) and discrete actions (adapted from data in Lichty, 1986, and Cohen, Sandler, & Schroeder, 1987).

without rehearsal as a precursor), and as much so for elderly as for young adults. Thus the age-related deficit in recall would really be a retrieval deficit. As noted earlier, retrieval from the episodic long-term store is an effortful process, and it should be susceptible to an age-related deficit regardless of the nature of the processes preceding retrieval. Some support for this position is obtained when we examine recognition scores for both previously performed activities and previously performed actions. Recognition memory tests have been given in several of our activity memory studies. A typical outcome of these tests (Lichty, Kausler, & Martinez, 1986) is shown in Figure 2.12. Note that there is essentially no age difference in hit rates (there is a modest age difference in false alarm rates, with elderly subjects having slightly greater rates). A comparable outcome was reported by Lichty (1986) in her study of action memory (see Fig. 2.12). Unfortunately, the probable ceiling effect present in these scores makes it difficult to interpret the negligible age differences. Other studies employing much longer series of activities and actions are needed in order to bypass the ceiling effect problem.

SUMMARY AND CONCLUSIONS

My review of laboratory studies has emphasized the fact that the human memory system operates less proficiently in late adulthood than in earlier adulthood. How extensive is the impairment in memory proficiency that accompanies normal aging? The answer depends not only on the specific component of memory

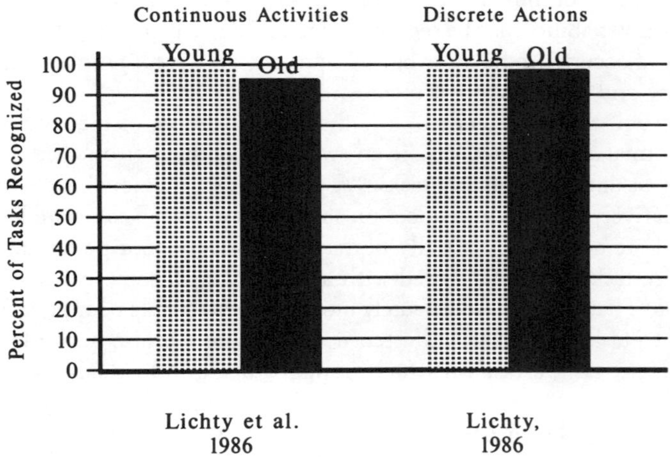

FIGURE 2.12 Adult age differences in recognition of continuous activities (adapted from data in Lichty, Kausler, & Martinez, 1986) and discrete actions (adapted from data in Lichty, 1986).

involved in the memory task at hand, but also on the specific characteristics of that task.

For generic memory, the extent of impairment is slight and appears to be limited largely to the retrieval of words needed to express thoughts. For episodic memory, the picture is considerably more complex. For retrieval-dependent memory, the extent of impairment with normal aging is surely greater for long-term memory than for short-term memory. This conclusion is obvious from the evidence provided by many studies over the years. The magnitude of the disparity between short-term and long-term memory impairment is especially apparent when a comparison on the same subjects is possible, as in the Salthouse, Kausler, and Saults (1988a) study. This comparison is shown in Figure 2.13. Here performance on each task for both middle-aged and elderly subjects is expressed as a percentage loss relative to the performance scores of young adults. Note that by late adulthood the loss is substantially greater for the long-term memory task (paired-associate learning) than for either of the short-term tasks. However, even within the single domain of short-term memory there is substantial variability, with the extent of impairment being contingent on task content. That is, the loss is considerably greater for spatial content than for verbal content.

The contrast between rehearsal-dependent and rehearsal-independent long-term memory is even more striking. Many studies employing tasks other than paired-associate learning (e.g., free recall) have revealed losses in proficiency of recall comparable to the decline apparent in Figure 2.13. For rehearsal-independent tasks (at least those tasks commonly postulated to be rehearsal-independent), the variability in degree of impairment is considerably more pronounced. A striking example of this variability may be seen in Figure 2.13. The percentage loss is slight for frequency-of-occurrence memory but substantially greater for both activity temporal memory and word temporal memory.

In my opinion, the assessment of any individual's degree of memory impairment with normal aging should require an evaluation of that person's performance on a number of different memory tasks. "A memory is a memory" is clearly not the case. Relatively poor performances on such tasks as paired-associate learning and temporal memory are essentially normal. Excessively poor performance on either of these tasks could be viewed with alarm and with some concern about true dementia. That concern would surely intensify if excessively poor performance occurs for both tasks—and it would intensify even more if it also occurs for a frequency judgment task, a task on which normally aging individuals should perform quite well (and Alzheimer's patients perform very poorly). I am not in the "diagnosis business," but if I were, I would want a profile of my clients' performances on many memory tasks involving both rehearsal-dependent and rehearsal-independent forms of memory. Unfortunately, the huge void in normative data for memory tasks of all kinds makes this profile evaluation virtually impossible to conduct. What is badly needed are major efforts to develop age norms for many memory tasks, norms that are comparable to those available for intelligence tests. The data gathered by Salthouse, Kausler, and Saults (1988a) could provide at least a start on this major endeavor. Stratified sampling did not enter into this study.

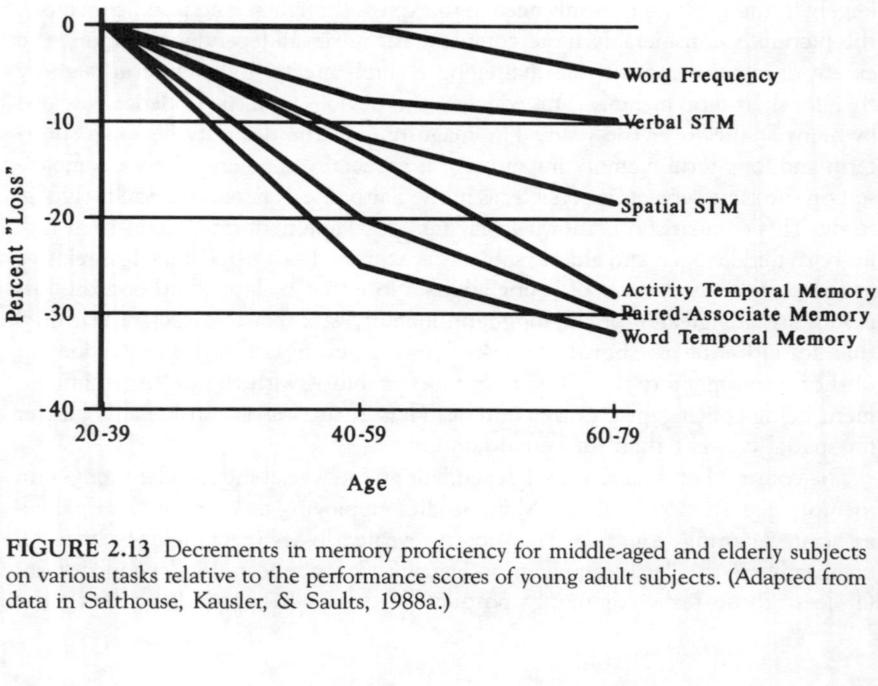

FIGURE 2.13 Decrements in memory proficiency for middle-aged and elderly subjects on various tasks relative to the performance scores of young adult subjects. (Adapted from data in Salthouse, Kausler, & Saults, 1988a.)

However, the subjects at every age level came from various socioeconomic levels and from both rural and urban communities.

Much of the emphasis of laboratory research has been on causative factors for memory impairment. While some investigators have searched for explanation in terms of factors other than aging *per se* (e.g., age differences in level of activity), others have searched for a general resource (e.g., working memory's capacity) that is adversely affected by normal aging. Neither search has been very successful thus far, nor have attempts to attribute memory impairment to a specific stage of information processing, that is, encoding/rehearsal or retrieval, been very satisfying. My best estimate at this time is that both encoding/rehearsal and retrieval are age sensitive, but with retrieval being more adversely affected by aging than encoding/rehearsal. Gerontological memory research needs less emphasis on theoretical issues and greater emphasis on the conditions that enhance memory performance of elderly adults.

For rehearsal-dependent memory, these conditions center largely on training and/or practice. We now know that training/practice can alter significantly the performance of elderly adults on rehearsal-dependent tasks. This outcome is nicely demonstrated in the research cited earlier on mnemonic training. The improvement in memory performance following such training may not be permanent, but there is always the possibility of introducing "booster shots" of further training. It is also demonstrated in the pronounced improvement in memory scanning rates manifested by older individuals following extensive practice on a Sternberg task (Salthouse & Somberg, 1982). Of course, age differences are essentially unaffected by training/practice. That is, young adults benefit as much as do elderly adults, resulting in age differences that are basically unchanged from pre- to post-training/practice. This should be of little concern, however. What is important is the discovery of ways to improve the older individual's memory proficiency. We also have good reason to believe that at least part of the older adult's problems with rehearsal-dependent memory tasks often stems from less than realistic metamemorial operations. Surely metamemorial problems are capable of being corrected with effective counseling of the older adult.

We face a greater challenge in our attempts to improve the older person's proficiency for rehearsal-independent forms of memory. By their very nature, these forms of memory are likely to be resistant to improvement in proficiency brought about by standard training/practice procedures. Nevertheless, there are likely to be conditions yet to be identified fully that enhance proficiency on rehearsal-independent memory tasks. In my laboratory, we are currently focusing on "forced retrieval" as a means of improving memory for activities. Our procedure calls for requiring subjects to recall, after every three activities, the activities that had just been performed, rather than delaying recall until the entire series is completed. Our preliminary results (Kausler & Phillips, 1988) indicate that temporal memory for activities is particularly affected by this procedure. In fact, scores of elderly subjects improve dramatically and approximate those of young adults. Gerontological memory research has always had its fair share of resourceful and clever investigators. My hope is that many of them will direct some of their effort away from theoretical issues concerning the reasons for age-related memory deficits to the more practical issue of what to do about those deficits.

REFERENCES

Attig, M., & Hasher, L. (1980). The processing of frequency of occurrence information by adults. *Journal of Gerontology*, 35(1):66–69.

Bäckman, L., & Nilsson, L-G. (1984). Aging effects in free recall: An exception to the rule. *Human Learning*, 3:53–69.

Bäckman, L., & Nilsson, L-G. (1985). Prerequisites for the lack of age differences in memory performance. *Experimental Aging Research*, 11(2):67–73.

Bahrick, H. P. (1979). Maintenance of knowledge: Questions about memory we forgot to ask. *Journal of Experimental Psychology: General*, 108(3):296–308.

Bahrick, H. P. (1984). Semantic memory content in permastore: Fifty years of memory for Spanish learned in school. *Journal of Experimental Psychology: General*, 113(1):1–29.

Bahrick, H. P., Bahrick, P. O., & Wittlinger, R. P. (1975). Fifty years of memory for names and faces: A cross-sectional approach. *Journal of Experimental Psychology: General*, 104(1):54–75.

Balota, D. A., & Duchek, J. M. (1989). Age related differences in lexical access, spreading activation and simple pronunciation. *Psychology and Aging*, 4(1), 3-9.

Bowles, N. L., & Poon, L. W. (1985). Aging and retrieval of words in semantic memory. *Journal of Gerontology*, 40(1):71–77.

Brown, J. (1958). Some tests of the decay theory of immediate memory. *Quarterly Journal of Experimental Psychology*, 10:12–21.

Bugelski, B. R., Kidd, E., & Segman, J. (1968). Image as a mediator in one-trial paired-associate learning. *Journal of Experimental Psychology*, 76(1):69–73.

Burke, D. M., & Light, L. L. (1981). Memory and aging: The role of retrieval processes. *Psychological Bulletin*, 90(3):513–546.

Burke, D. M., & Peters, L. (1986). Word associations in old age: Evidence for consistency in semantic encoding during adulthood. *Psychology and Aging*, 1(4):283–292.

Burke, D. M., White, H., & Diaz, D. L. (1987). Semantic priming in young and older adults: Evidence for age-constancy in automatic and attentional processes. *Journal of Experimental Psychology: Human Perception and Performance*, 13:79–88.

Burke, D. M., Worthley, J., & Martin, J. (1987). *I'll never forget what's-her-name: Aging and tip of the tongue experiences in everyday life.* Paper presented at the Second International Conference on Practical Aspects of Memory, Swansea, Wales.

Butters, N. (1987). Procedural learning in dementia: A double dissociation between Alzheimer and Huntington's disease patients on verbal priming and motor skill learning. *Journal of Clinical and Experimental Neuropsychology*, 9:68–69.

Chiarello, C., & Hoyer, W. J. (1988). Adult age differences in implicit and explicit memory: Time course and encoding effects. *Psychology and Aging*, 3(4), 358–366.

Cohen, N. J. (1984). Preserved learning capacity in amnesia: Evidence for multiple memory systems. In L. R. Squire & N. Butters (eds.), *Neuropsychology of memory* (pp. 83-103). New York: Guilford Press.

Cohen, R. L. (1983). The effects of encoding variables on the free recall of words and action events. *Memory & Cognition*, 11(6):575–582.

Cohen, R. L., Sandler, S. P., & Schroeder, K. (1987). Aging and memory for words and action events: The effects of item repetition and list length. *Psychology and Aging*, 2(3):280–285.

Craik, F. I. M. (1977). Age differences in human memory. In J. E. Birren & K. W. Schaie (eds.), *Handbook of the Psychology of Aging* (pp. 384-420). New York: Van Nostrand Reinhold.

Craik, F. I. M., & Byrd, M. (1982). Aging and cognitive deficits: The role of attentional resources. In F. I. M. Craik & S. Trehub (eds.), *Aging and Cognitive Processes* (pp. 191-211). New York: Plenum Press.

Craik, F. I. M., Byrd, M., & Swanson, J. M. (1987). Patterns of memory loss in three elderly samples. *Psychology and Aging*, 2(1):79–86.

Craik, F. I. M., & McDowd, J. M. (1987). Age differences in recall and recognition. *Journal of Experimental Psychology: Learning, Memory, and Cognition*, 13(3):474–479.

Craik, F. I. M., & Simon, E. (1980). Age differences in memory: The roles of attention and depth of processing. In L. W. Poon et al. (eds.), *New Directions in Aging and Memory* (pp. 95-112). Hillsdale, NJ: Lawrence Erlbaum.

Crook, T., Bartus, R. T., Ferris, S. H., Whitehouse, P., Cohen, G. D., & Gershon, S. (1986). Age-associated memory impairment: Proposed criteria and measures of clinical change. *Developmental Neuropsychology*, 2:1–12.

Daneman, M., & Carpenter, P. A. (1980). Individual differences in working memory and reading. *Journal of Verbal Learning and Verbal Behavior*, 19(4):450–466.

Erber, J. T. (1974). Age differences in recognition memory. *Journal of Gerontology*, 29(2), 177–181.

Gilewski, M. J., & Zelinski, E. M. (1986). Questionnaire assessment of memory complaints. In L. W. Poon, T. Crook, K. L. Davis, C. Eisdorfer, B. J. Gurland, A. W. Kaszniak, & L. W. Thompson (eds.), *Handbook for Clinical Memory Assessment of Older Adults* (pp. 93-107). Washington, DC: American Psychological Association.

Greene, R. L. (1986). Effects of intentionality and strategy on memory for frequency. *Journal of Experimental Psychology: Learning, Memory, and Cognition*, 12(4), 489–495.

Hartley, J. T. (1986). Reader and text variables as determinants of discourse memory in adulthood. *Psychology and Aging*, *1*(2):150–158.

Hasher, L., & Zacks, R. T. (1979). Automatic and effortful processes in memory. *Journal of Experimental Psychology: General*, *108*, 356–388.

Hasher, L., & Zacks, R. T. (1984). Automatic processing of fundamental information: The case of frequency of occurrence. *American Psychologist*, 39(12) 1372–1388.

Howe, M. L. (1988). Measuring memory development in adulthood: A model based approach to disentangling storage-retrieval contributions (pp. 39-64). In M. L. Howe & C. J. Brainerd (eds.), *Cognitive Development in Adulthood: Progress in Cognitive Development Research*. New York: Springer-Verlag.

Hulicka, I. M., & Grossman, J. L. (1967). Age-group comparisons for the use of mediators in paired-associate learning. *Journal of Gerontology*, 22(1):46–51.

Kaszniak, A. W., Poon, L. W., & Riege, W. (1986). Assessing memory deficits: An information processing approach. In L. W. Poon et al. (eds.), *Handbook for Clinical Assessment of Older Adults* (pp. 168-188). Washington, DC: American Psychological Association.

Kausler, D. H. (1970). Retention-forgetting as a nomological network for developmental research. In L. R. Goulet & P. B. Baltes (eds.), *Life-span Developmental Psychology: Research and Theory* (pp. 305-353). New York: Academic Press.

Kausler, D. H. (1982). *Experimental Psychology and Human Aging*. New York: John Wiley & Sons.

Kausler, D. H. (1985). Episodic memory: Memorizing performance. In N. Charness (eds.), *Aging and Human Performance* (pp. 101-141). Chichester: John Wiley & Sons.

Kausler, D. H. (1987). Interference. In G. L. Maddox, R. C. Atchley, L. W. Poon, G. S. Roth, I. C. Siegler, R. M. Steinberg, & R. J. Corsini (eds.), *The Encyclopedia of aging* (p. 359). New York: Springer.

Kausler, D. H. (in press). Comments on aging memory and its everyday operations. In L. W. Poon, D. C. Rubin, & B. A. Wilson (eds.), *Everyday Cognition in Adulthood and Aging*. New York: Cambridge University Press.

Kausler, D. H., & Hakami, M. K. (1983). Memory for activities: Adult age differences and intentionality. *Developmental Psychology, 19*(6), 889–894.

Kausler, D. H., & Lichty, W. (1988). Memory for activities: Rehearsal-independence and aging (pp. 93-131). In M. L. Howe & C. J. Brainerd (eds.), *Cognitive development in adulthood: Progress in cognitive development research*. New York: Springer-Verlag.

Kausler, D. H., Lichty, W., & Davis, R. T. (1985). Temporal memory for performed activities: Intentionality and adult age differences. *Developmental Psychology, 21*(6), 1132-1138.

Kausler, D. H., Lichty, W., & Freund, J. S. (1985). Adult age differences in recognition memory and frequency judgments for planned versus performed activities. *Developmental Psychology*, 21(4), 647–654.

Kausler, D. H., Lichty, W., & Hakami, M. K. (1984). Frequency judgments for distractor items in a short-term memory task: Instructional variation and adult age differences. *Journal of Verbal Learning and Verbal Behavior, 23*(5), 660-668.

Kausler, D. H., Lichty, W., Hakami, M. K., & Freund, J. S. (1986). Activity duration and adult age differences for activity performance. *Psychology and Aging*, 1(1), 80–81.

Kausler, D. H., & Phillips, P. L. (1988). Instructional variation and adult age differences in activity memory. *Experimental Aging Research, 14*, 195-199.

Kausler, D. H., & Puckett, J. M. (1980). Frequency judgments and correlated cognitive abilities in young and elderly adults. *Journal of Gerontology* 35(3), 376–382.

Kausler, D. H., & Puckett, J. M. (1981). Adult age differences in memory for sex of voice. *Journal of Gerontology, 36*(1), 44-50.

Kausler, D. H., Salthouse, T. A. & Saults, J. S. (1987). Frequency-of-occurrence memory over the adult lifespan. *Experimental Aging Research*, 13(3), 159–161.

Kausler, D. H., Salthouse, T. A., & Saults, J. S. (1988). Temporal memory over the adult lifespan. *American Journal of Psychology, 101*(2), 207–215.

Kral, V. A. (1962). Senescent forgetfulness: Benign and malignant. *Journal of the Canadian Medical Association,* 86, 257–260.

Lehman, E. B., & Mellinger, J. C. (1984). Effects of aging on memory for presentation modality. *Developmental Psychology,* *20*(6), 1210–1217.

Lehman, E. B., & Mellinger, J. C. (1986). Forgetting rates in modality memory for young, mid-life, and older women. *Psychology and Aging,* 1(2), 178–179.

Lichty, W. (1986). *Aging and memory for activities*. Doctoral dissertation, University of Missouri, Columbia.

Lichty, W., Kausler, D. H., & Martinez, D. R. (1986). Adult age differences in memory for motor versus cognitive activities. *Experimental Aging Research,* *12*(4), 227–230.

Light, L. L., & Anderson, P. A. (1985). Working-memory capacity, age, and memory for discourse. *Journal of Gerontology,* *40*(6), 737–747.

Light, L. L., & Burke, D. M. (in press). Patterns of language and memory in old age. In L. L. Light & D. M. Burke (eds.), *Language, Memory, and Aging.* Cambridge: Cambridge University Press.

Light, L. L., & Singh, A. (1987). Implicit and explicit memory in young and older adults. *Journal of Experimental Psychology: Learning, Memory, and Cognition* *13*(4), 531–541.

Light, L. L., Singh, A., & Capps, J. L. (1986). Dissociation of memory and awareness in young and older adults. *Journal of Clinical and Experimental Neuropsychology* 8(1), 62–74.

Light, L. L., Zelinski, E. M. (1983). Memory for spatial information in young and old adults. *Developmental Psychology,* *19*(6), 901-906.

Macht, M. L., & Buschke, H. (1983). Age differences in cognitive effort in recall. *Journal of Gerontology,* *38*(3), 695–700.

McCormack, P. D. (1981). Temporal coding by young and elderly adults: A test of the Hasher-Zacks model. *Developmental Psychology* *17*(4), 509–515.

McIntyre, J. S., & Craik, F. I. M. (1987). Age differences in memory for item and source information. *Canadian Journal of Psychology,* *41*(2), 175–192.

Milligan, W. L., Powell, D. A., Harley, C., & Furchtgott, E. (1984). A comparison of physical health and psychosocial variables as predictors of reaction time and serial learning performance in elderly men. *Journal of Gerontology* *39*(6), 704–710.

Murphy, M. D., Schmitt, F. A., Caruso, M. J., & Sanders, R. E. (1987). Metamemory in older adults: The role of monitoring in serial recall. *Psychology and Aging,* *2*(4):331–339.

Nebes, R. D., & Madden, D. J. (1988). Different patterns of cognitive slowing produced by Alzheimer's disease and normal aging. *Psychology and Aging,* *3*(1), 102-104.

Park, D. C., Royal, D., Dudley, W., & Morrell, R. (1988). Forgetting of pictures over a long retention interval in young and older adults. *Psychology and Aging,* *3*(1), 94-95.

Parkinson, S. R., Inman, V. W., & Dannenbaum, S. E. (1985). Adult age differences in short-term forgetting. *Acta Psychologica,* 60(1), 83–101.

Parks, C. W., Jr., Mitchell, D. B., & Perlmutter, M. (1986). Cognitive and social functioning across adulthood: Age or student status differences? *Psychology and Aging,* *1*(3), 248–254.

Peterson, L. R., & Peterson, M. J. (1959). Short-term retention of individual verbal items. *Journal of Experimental Psychology,* 58(3), 193-198.

Puckett, J. M., Stockburger, D. W. (1988). Absence of age-related proneness to short-term retroactive interference in the absence of rehearsal. *Psychology and Aging,* *3*(4): 342-247.

Ratner, H. H., Schell, D. A., Crimmins, A., Mittelman, D., & Baldinelli, L. (1987). Changes in adults' prose recall: Aging or cognitive demands? *Developmental Psychology, 23*, 521-525.

Rybarczyk, B. D., Hart, R. P., & Harkins, S. W. (1987). Age and forgetting rate with pictorial stimuli. *Psychology and Aging, 2*(4), 404–406.

Salthouse, T. A. (1982). *Adult Cognition: An Experimental Psychology of Human Aging*. New York: Springer.

Salthouse, T. A. (1985). *A Theory of Cognitive Aging*. Amsterdam: North Holland.

Salthouse, T. A., Kausler, D. H., Saults, J. S. (1988a). Investigation of student status, background variables, and feasibility of standard tasks in cognitive aging research. *Psychology and Aging, 3*(1): 29-37.

Salthouse, T. A., Kausler, D. H., & Saults, J. S. (1988b). Utilization of path analytic procedures to investigate the role of processing resources in cognitive aging. *Psychology and Aging, 3*(2), 158–166.

Salthouse, T. A., & Somberg, B. L. (1982). Skilled performance: Effects of adult age and experience on elementary processes. *Journal of Experimental Psychology: General, 111*(2), 176-207.

Schonfield, D., & Robertson, B. A. (1966). Memory storage and aging. *Canadian Journal of Psychology*, 20(2), 228–236.

Shimamura, A. P. (1986). Priming effects in amnesia: Evidence for a dissociable memory function. *Quarterly Journal of Experimental Psychology, 38A*, 619–644.

Smith, A. D. (1980). Age differences in encoding, storage, and retrieval. In L. W. Poon et al. (eds.), *New Directions in memory and aging* (pp. 23-45). Hillsdale, NJ: Lawrence Erlbaum Associates.

Stine, E. L., & Wingfield, A. (1987). Process and strategy in memory for speech among younger and older adults. *Psychology and Aging*, 2(3):272–279.

Storandt, M., Botwinick, J., & Danziger, W. L. (1986). Longitudinal changes: Patients with mild SDAT and matched healthy controls. In L. W. Poon et al. (eds.), *Handbook for Clinical Memory Assessment of Older Adults* (pp. 277-284). Washington, DC: American Psychological Association.

Strauss, M. E., Weingartner, H., & Thompson, K. (1985). Remembering words and how often they occurred in memory-impaired patients. *Memory & Cognition*, 13(6), 507-510.

Thorndike, E. L., Bregman, E. O., Tilton, J. W., & Woodyard, E. (1928). *Adult Learning*. New York: Macmillan.

Toglia, M. P., & Kimble, G. A. (1976). Recall and use of serial position information. *Journal of Experimental Psychology: Human Learning and Memory*, 2(4):431–445.

Tulving, E. (1972). Episodic and semantic memory. In E. Tulving & W. Donaldson (eds.), *Organization of memory* (pp. 381-403). New York: Academic Press.

Tulving, E. (1985). How many memory systems are there? *American Psychologist*, 40(4), 385–398.

Yesavage, J. A., Rose, T. L., & Bower, G. H. (1983). Interactive imagery and affective judgments improve face-name learning in the elderly. *Journal of Gerontology*, 38(2), 197-203.

Zacks, R. T., Hasher, L., Alba, J. W., Sanft, H., & Rose, K. C. (1984). Is temporal order encoded automatically? *Memory & Cognition, 12*(4), 387–394.

Zelinski, E. M., & Light, L. L. (1988). Young and older adults' use of context in spatial memory. *Psychology and Aging, 3*(1), 99–101.

Zivian, M. T., & Darjes, R. W. (1983). Free recall by in-school and out-of-school adults: Performance and metamemory. *Developmental Psychology*, 19(4), 513-520.

3

Everyday Memory Problems of Healthy Older Adults: Characteristics of a Successful Intervention

Robin L. West and Adrian Tomer

It is very common for older adults to complain about memory problems and to endorse statements saying that aging leads to memory declines and more forgetting (Chaffin & Herrmann, 1983; Sunderland, Watts, Baddeley, & Harris, 1986). It is much less common for the scientific community to explore the precise nature of these deficits. With the exception of self-report questionnaires, the investigation of everyday memory is relatively new. Systematic studies have begun to identify ways in which practical memory may be different from traditional laboratory tests (West, 1986), but we still know relatively little about intervention. Only a handful of memory training studies have used memory tasks in which the information content (e.g., names and faces, grocery lists), encoding, and retrieval conditions were comparable to those typically present in everyday environments (Anschutz, Camp, Markley, & Kramer, 1985; Scogin, Storandt, & Lott, 1985; Yesavage & Sheikh, in press). Nevertheless, there is much to be learned about successful intervention from the existing literature. This review will consider assessment, specific strategies that can be used, and the overall design of a training program, with emphasis on methods to maximize the effectiveness of interventions.

ASSESSMENT

There are a number of excellent reviews discussing the assessment process and the design of memory assessments for older adults, including methods for examining memory skills as well as individual difference factors (Poon, Fozard, & Treat, 1978; Poon, 1980; Poon, 1986). The breadth of the assessment will depend on the goals of the intervention. An intervention could be designed solely to improve memory scores, and an appropriate assessment would include one or more memory tests. Another intervention could be designed to change older adults' attitudes, attributions, or memory self-concept as well as performance, in which case measures of these characteristics would need to be included. The assessment could be designed as a selective tool to identify appropriate individuals for a training program and/or as a means to evaluate program accomplishments.

Everyday Memory Assessment

Potentially useful assessment devices include laboratory analogues of everyday memory. The existing batteries of everyday memory tests show considerable variation in difficulty level, ranging from the Rivermead Behavioral Memory Test (RBMT; young normals typically score 100%) to the Everyday Memory Interview (EMI; young normals score 100% on some subtests) to the more difficult computerized battery developed by Crook and Larrabee (1988) (Table 3.1).

All of the everyday batteries tap several different dimensions of memory skill and are able to discriminate between adults with deficits and those without deficits. The Rivermead Behavioral Memory Test (RBMT) has been investigated with young normals, head injury patients, and older adults. The overall score clearly discriminates between those with deficits and those without (Wilson, 1984; Wilson, Baddeley, & Hutchins, 1984). The MAC computerized battery has been used in longitudinal drug trial studies. Piloting on subtests was completed to develop a set of final tests that discriminates age groups by decades, as seen in Table 3.2 (Larrabee & Crook, 1989). Principal component analysis indicates that the MAC assessment includes visual and verbal memory, attention, and psychomotor speed, with comparable factors across age groups.

Multivariate discriminant analyses with the EMI (West, in press-a) indicate that several tests are sensitive to age differences, distinguishing between young (18–39 years), middle-aged (40–59 years), young-old (60–75 years), and old-old (75–90 years) groups (Table 3.3). On the immediate recall tests, discriminant analysis resulted in correct classification of group membership for 59% of the sample (Wilks' lambda $= 0.45$, $\chi^2 = 121.8$, $df = 21$, $p < 0.0001$), and on the delayed recall tests, there was 67% correct age group classification (Wilks' lambda $= 0.35$, $\chi^2 = 157.5$, $df = 30$, $p < 0.0001$). All of the immediate recall tests in the battery and all of the delayed recall tests (except for the single-item name recall test) discriminate healthy

TABLE 3.1 Outline of Items to Recall on Everyday Memory Batteries*

Items	Crook (MAC)	Wilson & Baddeley (RBMT)	West (EMI)
Everyday memory tasks	Names (many) Faces Grocery list Newscast Object locations Name-city association Telephone numbers Traffic and weather reports	Name Faces Pictures News story Hidden object Route (errand) Skill completion Prospective task Orientation (date, etc.)	Name Photographs Personal list Prose recall Object location Route Activity series Prospective task Conversation Doctor's instructions Interview tasks
Other test items	Driving reaction time	Digit span Paired associates	

* Batteries include immediate and delayed recall; serial, free, and cued recall; recognition (not EMI); incidental memory (not RBMT) and intentional memory; verbal, visual, and spatial tasks; timed (not EMI and RBMT) and self-paced tests.

individuals of all ages from those with self-reported poor health (78% correct classification of health status using immediate or delayed test scores).

Other Kinds of Assessment

Another approach that may be very productive is to assess strategy usage per se. The advantages of this type of assessment are (1) to identify individuals for training who do not initially use the strategy or use it poorly and (2) to examine training effectiveness in light of strategy usage instead of focusing only on performance (West, in press-a). Studies that have followed this suggestion have been highly informative about the underlying dynamics of training (Anschutz et al., 1985; DeLeon, 1974; Hellebusch, 1976; Pratt & Higbee, 1983; Roberts & Wilson, 1986; Schmitt, Murphy, & Sanders, 1981). Behavioral checklists and other forms of self-report may be used to acquire this type of data (Camp, Markley, & Kramer, 1983), as well as direct measures of rehearsal and organization (Schmitt, Murphy, & Sanders, 1981).

Tasks can be divided into subcomponents. The ability to perform each subcomponent could be assessed before and after training. This could be done with many

TABLE 3.2 Differentiation of Age Groups on the EMI with 160 Healthy Subjects

Test	Young	Middle-Aged	Young-Old	Old-Old
Immediate recall				
Photographs (50)	34.0	34.9	31.8	27.3
Route (12)	11.8	11.8	11.5	10.8
Activity series (20)*	15.9	14.0	13.6	12.1
Doctor's instructions (24)*	12.2	12.6	9.8	7.1
Cued recall (11)* (doctor's, prose)	6.1	6.8	4.8	3.1
Delayed recall				
Photographs (8)*	6.7	6.6	6.0	5.5
Personal list (100)*	86.9	82.7	74.7	66.6
Object location (10)	8.8	8.8	8.5	7.3
Activity series (20)*	18.2	17.4	14.9	11.5
Prospective task (6)	5.1	5.2	3.5	2.5
Conversation (100)	75.1	71.8	59.8	50.6
Doctor's instructions (24)*	11.9	13.0	9.7	6.3
Interview tasks (100)*	73.8	72.3	56.3	49.2

Note: A single significant discriminant function is needed to separate subjects into the identified groups on their immediate recall and delayed recall scores. A * notes those tests that show a significant difference between groups on univariate *F* ratios ($df = 3/156$, $p < 0.001$). The maximum score on each test is noted in parentheses.

TABLE 3.3 Age Group Comparisons on MAC, Means and Correlations with Age

Test	18–39 years	40–49 years	50–59 years	60–69 years	70+ years	Correlation
Name-face association (14)						
immediate	11.6	10.5	9.7	8.5	6.6	−0.38
delayed	11.3	10.1	9.1	7.9	6.0	−0.39
First-last names (6)	5.2	4.7	4.3	4.3	3.3	−0.29
Object locations (20)	14.3	14.1	12.8	11.5	10.3	−0.39
Telephone numbers (10)	7.7	7.5	7.2	6.7	6.4	−0.28

Note: All tests show a significant univariate *F* ratio for age group differences. The number of persons per age group varies from test to test. The maximum score on each test is noted in parentheses.

complex memory strategies such as the peg system, and some researchers have divided their training programs into subcomponents in this way (Kliegl, Smith, & Baltes, 1986; Schmitt, Murphy, & Sanders, 1981; Yesavage, Rose, & Bower, 1983). Subcomponent assessments could be used within a training program to examine individual progress on one component before moving on to the next step in training.

INDIVIDUAL DIFFERENCES

There are several perspectives on the issue of individual differences. First, it was recognized that the specific needs, motivations, and abilities of the participants should be taken into consideration in order to maximize the effectiveness of a memory training program (Treat, Poon, Fozard, & Popkin, 1978; Poon, Walsh-Sweeney, & Fozard, 1980; Yesavage and Sheikh, in press). Second, individual differences have been recognized as an obstacle to an adequate evaluation of memory programs. The heterogeneity commonly found in group settings makes it difficult to avoid ceiling effects for some of the participants and/or floor effects for others (Yesavage and Sheikh, in press; Zarit, Cole, & Guilder, 1981). Also, interindividual variability may obscure treatment effects (Schaffer & Poon, 1982). Third, the issue of differential improvement poses challenging scientific questions regarding the causes for variability and its relevance to theories about the plasticity of cognitive abilities (Willis & Baltes, 1980) and disuse (Salthouse, 1982).

Practitioners and scientists are interested in the way individual difference variables interact with each other and with program characteristics to influence outcome. Nevertheless, only modest progress has been made in identifying the relevant variables and their effects on memory. We will review the evidence, considering relationships with memory performance, memory gains, and maintenance and generalization effects.

In training studies, significant correlations with memory have been reported for a number of variables. Verbal ability and education have been found to correlate positively with memory performance (Perlmutter, Tenney, & Smith, 1980; Schaffer & Poon, 1982). On the other hand, negative correlations have been found for age (Schaffer & Poon, 1982), and depression (Perlmutter, Tenney, & Smith, 1980; Schaffer & Poon, 1982).

Individuals may also vary in memory self-evaluation. Quite surprisingly, memory complaints do not correlate with memory performance in most of the training studies (Flynn, 1986; Kahn et al., 1975; Perlmutter, Tenney, & Smith, 1980; Scogin, Storandt, & Lott, 1985; Zarit, Cole, & Guider, 1981), and in one case, complaints were correlated negatively with performance (Schaffer & Poon, 1982). Such results may occur because highly educated individuals with excellent memory skills tend to have more stringent criteria for self-assessment (Flynn, 1986; Schaffer & Poon, 1982) or because depression influences complaints more than performance (Zarit, Gallagher, & Kramer, 1981). In addition, problems may result from using laboratory tests to assess the predictive validity of memory complaints (Gilewski & Zelinski, 1986; West, Berry, & Dennehy, 1987).

Memory gains or changes seem to be related to initial memory performance, with low performers tending to improve and high performers tending to decline or to remain stable, irrespective of type of training (Schaffer & Poon, 1982). However, a regression toward the mean might be an alternative explanation for this trend, since the trend was apparent in the control group as well as the training groups.

Personality traits may also be related to memory gains. Preliminary data reported by Yesavage and Sheikh (in press) suggest that elderly participants who scored higher on the "intuitive" scale of the Myers-Briggs Jungian Personality Indicator improved more than those who scored higher on the "sensing" scale. In the same vein, anxiety reduction techniques have been found to facilitate memory in subjects who begin with high anxiety levels (Yesavage, Rose, & Spiegel, 1982), but not in others.

In another personality measure, Erber, Abello, and Moninger (1988) found that Locus of Control (measured on the Rotter Scale) was not related to memory gains following imagery mnemonic instructions for older adults. Externally-controlled young adults, however, benefited more from imagery instructions than internally-controlled young adults.

Individual differences are reflected also in the fact that memory performance changes after training are not always correlated with changes in memory complaints (Scogin, Storandt, & Lott, 1985; Zarit, Gallagher, & Kramer, 1981). The motivation of elderly subjects interested in participation in a memory training program should therefore be considered when establishing the goals or the potential benefits of the program for the participants. A person with excellent memory skills may not improve his memory performance (Schaffer & Poon, 1982) but can still be expected to improve his self-assessment and satisfaction with his memory ability (Flynn, 1986; Zarit, Cole, & Guider, 1981; Zarit, Gallagher, & Kramer, 1981).

Individual differences might be especially important in the context of maintaining memory performance and/or generalizing strategies to different memory tasks. There is some evidence that participants who do not modify newly-learned strategies are more likely to show long-term maintenance and generalization (Anschutz et al., 1985), but the antecedents of this differential inclination to maintain strategies is unclear. Individuals can also develop and use a strategy independently of instructions given to them, and maintenance and generalization effects have been found in these cases (DeLeon, 1974). At the same time, significant correlations between strategy usage *per se* and demographic variables have not been reported.

Other motivational and cognitive variables that could potentially affect either gains or maintenance and generalization need to be studied. In particular, it is important to study cognitive style variables (for example, the tendency to use a certain strategy), which may eventually determine the success of a program for a certain individual.

Given the scarcity of data regarding interindividual differences, it might be useful to mention several difficulties that appear to have slowed the development of a systematic body of knowledge: Most of the studies do not analyze and/or report results at the level of interindividual differences. Also, there are notorious difficulties in measuring change (Harris, 1963). An evaluation of the significance of change for an individual can be done only against a longitudinal baseline (Willis, 1985). It is possible that either more complex variables and/or a multitude of variables should be considered together in order to successfully predict memory change for individuals. Large samples are required for this last purpose.

While some of these problems may be expected to continue to plague the investigation of interindividual differences in the near future, some significant progress may be anticipated. Models to assess change (usually requiring more than two time points) have become available (Bryk & Raudenbush, 1987). The advantages of conducting a training study in the framework of a larger (and preferably longitudinal) study have been demonstrated (Willis & Schaie, 1986). An investigation of more complex personality variables is also under way (Yesavage & Sheikh, in press).

STRATEGIES

Although it is clear that older adults make use of external aids to support memory (Cavanaugh, Grady, & Perlmutter, 1983; Lovelace, 1984), it is not possible for individuals to carry a notebook everywhere nor is it easy to record everything of importance in a notebook. Memory success also requires the application of internal memory strategies. This section will focus on internal methods of remembering. (Such training can increase successful application of external aids even though they are already commonly used; see Harris, 1978, 1980, 1984).

What strategy should be selected for training? The choices are endless. Techniques that enhance long-term memory can generally be divided into those that rely on imagery, verbal elaboration, organization, or retrieval practice. Several books and articles have attempted a comprehensive description of these strategies (West, 1985; Wilson & Moffat, 1984a). Some focus mainly on imagery (Higbee, 1977; Lapp, 1987; Lorayne & Lucas, 1974), and a few include verbal association methods (Cermak, 1975; Higbee, 1977). Specific techniques can also be recommended for particular everyday memory tasks (West, in press-a). A variety of strategies have been used with students (Bellezza, 1983; Morris, 1979) and with adult patient populations (Grafman, 1984; Moffat, in press; Schacter & Glisky, in press; Wilson & Moffat, 1984a, 1984b). The most commonly examined technique with older adults is imagery (Poon, Walsh-Sweeney, & Fozard, 1980).

Organization

Many of the methods based on organization (such as the PQRST method, outlining, and tree diagrams) are primarily used for remembering prose and are appropriate for students, although they have also been recommended for older adults (West, 1985) and head injury patients (Wilson & Moffat, 1984b). Organization according to first letters is sometimes employed (Harris, 1980; Lovelace, 1984), but it did not improve recall in training studies (Hellebusch, 1976; Hultsch, 1969). Chunking of numbers is also a useful organizational technique (Kliegl, Smith, & Baltes, 1986; Taub, 1973).

Older adults do not use organization as consistently or as effectively as the young (Hultsch, 1971, 1974; Rankin, Karol, & Tuten, 1984; Sanders et al., 1980; Worden & Meggison, 1984). In spontaneous sorting of *objects* into meaningful groups, older adults do not use the same categories as the young (Cicirelli, 1976), but they appear to organize *words* into the same categories (Howard, 1980). Research data show that organization could facilitate many practical memory tasks (West, 1986), and that older adults can be trained to organize lists for improved recall (Flynn, 1986; Bäckman & Karlsson, 1986; Schmitt, Murphy, & Sanders, 1981; Scogin, Storandt, & Lott, 1985; Zarit, Cole, & Guider, 1981; Zarit, Gallagher, & Kramer, 1981), but recall improvements have not occurred under all conditions (Hultsch, 1969; Rankin, Karol, & Tuten, 1984).

Retrieval

Although there is definite evidence that age-related retrieval deficits exist (Burke & Light, 1981; Kausler, 1982), no one has focused their efforts on retrieval training, except to the extent that encoding strategies such as organization and the method of loci contain embedded retrieval plans (Bower, 1970, 1972; Poon, 1980). Older adults may be receptive to retrieval training since the most common internal strategy for practical memory is mental retracing, a retrieval method (Harris, 1980; Lovelace, 1984). Training could emphasize regular rehearsal, mental retracing, selective testing, distributed practice, encoding specificity (reinstating encoding conditions), or expanded intervals for review (West, 1985, in press-a). The expanded interval technique has been used successfully with head injury patients (Schacter, Rich, & Stampp, 1985) and Alzheimer's patients (Camp, Chapter 10). Also, older adults could potentially be taught to make use of association networks to overcome retrieval blocks (see Reason & Lucas, 1984).

Imagery

Imagery has been studied more than any other internal strategy. Older adults show clear deficits in the use of imagery, and imagery training can be effective as indicated by reviews in Poon, Walsh-Sweeney, and Fozard, 1980; Yesavage and Sheikh, in press; and other recent studies (Anschutz et al., 1985; Rebok & Balcerak, 1986; Erber, Abello, & Moninger, 1987; Flynn, 1986; Poon & Walsh-Sweeney, 1981; Roberts & Wilson, 1986; Scogin, Storandt, & Lott, 1985; Sheikh et al., 1986; Treat, Poon, & Fozard, 1981; Yesavage, 1984; Yesavage & Jacob, 1984; Yesavage & Rose, 1984a, 1984b; Hill, Sheikh, & Yesavage, 1988).

Imagery methods include interactive imagery (Poon & Walsh-Sweeney, 1981), and chaining images in sequence (Zarit, Cole, & Guider, 1981). Some complex methods, such as the peg system (Pratt & Higbee, 1983), the keyword method (Roberts & Wilson, 1986), the method of loci (Robertson-Tchabo, Hausman, & Arenberg, 1976) and the image-name match method (Yesavage, Rose, & Bower, 1983) have also been taught to older adults, with mixed success. There are indications that older adults are not receptive to imagery training using bizarre images (J. A. Yesavage, personal communication, March, 1985; Poon & Walsh-Sweeney, 1981). However, there are no apparent-age differences in imagery ratings of words (Kausler, 1980), or the quality of imagery overall (Hartley, 1982).

Verbal Elaboration

Some scholars have argued that verbal elaboration would be more appropriate than imagery for training because verbal mediation training has led to memory improvements (Catino, Taub, & Borkowski, 1977; DeLeon, 1974; Hellebusch, 1976; Hulicka & Grossman, 1967), and because older adults are likely to apply verbal mnemonics (Hulicka, Sterns, & Grossman, 1967; Rowe & Schnore, 1971; Treat, Poon, & Fozard, 1981; Weinstein et al., 1981). Older adults may be more successful with verbal than imaginal mediators for a variety of reasons (Cermak, 1980; West, in press; Winograd & Simon, 1980). There is evidence that verbal skills remain intact as individuals age (Botwinick, 1982), and there are no age changes in verbal association networks (Howard, 1980; Lovelace & Cooley, 1982). At the same time, older adults' verbal elaborations are often not as precise as those of younger adults (Perlmutter, 1979; Puglisi, Park, & Smith, 1987; Rabinowitz & Ackerman, 1982; Rankin & Collins, 1985) so training efforts should probably focus on the formation of distinctive associates that have personal meaning.

Methods based on verbal memory include simple association between items (Hulicka & Grossman, 1967), sentence generation, and first-letter associations (Hellebusch, 1976). Among the complex methods, the figure alphabet (a phonetic system for number recall) has been used with older adults in training (Smith et al., 1984) as well as name sentences.

A recent study completed in this laboratory shows that verbal elaboration training can lead to generalizable memory improvement for older adults. The EMI was used as a pre-assessment, and an alternate form of the EMI was administered after all training sessions to 22 older adults. A waiting list group of comparable size completed both assessments without intervening training. Training was administered in groups of six to ten persons. In the initial session, age-related memory changes were described, and first-letter association was used to remember these changes. In each of the next three sessions (2 days apart), one memory task was defined along with some discussion of how memory failures occur. This was followed by extensive practice of one verbal elaboration technique: simple association was taught for recalling object locations, name sentences were applied to remember names and faces, and first-letter association was used for remembering text.

To examine the results, measures on the EMI were divided into immediate and delayed tests, free recall, and cued recall. A multivariate analysis examined the impact of group (trained or control) and test (pretest or posttest). Tests with ceiling effects on the pretest or posttest were eliminated from the analysis (name, object location, route, prospective task). If the impact of training was strong, the trained group should show improvement relative to the control group on immediate learning as well as delayed, and on free recall as well as cued recall tests. Instead, posttest scores were higher for both groups on all measures, and the results reflected a significant group by test interaction only on the delayed cued recall tests. The gains made by the training group reflected generalization of the verbal elaboration strategy, at least when retrieval support was present, in the form of cues. The smallest gains for the trained group, relative to the control group, were on the immediate free recall tests. These results suggest that verbal elaboration may have potential value for long-term retention of information, especially when retrieval cues are present (as they often are in normal everyday environments).

All of these available techniques could potentially be effective for both laboratory and everyday memory tasks. Strategy selection should be guided by the potential application of the strategy to a wide range of practical memory tasks, the motivation of participants to master specific kinds of memory tasks (some tasks, such as remembering lists of groceries or errands, could probably be improved with any of the existing memory techniques), expectations about the existing strategy skill level of participants, and the amount of time available to devote to complex training methods such as the peg system or image-name match method.

DESIGNING AN INTERVENTION

Interventions should identify memory techniques that lead to improvements in performance. Ideally, the trained strategies will be useful for all individuals or a defined subset of the population, they will lead to performance improvements over and above those resulting from practice alone, and they will become integrated with the memory system. If the strategies are integrated, they will be applied spontaneously to more than one specific task domain (when it is appropriate), and they will not be quickly abandoned. An intervention could lead to immediate and significant memory improvements on a specific task and be deemed successful, but the limits of that success would become apparent if the improvement was short-lived (not maintained over time) or was not evident on other tests (no generalization occurs).

Maintenance

Several different types of research have addressed the issue of maintenance (Poon, Walsh-Sweeney, & Fozard, 1980; Treat et al., 1978; West, in press-a). One indication that a strategy has been maintained is that an individual will use it spontaneously in a memory testing situation, without being instructed to do so. Also, if posttest scores are higher than pretest scores and the gain is maintained on later tests, strategy maintenance is assumed. Some researchers avoid this issue by instructing subjects to use newly learned strategies or by providing a specific mnemonic to the subject (Poon & Walsh-Sweeney, 1981; Yesavage & Rose, 1984a). In a recent study, adults instructed to use their trained strategies were compared with those who were not so instructed; persons who were not told to use the strategies on the last test performed no better than control subjects who had never been trained (Roberts & Wilson, 1986).

A less common way to evaluate maintenance is to see if specific information learned with a strategy is still remembered some time later. This provides an examination of the long-term effectiveness of the strategy. It might be the case, for instance, that people can retain information for short periods of time regardless of training, but that strategic processing allows a person to retain material for longer delays. Investigators have generally found that strategy training increases the abilty to retain specific information over time, although this particular benefit has not always been evident for older adults (Hellebusch, 1976; Poon & Walsh-Sweeney, 1981; Thomas & Ruben, cited in Poon, Walsh-Sweeney, & Fozard, 1980; Yesavage, Rose, & Bower, 1983).

A number of investigators have taken older adults who have received memory training and have given them a subsequent opportunity to use a learned strategy, a typical way to examine maintenance. Although in some cases older adults will spontaneously use a trained strategy over a number of trials (Schmitt, Murphy, & Sanders, 1981) or will maintain performance levels achieved immediately after training (Flynn, 1986; Scogin, Storandt, & Lott, 1985; Smith et al., 1984; Zarit, Gallagher, & Kramer, 1981), often they do not (Erber, Abello, & Moninger, 1988; Hellebusch, 1976; Pratt & Higbee, 1983; Robertson-Tchabo, Hausman, & Arenberg, 1976; Schaffer & Poon, 1982; Treat, Poon, & Fozard, 1981). Studies with other types of cognitive training have rarely examined maintenance and have shown mixed results (Bleiszner, Willis, & Baltes, 1981; Plemons, Willis, & Baltes, 1978; Willis, Bleiszner, & Baltes, 1981). The time period has had little impact on the results, although there is some indication that the method of loci will be maintained by some individuals for longer periods than others (Anschutz et al., 1985; Smith et al., 1984). Most of the studies demonstrating maintenance were ones in which many memory strategies were trained, and any one, or all, of the techniques could have been applied during the final testing sessions to enhance performance.

These data on maintenance are inconclusive because they fail to indicate the reasons for successful maintenance. Performance gains may have been maintained without trainees applying the learned strategies (DeLeon, 1974). Also, it is important to realize that no one as yet knows the impact of regular refresher courses. Because of insufficient evidence, it is not known if the same maintenance problem will occur after training on everyday memory tasks (Anschutz et al., 1985; Anschutz, Camp, Markley, & Kramer, 1987; Flynn, 1986).

Generalization

Generalization refers to the extent to which a method learned in one context can be applied by the learner in a new context. There has been considerable disagreement about whether or not it is desirable to try to achieve generalization. In fact, many rehabilitation psychologists have argued that individuals with serious memory problems can only use strategies to learn specific information, and only when the strategy application is guided by the psychologist (Schacter & Glisky, in press; Wilson, 1989; Wilson & Moffat, 1984b). With this approach, there is no attempt to teach the strategy per se. Individuals are taught to remember "Robin West" by saying "the robin is flying west." They are not trained in the general method of remembering names by connecting first and last names with some kind of verbal association, and there is no expectation that the technique will be applied by the learner to any other name.

Practitioners are very interested in this issue. If no generalization occurs, individuals who have learned to use association to recall names cannot use association to recall lists, to remember to take medicines, or to meet social obligations. A technique that should not be domain-specific becomes domain-specific if no generalization occurs (West, in press-a).

As in the case of maintenance, the issue of generalization is often avoided by examining strategy usage only on a single task (Hultsch, 1969; Mason & Smith, 1977). With one test, older adults who have not been given the strategy typically do not perform as well as those who have been exposed to it (Canestrari, 1968; Hulicka & Grossman, 1967; Treat & Reese, 1976; Yesavage & Rose, 1984a, 1984b).

There are several levels of generalization that could potentially occur after training. The trainee could subsequently be able to use the newly learned technique on a set of to-be-remembered information that is similar, but not the same, as the set used during training. One example of this "near" generalization is learning how to use a technique to recall word pairs and later applying it to picture pairs. This type of generalization has not been demonstrated (Hellebusch, 1976; Roberts & Wilson, 1986). With other types of cognitive training, near transfer (training impact on tasks defined as involving the same factor) has been demonstrated (Bleiszner, Willis, & Baltes, 1981; Willis & Schaie, 1986). Although near generalization is an important indication of how well a strategy has been learned, the strategy is still domain-specific because the basic task requirements have not changed.

A broader type of generalization occurs when a technique taught as an approach to one particular type of memory situation can be transferred to another type of memory situation. When the strategy can be applied to a memory task with different task demands than the one used for training, it is an indication of "far" generalization. This represents the ideal goal for the memory trainer who wants the client to be able to go home and use newly learned techniques to improve his overall memory success. There is mixed evidence for this type of generalization after memory training (Anschutz et al., 1985; DeLeon, 1974; Yesavage & Rose, 1983), and it has not been demonstrated with other types of cognitive training (Denney, 1982). Basically, there are few demonstrations of either type of generalization. Whereas some would argue that far generalization should not be expected (Baltes & Willis, 1982), it may be premature to abandon the attempt.

Practice Effects

There is considerable evidence that practice, by itself, will improve the memory scores of many older adults (Treat et al., 1978), as well as scores on other intellectual measures (Labouvie-Vief & Gonda, 1976; Willis, Bleiszner, & Baltes, 1981). Posttest memory scores are often higher for the untrained subjects as well as for those subjects receiving training (Erber, Abello, & Moninger, 1988; Perlmutter, Tenney, & Smith, 1980; Schaffer & Poon, 1982; West, Boatwright, & Schleser, 1984). This can be positive news for the practitioner, whose primary goal is to see that training leads to improvements. If practice alone will result in better memory scores, then an effective intervention may consist of considerable practice (Taub & Long, 1972; Treat, Poon, & Fozard, 1981) and does not require the training of sophisticated strategic techniques.

Unfortunately, practice effects create problems for designing and interpreting memory training studies. The presence of significant practice effects means that no study is adequate without a control group that receives a pretest and posttest without intervening training. By this standard, a number of studies are inadequate because they simply show that people who get training will achieve higher scores on a subsequent test (Rose & Yesavage, 1983; Smith et al., 1984). They do not show that people with training achieve higher scores on a second test than people who did not have training. The exceptions, demonstrating training impact over and above control groups with practice, are few (Rebok & Balcerak, 1986; Roberts & Wilson, 1986; Scogin, Storandt, & Lott, 1985; Yesavage, Rose, & Bower, 1983; Zarit, Cole, & Guider, 1981; Zarit, Gallagher, & Kramer, 1981).

Pacing

There is ample evidence that older adults take longer to learn than younger people (Kausler, 1982). Although providing a specific mnemonic for a specific item will enhance its recall (Poon & Walsh-Sweeney, 1981), this is not sufficient for training older adults in a strategy that they may be able to apply on their own at home. For that, extensive practice is required to make the method relatively easy to apply. Practice should be combined with feedback showing the effectiveness of the mnemonic and with encouragement to practice at home. The research evidence shows that intervention programs that are longer and more thorough in their approach tend to be more effective (Yesavage & Sheikh, in press). One of the most successful programs involved a self-paced written training manual (Scogin, Storandt, & Lott, 1985). Also, training effects may be evident only if sufficient time is given for encoding and retrieval (Hulicka, Sterns, & Grossman, 1967; Treat & Reese, 1976). Memory training needs to be sensitive to the speed decrements associated with aging.

Social-Cognitive Processes

Another factor that may affect intervention success is older adults' attributions about declining memory. Training may not lead to lasting improvements if older adults believe that age, per se, is the true cause for experienced memory problems. Blaming memory failure on age means that one's attributions about memory are internal (age is a characteristic of the individual and not the environment), stable (one never gets younger), and global (age is expected to affect many different aspects of the individual's life, not just memory). Although older adults' attributions do not always fit this model, attributions of this kind are likely to result in further performance deterioration (Lachman & Jelalian, 1984; Lachman & McArthur, 1986; Lachman, Steinberg, & Trotter, 1986). A recent interview study by Cavanaugh and Morton (1988) indicates that those individuals who are most likely to attribute memory changes to age—those with internal locus of control—are also the least likely to employ memory strategies.

Changing the focus of the attribution to "blame" problems consistently on lack of effort, task difficulty, and/or lack of environmental stimulation, and to attribute successes to ability and effort, may be a requisite first step toward memory improvement. Consistent with this argument, interventions can be designed to improve memory self-efficacy, under the assumption that a higher memory self-concept and less focus on negative self-evaluation may facilitate memory improvement

(Rebok & Balcerak, 1986; Berry, 1986; Flynn, 1986; Lachman & Dick, 1987). It is apparent that memory training can temporarily reduce memory complaints (Richardson & Pratt, 1981; Scogin, Storandt, & Lott, 1985; Zarit, Cole, & Guider, 1981; Zarit, Gallagher, & Kramer, 1981), although its impact on long-term self-evaluative processes is not clear. Cognitive behavior modification or attribution retraining may prove to be useful for facilitating long-term reevaluation, but these methods have not been tested extensively with older adults (see Labouvie-Vief & Gonda, 1976; Reynolds & Stark, 1983).

Metacognitive Processes

If older adults are to apply training consistently in practical memory situations, they may need additional metacognitive knowledge. If an individual is unaware of not having learned an item, he or she is not likely to make an effort to learn it through strategic processing. The same lack of strategic effort will be evident if the individual does not know that strategy usage improves recall.

Although questionnaire data on metamemory reveals no consistent age deficits in basic knowledge about memory (Dixon, in press), studies of monitoring provide mixed evidence for age-related change. Older adults are often not as careful as young people in monitoring the contents of memory; for example, their estimates of the amount of study time needed to promote good recall are often incorrect (Murphy et al., 1981). On the other hand, when older adults make feeling-of-knowing judgments after studying to-be-remembered items, their judgments are usually as accurate as those of young adults (West, 1984). Also, older adults are just as proficient as young people in assessing the accuracy of their retrieval (Baumler & Erber, 1986) or their potential to recognize unrecallable information (Lachman & Lachman, 1980).

Given this mixed evidence, it is possible that age-related metacognitive deficits may contribute to older adults' failure to use strategies. Training could include practice with self-testing and monitoring skills (Murphy et al., 1987) that focus on evaluating the contents of memory: How much do I know about this topic? This type of monitoring is critical to the effective planning and application of strategic effort. Metacognitive training could also focus on providing trainees with more information about when to use a particular strategy and direct feedback about the increased performance that results from strategy usage (West, in press-a).

Environmental Press

The long-range impact of an intervention may be related also to environmental stimulation. Older adults have made tremendous improvements in memory performance as a function of practice, and in some cases, these improvements have been maintained over long periods of time (Taub & Long, 1972). One reason that practice may help is because it changes, at least temporarily, the environmental press (Fozard & Popkin, 1978; Langer & Rodin, 1976; Lawton & Nahemow, 1973; Rodin & Langer, 1977). Testing focuses attention on the memory process and encourages older adults to work hard to perform better. When the older adult returns to his normal, less challenging home environment, hard-won gains may easily be lost. Regular testing and/or review sessions may be critical for maintenance. There are no studies employing regular review sessions, although multiple testing sessions over several months have been used to study maintenance of specific to-be-remembered information (Thomas & Ruben, cited in Poon, Walsh-Sweeney, & Fozard, 1980) or strategies (Anschutz et al., 1985).

GENERAL APPROACH TO TRAINING

The most effective memory training packages have been those in which investigators have provided extensive training (at least 1 hour) on one very difficult, narrowly defined memory task, with a test on that task before and after training. The best example of this is Yesavage's training program for name recall. His training has consistently led to gains on posttests, and higher gains have been achieved for more thorough training packages in which complex techniques were trained over multiple sessions (Yesavage & Sheikh, in press). In other laboratories, immediate posttest gains (exceeding practice effects) have occurred when multiple training sessions have focused on different strategies, as long as each session was keyed to one particular memory technique, with a pretest and posttest within each session (Zarit, Cole, & Guider, 1981; Zarit, Gallagher, & Kramer, 1981). Short-term training on complex techniques, however, has not been effective (Mason & Smith, 1977). Also, when investigators have trained multiple strategies over several sessions, reliable performance improvements resulting from training have not been evident on posttests occurring after the completion of the total training package (Perlmutter, Tenney, & Smith, 1980; Schaffer & Poon, 1982; West, Boatwright, & Schleser, 1984) except when the training was in written form (Flynn, 1986; Scogin, Storandt, & Lott, 1985).

Thus the most successful design for creating immediate test score gains is to select one strategy and one task, and spend 1–3 hours teaching older adults to use that strategy. During that time, there would be extensive strategy practice. A difficult laboratory pretest would be given, with one test during training (to provide feedback on strategy usefulness), and a posttest after training. Strategy-trained subjects would be instructed to use the training method on all tests, and the intervention would "teach to the test." The control group would not meet, or would meet only to discuss the aging process and general ways to adjust to age-associated memory impairment (AAMI). Based on the literature, the trained group would probably perform better on the final posttest than the control group.

Although this approach clearly leads to posttest gains, it does not permit us to examine maintenance or generalization. It might be better to develop memory training programs that encourage older adults to evaluate everyday memory tasks from a strategic point of view (why remembering can be difficult under certain conditions, ways to make remembering easier) and teach them how to adapt a single strategy (e.g., imagery or verbal elaboration) to fit a variety of memory tasks. In this way, generalization and maintenance are incorporated in the training program, and trainees are given the tools to be successful memorizers in everyday situations (West, in press-a). Although an intervention of this kind can be over-ambitious (failure can result if investigators train too many different, complex strategies), the most productive future studies are likely to be those that explore the maintenance and generalization of effects obtained in broad-based interventions, including multiple training sessions (Zarit, Cole & Guider, 1981) or written training manuals offering self-paced practice in the home (Scogin, Storandt, & Lott, 1985). To give us a better picture of what works, treatment impact should be evaluated with respect to numerous individual difference variables (e.g., Schaffer & Poon, 1982).

Gerontologists have much to learn about the effects of memory training on everyday memory. Objective assessments of everyday memory skill are new and have not been used in most of the memory training studies. There are many potential strategies to train. Although providing a specific mnemonic for a specific item will enhance its recall (Poon & Walsh-Sweeney, 1981) this is not sufficient for training older adults in a strategy that they may be able to apply on their own at home. For that, extensive practice (including practice at home) is required. Research evidence shows that intervention programs that are longer and more thorough in their approach tend to be more effective (Yesavage & Sheikh, in press). Successful memory training also takes time, motivation, and effort by the learner to change poor but very well-established methods of memorizing. As gerontologists investigate a wider range of training methods, we will hopefully determine that intervention for everyday memory problems is well worth the effort.

REFERENCES

Anschutz, L., Camp, C., Markley, R. P., & Kramer, J. J. (1987). Remembering mnemonics: A three-year follow-up on the effects of mnemonics training in elderly adults. *Experimental Aging Research, 13*, 141–144.

Anschutz, L., Camp, C. J., Markley, R. P., & Kramer, J. J. (1985). Maintenance and generalization of mnemonics for grocery shopping by older adults. *Experimental Aging Research, 11*, 157–160.

Bäckman, L., & Karlsson, T. (1986). Episodic remembering in young adults, 73-year-olds, and 82-year-olds. *Scandinavian Journal of Psychology, 27*, 320–325.

Baltes, P. B., & Willis, S. L. (1982). Enhancement (plasticity) of intellectual functioning in old age: Penn State's Adult Development and Enrichment Project (ADEPT). In F. I. M. Craik & S. Trehub (Eds.), *Aging and cognitive processes* (pp. 353–389). New York: Plenum Press.

Baumler, M., & Erber, J. T. (1986, August). Age and self-efficacy: Competence on a cognitive task. Paper presented at the meeting of the American Psychological Association, Washington, DC.

Bellezza, F. S. (1983). Mnemonic-device instruction with adults. In M. Pressley & J. R. Levin (Eds.), *Cognitive strategy research* (pp. 51-73). New York: Springer-Verlag.

Berry, J. M. (1986). Memory complaint and performance in older women: A self-efficacy and causal attribution model. Unpublished doctoral dissertation, Washington University, St. Louis.

Blieszner, R., Willis, S. L., & Baltes, P. B. (1981). Training research in aging on the fluid ability of inductive reasoning. *Journal of Applied Developmental Psychology*, 2, 247-265.

Botwinick, J. (1982). *Aging and behavior* (3rd Ed.). New York: Springer.

Bower, G. H. (1970). Organizational factors in memory. *Cognitive Psychology, 1*, 18–46.

Bower, G. H. (1972). A selective review of organizational factors in memory. In E. Tulving & W. Donaldson (Eds.), *Organization and memory*. (pp. 93-145). New York: Academic Press.

Bryk, A. S., & Raudenbush, S. W. (1987). Application of hierarchical linear models to assessing change. *Psychological Bulletin, 1*, 147-158.

Burke, D. M., & Light, L. L. (1981). Memory and aging: The role of retrieval processes. *Psychological Bulletin*, 90 513–546.

Camp, C. J., Markley, R. P., & Kramer, J. J. (1987). Spontaneous use of mnemonics by elderly individuals. *Educational Gerontology*, 9, 57–71.

Canestrari, R. E., Jr. (1968). Age changes in acquisition. In G. A. Talland (Ed.), *Human aging and behavior* (pp. 169-188) New York: Academic Press.

Catino, C., Taub, S. I., & Borkowski, J. G. (1977). Mediation in children and the elderly as a function of memory capabilities. *The Journal of Genetic Psychology*, 130, 35–47.

Cavanaugh, J. C., Grady, J. G., & Perlmutter, M. (1983). Forgetting and use of memory aids in 20- to 70-year-olds' everyday life. *International Journal of Aging and Human Development, 17*, 113–122.

Cavanaugh, J. C., & Morton, K. R. (1988). Older adults' attributions about everyday memory. In M. Gruneberg, R. Sykes, & P. E. Morris (Eds.), *Practical aspects of memory: Current research and issues*, vol. 1. London: John Wiley.

Cermak, L. S. (1975). *Improving your memory*. New York: McGraw-Hill.

Cermak, L. S. (1980). Comments on imagery as a therapeutic mnemonic. In L. W. Poon, J. L. Fozard, L. S. Cermak, D. Avenberg, & L. W. Thompson (Eds.), *New directions in memory and aging: Proceedings of the George A. Talland memorial conference* (pp. 507–510), Hillsdale, NJ: Lawrence Erlbaum.

Chaffin, R., & Herrmann, D. J. (1983). Self reports of memory abilities by old and young adults. *Human Learning, 2*, 17–28.

Cicirelli, V. G. (1976). Categorization behavior in aging subjects. *Journal of Gerontology, 31*(6), 676-680.

Crook, T. H., & Larrabee, G. H. (1988). Interrelationships among everyday memory tests: Stability of factor structure with age. *Neuropsychology, 2*, 1-12.

DeLeon, J. M. (1974). *Effects of training in repetition and mediation on paired-associate learning and practical memory in the aged*. Unpublished Ph.D. dissertation, University of Hawaii.

Denney, N. W. (1982). Aging and cognitive changes. In B. B. Wolman (Ed.), *Handbook of developmental psychology* (pp. 807-827). Englewood Cliffs, NJ: Prentice-Hall.

Dixon, R. A. (in press). Questionnaire research on metamemory and aging: Issues of structure and function. In L. W. Poon, D. C. Rubin, & B. A. Wilson (Eds.), *Everyday cognition in adulthood and late life*. Cambridge, England: Cambridge University Press.

Erber, J. T., Abello, S., & Moninger, C. (1988). Age and individual differences in immediate and delayed effectiveness of imagery mnemonic instructions. *Experimental Aging Research, 14*, 119–124.

Flynn, T. (1986, November). Memory performance, memory complaint and self-efficacy in older adults. Paper presented at the meeting of the Gerontological Society of America, Chicago.

Fozard, J. L., & Popkin, S. J. (1978). Optimizing adult development: Ends and means of an applied psychology of aging. *American Psychologist, 33*, 975–989.

Gilewski, M. J., & Zelinski, E. M. (1986). Questionnaire assessment of memory complaints. In L. W. Poon (Ed.), *Handbook for clinical memory assessment of older adults* (pp. 93-107). Washington, DC: American Psychological Association.

Grafman, J. (1984). Memory assessment and remediation in brain-injured patients. In B. A. Edelstein & E. T. Couture (Eds.), *Behavioral assessment and rehabilitation of the traumatically brain damaged* (pp. 151-189). New York: Plenum Press.

Harns, C. W. (Ed.) (1963). *Problems in the measurment of change*. Madison: University of Wisconsin Press.

Harns, J. E. (1978). External memory aids. In M. M. Gruneberg, P. E. Morris, & R. N. Sykes (Eds.), *Practical aspects of memory* (pp. 172-179). London: Academic Press.

Harris, J. E. (1980). Memory aids people use: Two interview studies. *Memory & Cognition, 8*, 31-38.

Harris, J. (1984). Methods of improving memory. In B. A. Wilson & N. Moffat (Eds.), *Clinical management of memory problems* (pp. 46-62). Rockville, MD: Aspen.

Hartley, J. T. (1982, November). Semantic characteristics of older and younger persons' visual images. Paper presented at the meeting of the Gerontological Society of America, Boston.

Hellebusch, S. J. (1976). *On improving learning and memory in the aged: The effects of mnemonics on strategy, transfer, and generalization*. Dissertation Abstract (1459-B Order No. 76-19, 465), University of Notre Dame.

Higbee, K. L. (1977). *Your memory: How it works and how to improve it*. Englewood Cliffs, NJ: Prentice-Hall.

Hill, R. D., Sheikh, J. I., & Yesavge, J. A. (1988). Pretraining enhances mnemonic training in elderly adults. *Experimental Aging Research, 14*, 207–211.

Howard, D. V. (1980). Category norms: A comparison of the Battig and Montague (1969) norms with the responses of adults between the ages of 20 and 80. *Journal of Gerontology, 35*(2), 225-231.

Hulicka, I. M., & Grossman, J. L. (1967). Age group comparisons for the use of mediators in paired-associate learning. *Journal of Gerontology, 22*, 46-51.

Hulicka, I. M., Sterns, H., & Grossman, J. (1967). Age-group comparisons of paired-associate learning as a function of paced and self-paced association and response times. *Journal of Gerontology, 22*, 274-280.

Hultsch, D. F. (1969). Adult age differences in the organization of free recall. *Developmental Psychology, 1*, 673-678.

Hultsch, D. F. (1971). Organization and memory in adulthood. *Human Development, 14*, 16-29.

Hultsch, D. F. (1974). Learning to learn in adulthood. *Journal of Gerontology, 29*(3), 302-308.

Kahn, R. L., Zarit, S. H., Hilbert, N. M., & Niederehe, M. A. (1975). Memory complaint and impairment in the aged: The effect of depression and altered brain function. *Archive of General Psychiatry, 32*, 1569-1573.

Kausler, D. H. (1980). Imagery ratings for young and elderly adults. *Experimental Aging Research, 6*, 185-188.

Kausler, D. H. (1982). *Experimental psychology and human aging*. New York: John Wiley.

Kliegl, R., Smith, J., & Baltes, P. B. (1986). Testing-the-limits, expertise, and memory in adulthood and old age. In F. Klix & H. Hagendorf (Eds.), *Human memory and cognitive capabilities* (pp. 395-407). North-Holland: Elsevier Science Publishers.

Labouvie-Vief, G., & Gonda, J. N. (1976). Cognitive strategy training and intellectual performance in the elderly. *Journal of Gerontology, 31*, 327-332.

Lachman, J. L., & Lachman, R. (1980). Age and the actualization of world knowledge. In L. W. Poon, J. L. Fozard, L. S. Cermak, D. Arenberg, & L. W. Thompson (Eds.), *New directions in memory and aging: Proceedings of the George A. Talland Memorial Conference* (pp. 285-311). Hillsdale, NJ: Lawrence Erlbaum Associates.

Lachman, M. E., & Dick, L. (1987, November). Does memory training influence self-conceptions of memory aging? Paper presented at the meeting of the Gerontological Society of America, Washington, DC.

Lachman, M. E., & Jelalian, E. (1984). Self-efficacy and attributions for intellectual performance in young and elderly adults. *Journal of Gerontology, 39*, 577-582.

Lachman, M. E., & McArthur, L. Z. (1986). Adulthood age differences in causal attributions for cognitive, physical, and social performance. *Psychology and Aging, 1*(2), 127-132.

Lachman, M. E., Steinberg, E. S., & Trotter, S. D. (1986, November). The effects of control beliefs and attributions on memory self-assessments and performance. Paper presented at the meeting of the Gerontological Society of America, Chicago.

Langer, E. J., & Rodin, J. (1976). The effects of enhanced responsibility for the aged: A field experiment in an institutional setting. *Journal of Personality and Social Psychology, 34*, 191-198.

Lapp, D. C. (1987). *Don't forget*. New York: McGraw-Hill.

Larrabee, G. J., & Crook, T. H. (1989). Dimensions of everyday memory in age-associated memory impairment. *Psychological Assessment: A Journal of Consulting and Clinical Psychology, 1*, 92–97.

Lawton, M. P., & Nahemow, L. (1973). Ecology and the aging process. In C. Eisdorfer & M. P. Lawton (Eds.), *The psychology of adult development and aging* (pp. 619-674). Washington, DC: American Psychological Association.

Lorayne, H., & Lucas, J. (1974). *The memory book*. New York: Ballantine Books.

Lovelace, E. A. (1984, August). Reported mnemonics and perceived memory changes with aging. Paper presented at the meeting of the American Psychological Association, Toronto.

Lovelace, E. A., & Cooley, S. (1982) Free association of older adults to single words and conceptually related word triads. *Journal of Gerontology, 37*, 432-437.

Mason, S. E., & Smith, A. D. (1977). Imagery in the aged. *Experimental Aging Research*, 3, 17–32.

Moffat, N. (in press). Home based cognitive rehabilitation with the elderly. In L. W. Poon, B. Wilson, & D. Rubin (Eds.), *Everyday cognition in adulthood and late life*. Cambridge, England: Cambridge University Press.

Morris, P. E. (1979). Strategies for learning and recall. In M. M. Gruneberg & P. E. Morris (Eds.), *Applied problems in memory* (pp. 25-57). London: Academic Press.

Murphy, M. D., Sanders, R. E., Gabriesheski, A. S., & Schmitt, F. A. (1981). Metamemory in the aged. *Journal of Gerontology, 36*, 185-193.

Murphy, M. D., Schmitt, F. A., Caruso, M. J., & Sanders, R. E. (1987). Metamemory in older adults: The role of monitoring in serial recall. *Psychology and Aging, 2*, 331-339.

Perlmuter, L. C., Tenney, Y. J., & Smith, P. A. (1980). *The evaluation and remediation of memory problems in the aged* (Tech. Rep. No. 80-02). Boston: Veterans Administration Outpatient Clinic, Memory and Learning Clinic.

Perlmutter, M. (1979). Age differences in adults' free recall, cued recall, and recognition. *Journal of Gerontology, 34*, 533-539.

Plemons, J. K., Willis, S. L., & Baltes, P. B. (1978). Modifiability of fluid intelligence in aging: A short-term longitudinal training approach. *Journal of Gerontology, 33*, 224-231.

Poon, L. W. (1980). A systems approach for the assessment and treatment of memory problems. In J. M. Ferguson & C. B. Taylor (eds.), *The comprehensive handbook of behavioral medicine* vol. 1.(pp. 191-212), New York: Spectrum.

Poon, L. W. (1986). *Handbook for clinical memory assessment of older adults*. Washington, DC: American Psychological Association.

Poon, L. W., Fozard, J. L., & Treat, N. J. (1978). From clinical and research findings on memory to intervention programs. *Experimental Aging Research* 4, 235-253.

Poon, L. W., & Walsh-Sweeney, L. (1981). Effects of bizarre and interacting imagery on learning and retrieval of the aged. *Experimental Aging Research*, 7, 65–70.

Poon, L. W., Walsh-Sweeney, L., & Fozard, J. L. (1980). Memory skill training for the elderly: Salient issues on the use of imagery mnemonics. In L. W. Poon, J. L. Fozard, L. S. Cermak, D. Arenberg, & L. W. Thompson (Eds.), *New directions in memory and aging: Proceedings of the George A. Talland memorial conference* (pp. 461-484). Hillsdale, NJ: Lawrence Erlbaum Associates.

Pratt, J. D., & Higbee, K. L. (1983). Use of an imagery mnemonic by the elderly in natural settings. *Human Learning* 2, 227–235.

Puglisi, J. T., Park, D. C., & Smith, A. D. (1987). Picture associations among older and young adults. *Experimental Aging Research, 13*, 115–116.

Rabinowitz, J. C., & Ackerman, B. P. (1982). General encoding of episodic events by elderly adults. In F. I. M. Craik & S. Trehub (Eds.), *Aging and cognitive processes* (pp. 145-154). New York: Plenum.

Rankin, J. L., & Collins, M. (1985). Adult age differences in memory elaboration. *Journal of Gerontology, 40*, 451-458.

Rankin, J. L., Karol, R., & Tuten, C. (1984) Strategy use, recall, and recall organization in young, middle-aged, and elderly adults. *Experimental Aging Research* 10(4):193–196.

Reason, J. T., & Lucas, D. (1984) Using cognitive diaries to investigate naturally occurring memory blocks. In J. E. Harris & P. E. Morris (Eds.), *Everyday memory: Actions and absent-mindedness*. London: Academic Press, (pp. 53-70).

Rebok, G. W., & Balcerak, L. J., (in press). Memory, self-efficacy and performance in young and old adults: Effects of mnemonic training. *Developmental Psychology*.

Reynolds, W. M., & Stark, K. D. (1983). Cognitive behavior modification: The clinical application of cognitive strategies. In M. Pressley & J. R. Levin (eds.), Cognitive strategy research (pp. 221-226). New York: Springer-Verlag.

Richardson, L. M., & Pratt, M. A. (1981, November). Improving memory in the aged. Paper presented at the meeting of the Gerontological Society of America, Toronto.

Roberts, P., & Wilson, K. A. (1986, August). Verbal imagery training and usage in three adult age groups. Paper presented at the meeting of the American Psychological Association, Washington, DC.

Robertson-Tchabo, E. A., Hausman, C. P., & Arenberg, D. (1976). A classical mnemonic for older learners: A trip that works. *Educational Gerontology, 1*, 215–226.

Rodin, J., & Langer, E. (1977). Long-term effects of a control-relevant intervention among the institutionalized aged. *Journal of Personality and Social Psychology, 35*, 897–902.

Rose, T. L., & Yesavage, J. A. (1983). Differential effects of a list-learning mnemonic in three age groups. *Gerontology, 29*, 293–298.

Rowe, E. J., & Schnore, M. M. (1971). Item concreteness and reported strategies in paired-associate learning as a function of age. *Journal of Gerontology, 26*, 470–475.

Salthouse, T. A. (1982). *Adult cognition*. New York: Springer-Verlag.

Sanders, R. E., Murphy, M. D., Schmitt, F. A., & Walsh, K. K. (1980). Age differences in free recall rehearsal strategies. *Journal of Gerontology, 35*, 550–558.

Schacter, D. L., & Glisky, E. L. (in press). Memory remediation: Restoration, alleviation, and the acquisition of domain-specific knowledge. In B. Uzzell & Y. Gross (Eds.), *Clinical neuropsychology of intervention*. Boston: Martinus Nyhoff.

Schacter, D. L., Rich, S. A., & Stampp, M. S. (1985). Remediation of memory disorders: Experimental evaluation of the spaced-retrieval technique. *Journal of Clinical and Experimental Neuropsychology, 7*, 79–96.

Schaffer, G., & Poon, L. W. (1982). Individual variability in memory training with the elderly. *Educational Gerontology, 8*, 217–229.

Schmitt, F. A., Murphy, M. D., & Sanders, R. E. (1981). Training older adult free recall rehearsal strategies. *Journal of Gerontology, 36*(3), 329–337.

Scogin, F., Storandt, M., & Cott, L. (1985). Memory-skills training, memory complaints, and depression in older adults. *Journal of Gerontology, 40*, 562–568.

Sheikh, J., Hill, R., Decker-Tanke, E., & Yesavage, J. A. (1986, November). Individual differences in response to memory training: Verbal intelligence and state anxiety predict improvement. Paper presented at the meeting of the Gerontological Society of America, Chicago.

Smith, J., Heckhausen, J., Kliegl, R., & Baltes, P. B. (1984, November). Cognitive reserve capacity, expertise, and aging: Plasticity of digit span performance. Paper presented at the meeting of the Gerontological Society of America, San Antonio.

Sunderland, A., Watts, K., Baddeley, A. D., & Harris, J. E. (1986). Subjective memory assessment and test performance in elderly adults. *Journal of Gerontology, 41*, 376–384.

Taub, H. A. (1973). Memory span, practice & aging. *Journal of Gerontology, 28*, 335–338.

Taub, H. A., & Long, M. (1972). The effects of practice on short-term memory of young and old subjects. *Journal of Gerontology*, 27, 494-499.

Treat, N. J., Poon, L. W., & Fozard, J. L. (1981). Age, imagery, and practice in paired-associate learning. *Experimental Aging Research, 7*, 337–342.

Treat, N. J., Poon, L. W., Fozard, J. L., & Popkin, S. J. (1978). Toward applying cognitive skill training to memory problems. *Experimental Aging Research, 4*, 305–319.

Treat, N. J., & Reese, H. W. (1976). Age, pacing and imagery in paired-associate learning. *Developmental Psychology, 12*, 119–124.

Weinstein, C. E., Duffy, M., Underwood, V. L., MacDonald, J., & Gott, S. P. (1981). Memory strategies reported by older adults for experimental and everyday learning tasks. *Educational Gerontology, 7*, 205–213.

West, R. L. (1985). *Memory Fitness Over 40*. Gainesville, FL: Triad.

West, R. L. (1986). Everyday memory and aging. *Developmental Neuropsychology, 2*, 323–344.

West, R. L. (in press-a). Planning practical memory training for the aged. In L. W. Poon, B. Wilson, & D. Rubin (Eds.), *Everyday cognition in adulthood and late life*. Cambridge, England: Cambridge University Press.

West, R. L. (in press-b). Everyday memory and aging: Appropriate tests and tasks. In R. L. West & J. J. Sinnott (Eds.), *Everyday memory and aging: Current research and methodology*. New York: Springer-Verlag.

West, R. L., Berry, J., & Dennehy, D. (1987, August). Self-efficacy and memory performance: Measurement issues. Paper presented at the meeting of the American Psychological Association, New York.

West, R. L., Boatwright, L. K., & Schleser, R. (1984, May). The effects of practical memory training for the elderly. Paper presented at the meeting of the Southern Gerontological Society, Knoxville, TN.

Willis, S. L. (1985). Towards an educational psychology of the older adult learner: Intellectual and cognitive bases. In J. E. Birren & K. W. Schaie (Eds.), *Handbook of the psychology of aging* (2nd ed., pp. 818-847). New York: Van Nostrand Reinhold.

Willis, S. L., & Baltes, P. B. (1980). Intelligence in adulthood and aging: Contemporary issues. In L. W. Poon (Ed.), *Aging in the 1980's* (pp. 260-272). Washington, DC: American Psychological Association.

Willis, S. L., Blieszner, R., & Baltes, P. B. (1981). Intellectual training research in aging: Modification of performance on the fluid ability of figural relations. *Journal of Educational Psychology, 73*, 41-50.

Willis, S. L., & Schaie, K. W. (1986). Training the elderly on the ability factors of spatial orientation and inductive reasoning. *Psychology and Aging, 1*(3), 239-247.

Wilson, B. (1984). Memory therapy in practice. In B. A. Wilson & N. Moffat (Eds.), *Clinical management of memory problems* (pp. 89-111). Rockville, MD: Aspen.

Wilson, B. (in press). Designing memory therapy programmes. In L. W. Poon, B. Wilson, & D. Rubin (Eds.), *Everyday cognition in adulthood and late life*. Cambridge, England: Cambridge University Press.

Wilson, B. A., Baddeley, A. D., & Cockburn, J. (1988). Trials, tribulations and triumphs in the development of a test of everyday memory. In M. M. Gruneberg, P. E. Morris & R. N. Sykes, (Eds.), *Practical aspects of memory: Current research and issues*, (Vol. 2, pp. 249-254). John Wiley & Sons: Chichester, England.

Wilson, B., Baddeley, A., & Hutchins, H. (1984). *The Rivermead Behavioural Memory Test* (Tech. Rep. No. 84/1). Oxford, England: Rivermead Rehabilitation Centre.

Wilson, B. A., & Moffat, N. (1984a). *Clinical management of memory problems*. Rockville, MD: Aspen.

Wilson, B., & Moffat, N. (1984b). Rehabilitation of memory for everyday life. In J. E. Harris & P. E. Morris (Eds.), *Everyday memory, actions and absent-mindedness* (pp. 207–233), London: Academic Press.

Winograd, E., & Simon, E. W. (1980). Visual memory and imagery in the aged. In L. W. Poon, J. L. Fozard, L. S. Cermak, D. Arenberg, & L. W. Thompson (Eds.), *New directions in memory and aging: Proceedings of the George A. Tolland Memorial Conference* (pp. 485-506). Hillsdale, NJ: Lawrence Erlbaum Associates.

Worden, P. E., & Meggison, D. L. (1984). Aging and the category-recall relationship. *Journal of Gerontology, 39*, 322–324.

Yesavage, J. A. (1984). Relaxation and memory training in 39 elderly patients. *American Journal of Psychiatry, 141*, 778–781.

Yesavage, J. A., & Jacob, R. (1984). Effects of relaxation and mnemonics on memory, attention and anxiety in the elderly. *Experimental Aging Research, 10*, 211–214.

Yesavage, J. A., & Rose, T. L. (1983). Concentration and mnemonic training in elderly subjects with memory complaints: A study of combined therapy and order effects. *Psychiatry Research, 9*, 157–167.

Yesavage, J. A., & Rose, T. L. (1984a). The effects of a face-name mnemonic in young, middle-aged, and elderly adults. *Experimental Aging Research, 10*, 55–57.

Yesavage, J. A., & Rose, T. L. (1984b). Semantic elaboration and the method of loci: A new trip for older learners. *Experimental Aging Research, 10*, 155–159.

Yesavage, J. A., Rose, T. L., & Bower, G. H. (1983). Interactive imagery and affective judgments improve face-name learning in the elderly. *Journal of Gerontology*, 38, 197–203.

Yesavage, J. A., Rose, T. L., & Spiegel, D. (1982). Relaxation training and memory improvement in elderly normals: Correlation of anxiety ratings and recall improvement. *Experimental Aging Research, 8*, 195–198.

Yesavage, J. A., & Sheikh, J. I. (in press). Mnemonics as modified for use by the elderly. In L. W. Poon, B. Wilson, & D. Rubin (Eds.), *Everyday cognition in adulthood and late life*. Cambridge, England: Cambridge University Press.

Yesavage, J., Sheikh, J., & Hill, R. (1986, November). Preliminary training enhances effectiveness of memory mnemonics in the elderly. Paper presented at the meeting of the Gerontological Society of America, Chicago.

Zarit, S. H., Cole, K. D., & Guider, R. L. (1981). Memory training strategies and subjective complaints of memory in the aged. *The Gerontologist, 21*, 158–164.

Zarit, S. J., Gallagher, D., & Kramer, N. (1981). Memory training in the community aged: Effects on depression, memory complaint, and memory performance. *Educational Gerontology*, 6, 11–27.

4

The Translation of Laboratory Findings in Cognitive Aging to Clinical Application

Leonard W. Poon

The term "from lab to life" has received increasing attention and discussion in the last decade (for one review, see Poon, Rubin, & Wilson, in press). Its importance is underlined in all research proposals for federal funding in that all applicants must delineate the "significance" of the research not only in theoretical perspectives but also in its relevance in clinical and everyday applications. Although the need for translating laboratory findings to clinical applications is universally recognized, there is confusion on how the translation should be done.

This chapter focuses on issues related to the translation of laboratory findings in cognitive aging to clinical applications. The chapter examines (1) the needs and questions of clinicians, patients, and treatment personnel regarding cognitive functioning, (2) the steps necessary to translate laboratory findings to meet these needs and answer these questions, and (3) an example demonstrating the translation of laboratory findings to clinical application to illustrate the points.

NEEDED QUESTIONS

In cognition and aging, there are a number of ways to build a bridge between laboratory findings and clinical applications. One way is to evaluate the needs of the consumers in a clinical situation—that is, the needs of the patients, their families, clinicians, and treatment personnel. What information about cognition and aging do the consumers need to have in order to answer questions about their everyday memory problems or to make meaningful clinical diagnosis and treatment decisions? With an evaluation of needs, clinicians and researchers can then assess whether currently available laboratory-based information is adequate in its present form to meet the needs or whether new information is needed.

Erickson, Poon, and Walsh-Sweeney (1980) identified those questions by the consumers as "needed questions." They are defined as questions whose answers serve the immediate concerns of the patient, the patient's family, and the various treatment personnel (e.g., psychologists, physicians, rehabilitation specialists, speech pathologists, and physical and occupational therapists) in the intervention setting (hospital, rehabilitation center, outpatient clinic, etc.).

An elderly patient who has perceived some degree of memory loss needs to know what has gone wrong. The patient tends to be anxious about forgetting dates, names, faces, and appointments, the difficulty of learning new things, and the frustration that goes with misplacing things. These lapses often cause the patient inconvenience or embarrassment, and if the frequency of these lapses becomes intolerable, then the patient wants explanations, a prognosis, and perhaps remedial attention. One of the first questions from the patient is whether the perceived loss is normal or a symptom of either Alzheimer's disease or hardening of the arteries, both of which have been frequently and vividly portrayed in the news media.

The treatment personnel have "needed questions" also. They are interested in obtaining answers about the etiology of the complaints, potential strategies for the selection of treatment, and long-term prognosis. They may also have questions about the patients regarding (1) the patient's motivation to improve, (2) whether the patient is being manipulative, (3) what sort of treatment is consonant with the personality or style of the patient, (4) what sort of reinforcers are effective, (5) should they also change the environment, and (6) whether the family should assist in the treatment.

Questions asked by the patients and treatment personnel tend to be specific and pragmatic. An important from-lab-to-life issue is the evaluation and translation of laboratory findings to answer these questions.

SOURCES OF CONFUSION IN TRANSLATION

Concern for memory failure is one of two concerns frequently expressed by older adults (Lowenthal et al., 1967). When confronted with these concerns, clinicians need to be able to tell whether the concern is benign or a sign of a more serious problem. How can the clinician take advantage of the volumes of research on memory and aging (see Chapters 1 and 2) to assist in making a diagnosis and in recommending treatment?

There are three common sources of confusion in the use of laboratory findings for clinical memory assessment and in the selection of appropriate tests (Poon et al., 1986):

1. There are many under-developed tests available in the market.
2. There is confusion in the use of experimental procedures to predict behavior.
3. Generalization of experimental findings is often not established prior to their application.

Potpourri of Tests

Although there are numerous standardized memory test batteries in the market place, there is unfortunately no general concensus among researchers and clinicians on which battery is most appropriate in diagnosing memory and cognitive dysfunction with the elderly (Erickson, Poon, & Walsh-Sweeney, 1980). For example, the often-used Wechsler Memory Scale has been criticized for lacking a measure for long-term retention, for not differentiating modality-specific memory functions, and for not being validated for the elderly population (Erickson & Scott, 1977; Erickson, Poon, & Walsh-Sweeney, 1980). The Randt Memory Test (Randt, Brown, & Osborne, 1980) was found lacking in the measurement of nonverbal memory, and the Guild Memory Test (Gilbert & Levee, 1971) was found by some clinicians to be too complex for people with more than a mild deficit. The problem of test sensitivity and specificity is illustrated by the common complaint among clinicians that the results of some memory tests bear no resemblance to the everyday memory functioning and complaints of the patients. With the potpourri of tests in the market, it is understandable that there is confusion about the selection and use of tests.

Understanding and Predicting Memory Function

A major contributor toward the current proliferation of tests and confusion about their implementation is a frequent misunderstanding by both clinicians and researchers on the use of experimental procedures for understanding and predicting memory functioning. That is, many of the experiments on memory and aging summarized in Chapters 1 and 2 were designed to understand basic age-related differences in cognitive mechanisms. These experiments were conducted to test hypotheses on specific cognitive models or phenomena. In these experiments, some variables that show statistically significant effects, or significant interactions with age, may account for a small amount of the data variance. For example, in an experiment examining the usefulness of a memory paradigm to differentiate the performance of young and elderly adults, a statistically significant age effect was obtained, in that older persons performed at a lower level. However, the age variable could only account for 2% of the data variance. Because of the low proportion of variance that the age variable could account for, albeit a statistically significant one, the usefulness of this memory paradigm to differentiate age differences remains to be developed.

In contrast with experimental procedures, tests that make clinical diagnoses are designed to predict the absence, presence, or severity of a dysfunction or process. To make predictions, the tests must be reliable and valid in order to ensure accurate diagnosis of presence or absence of a dysfunction. Strictly speaking, a reliable and predictive test does not need to provide an understanding of basic mechanisms.

Procedures and tests that are designed to test hypotheses or to predict behavior could contain independent psychometric properties. On the one hand, an experimental paradigm that is an excellent tool for understanding a process may not be sufficient to make predictions. Further development is needed to demonstrate the paradigm's reliability and validity in predicting a dysfunction. On the other hand, an instrument that may be predictive of a dysfunction may not be useful in providing an understanding of the causes leading to the dysfunction. If information on causes or mechanisms contributing to the observed dysfunction are needed, then more laboratory/experimental, hypothesis-testing techniques are needed. A proper differentiation between tests and procedures that were designed for understanding basic mechanisms and for predicting an absence or presence of a dysfunction could clarify some of the current confusion in test selection.

Generalization

Finally, this issue is closely associated with the use of laboratory findings based on narrowly defined subject characteristics or stimuli sampling procedures. Before applying the finding to a similar or different sample or situation, the range of generalization of the obtained results should be defined or demonstrated. For example, a test that may be predictive of cognitive dysfunction in right hemisphere cerebrovascular accident (CVA) may not be predictive of left hemisphere CVA. Appropriate steps to evaluate the sensitivity and generalization from one situation to another are needed. This is a necessary but seldom followed measure to minimize confusion or misinterpretation using a new or untried procedure or using an established test in a new diagnostic situation.

To summarize the contents of the first two sections, the following are some common-sense ingredients that should enhance the use of laboratory findings or existing instruments for diagnostic applications:

1. An understanding of the processes underlying the dysfunction and the known interactions between the variable under examination and a number of concomitant variables;
2. An understanding of needed questions from the clinical perspective;
3. A clear objective for the evaluation;
4. A well-defined set of criteria for validation of the usefulness of the instrument to satisfy good psychometric practices; and
5. A little bit of luck and cooperation from the patient and/or the family to test different hypotheses about the dysfunction.

FROM LABORATORY FINDINGS TO CLINICAL APPLICATION

The remaining portion of this chapter will describe an effort to translate laboratory findings to clinical application. This section will first identify a clinical question commonly asked by clinicians. A description of laboratory-based investigation of underlying mechanisms will follow. Finally, steps in translating basic findings to a clinically useful technique will be described.

The Question

A question that seems to intrigue diagnosticians is, *why do tests that purport to measure the same process but vary in the level of difficulty provide different magnitudes of effects?* To illustrate, tests A and B both purport to measure process C. However, test A is more difficult than test B, and test A shows a larger magnitude of dysfunction than test B. The question by a diagnostician is: Which test should I use?

The Underlying Mechanisms

The underlying mechanism, called the *complexity phenomenon* (Cerella, Poon, & Williams, 1980), has been baffling to researchers in cognition and aging. In the 1950s and 1960s, pioneer researchers in cognition and aging, (Alan Welford from England and Jim Birren from the United States) noted that as the difficulty of a task increased, the elderly's cognitive performance tended to slow down in a disproportionate way. Welford (1965) suggested that there was a linear relationship in this disproportionate slowing. Birren (1965) summarized this phenomenon in a similar way: " . . . although present in simple skills, the slowing appears larger as one ascends a hierarchical ladder of complexity of process."

Two research questions immediately arise:

1. Is this a universal phenomenon in aging?
2. Could different tasks produce different complexity rates?

We attempted to answer these questions several years ago in reanalyzing data from a large number of experiments published in the literature across a number of cognitive tasks. This sort of analysis is called meta-analysis or meta-data analysis. If a phenomenon is universal, then it should show orderliness in data obtained across different laboratories, paradigms, and cognitive tasks. If different tasks consistently produce different complexity rates, then this phenomenon should also emerge in the analysis.

Figure 4.1 summarizes our effort (Cerella, Poon, & Williams, 1980) in examining the universality or regularity of the complexity or difficulty phenomenon in the published literature. Figure 4.1 contains 99 data points obtained from 18 studies of reaction time that attempt to manipulate task complexity or difficulty within each paradigm. These 18 studies came from eight different types of cognitive tasks, ranging from memory scan task to choice reaction time task to paired-associate learning and card sorting tasks. The relationship between difficulty and age differences seems to be linear with a correlation close to 0.90.

This plot provides some notion of the universality and regularity of the data. The regularity of the complexity effect across tasks is so striking that we thought there might be a simple underlying factor between the age groups that could explain the relationship. We then paired the mean latency for each task for the young and elderly groups and replotted the 99 data points (Figure 4.2).

Figure 4.2 shows an orderly linear relationship between the latencies of the young and old across a wide array of cognitive functions. The linear function shows that, regardless of the cognitive task, old latencies can be reliably predicted from young latencies, and that they are slower by a constant amount.

The equation OLD $= 1.36 \times$ YOUNG minus a negligible intercept describing the points in Figure 4.2 may provide a possible explanation for the complexity phenomenon. That is, older people suffer more in performance with increasing task complexity because they are slower and by a constant amount.

Table 4.1 shows our attempt to refine our explanations by examining the effects of different factors on the overall amount of variance and age-specific variance that could be accounted for by different combinations of variables.

The table shows the original linear equation (set I) and the amount of overall and age-specific variance that could be accounted for by the equation. Adding the information of age (set II) increased the amount variance accounted for in the equation. However, the knowledge of the task (set III) did not increase the cumulative variance. The largest amount of variance was accounted for by inserting the age of the subject and whether the task is a sensory motor task or a mental manipulation task (set V). This set of four linear equations shows that sensorimotor speed slows down negligibly with age (by a magnitude of about 1.25). However, mental manipulation speed slows down dramatically (by a factor of 1.66).

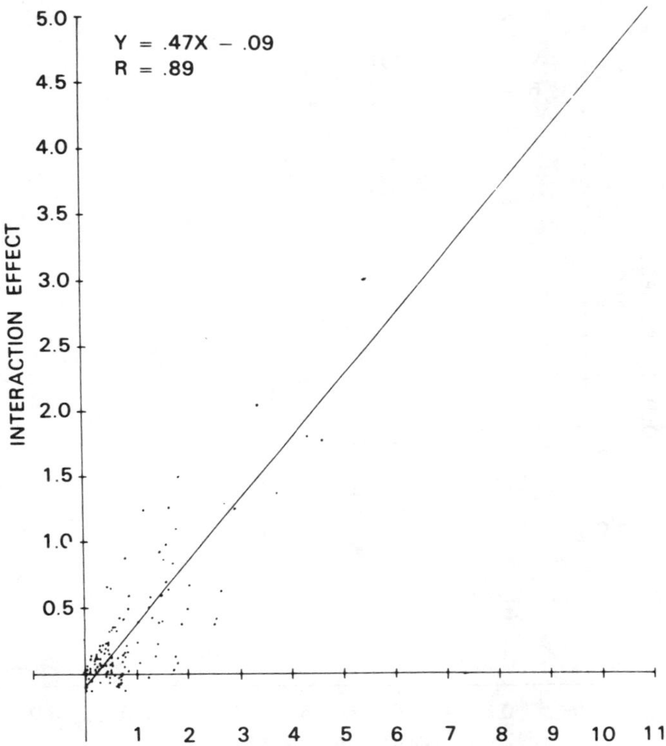

FIGURE 4.1 Data from eldely subjects and experimental tasks compared with data from young subjects and control tasks. The comparison shows that the magnitude of the age effect on a task (i.e., the age × task interaction) is proportional to the difficulty of the task (i.e., the condition effect).

This exercise has uncovered some understanding of the complexity phenomenon and offers the following postulations:

1. Older people perform poorly and in a linearly disproportionate way because they are slower and by a constant amount.
2. We have not explained why they are slower, but we have demonstrated that this seems to be a universal phenomenon with a wide variety of tasks.
3. The phenomenon seems to be robust and reliable. Two other laboratories have replicated our findings in their own meta-data analysis (Salthouse, 1982; Hale, Myerson, & Wagstaff, 1987).

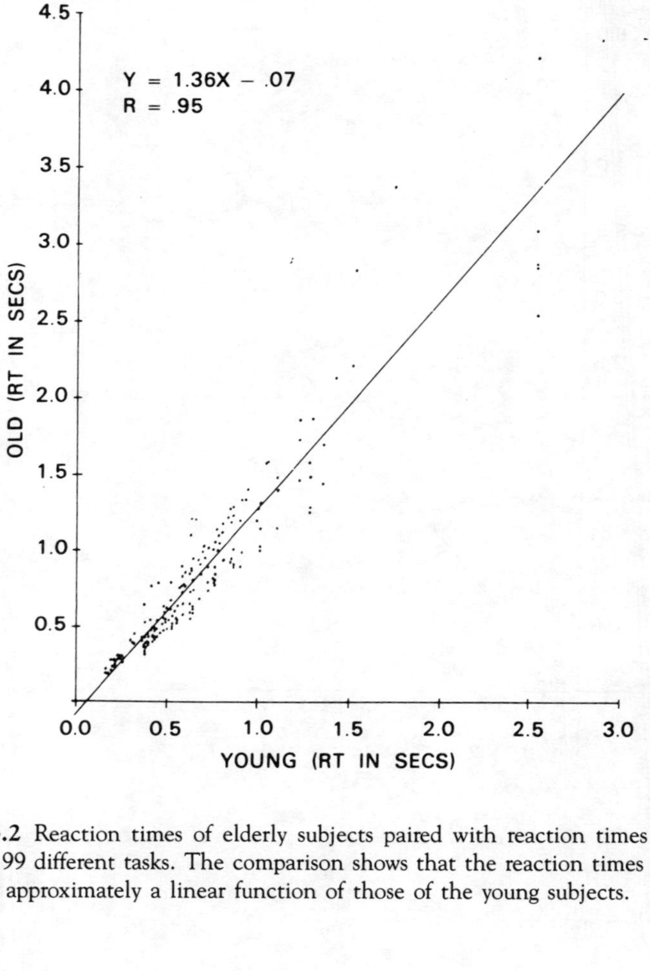

FIGURE 4.2 Reaction times of elderly subjects paired with reaction times of young subjects on 99 different tasks. The comparison shows that the reaction times of elderly subjects are approximately a linear function of those of the young subjects.

Clinical Application

The following is a description of an attempt to apply our understanding of the complexity phenomenon in a clinically relevant way (Poon et al., 1989).

We began by asking three questions:

1. If there is a constant amount of slowing in normal aging, would this slowing be exaggerated in early cases of Alzheimer's disease (AD) and in major depression?
2. Would the same linear function be evident with both patient groups?

TABLE 4.1 Effects of Different Factors on Elderly Subjects' Reaction Time

Independent variables	Interaction terms	Regression equations	Overall accountable variance (%)	Age-specific variance (%)
I. Standard RT		O = 1.36 Y – 0.07	90.2	40
II. Age and standard RT	a. Over 60	O = 1.62 Y – 0.13	96.4	78
	b. Under 60	O = 1.16 Y – 0.04		
III. Task and standard RT	a. Card sorting	O = 1.08 Y – 0.15	91.2	57
	b. Memory scanning	O = 1.40 Y – 0.16		
	c. S–R mapping	O = 1.32 Y – 0.03		
	d. Choice reaction time	O = 1.70 Y – 0.26		
	e. PI	O = 1.25 Y – 0.08		
	f. Miscellaneous	O = 1.50 Y – 0.12		
IV. Central/ peripheral and standard RT	a. Sensorimotor	O = 1.14 Y – 0.01	91.7	61
	b. Mental	O = 1.62 Y – 0.00		
V. Age and central/ peripheral and standard RT	a. Mental over 60	O = 1.66 Y – 0.00	96.1	81
	b. Mental under 60	O = 1.14 Y – 0.02		
	c. Sensory over 60	O = 1.24 Y – 0.00		
	d. Sensory under 60	O = 1.18 Y – 0.07		

3. Could we use this group analysis technique to describe the cognitive competence of an individual?

We answered these questions by measuring the cognitive performances on a wide range of reaction time tasks on three groups: (1) early demented (but not depressed) elderly subjects [mini-mental state exam (MMSE = 23)], (2) major depressives (but not demented) elderly [Hamilton Rating Scale (HRS = 12); Research Diagnostic Criteria (RDC = 14)], and (3) control subjects. (For a detailed description of subjects and subject selection procedures see Williams et al., 1988.) The reaction time tasks measured attention, decision making, memory scanning and retrieval, and semantic processing that had been shown to be sensitive to AD (American Psychiatric Association, 1980). (For a detailed description of the tasks and analysis technique, see Poon et al., 1989.) Figure 4.3 shows the results.

Figure 4.3 employs a technique similar to that used in Figure 4.2 in which the reaction times of the early AD and major depressive groups for each condition across the five cognitive tasks are plotted against the reaction times of the control subjects. The diagonal line represents the performance of the control group plotted against itself. This analysis provides a profile of cognitive performances across a range of cognitive abilities.

As expected, the cognitive speed profiles summarizing the performances of all cognitive tasks for the early AD and major depression groups were slower than the normal controls. However, as shown in our work in normal aging, the profiles of the performances of both early demented and major depressive patients could be parsimoniously summarized by linear functions as noted in Figure 4.2.

Comparison of the slopes of the three groups showed that the performances of the early AD and major depressive groups were significantly different than the controls. Further, the early demented group was significantly different than the major depressive group. (For detailed information on the profile analysis, see Poon et al., 1989.)

Our findings on cognitive speed profile from normal aging to early stages of Alzheimer's disease and major depression can be summarized as follows:

1. There was indeed detectable slowing of cognitive processes in early AD and major depression.
2. The nature of slowing seemed to be similar to normal slowing in that cognitive performances of both early AD and major depressives could be parsimoniously described by linear functions.
3. Significant differences among the three groups could be shown by changing the slopes of the linear functions.

Finally, in order to apply this technique for clinical assessment, it is necessary to demonstrate its utility to provide clinical profiles on individual patients.

Figure 4.4 displays the performance profiles of six subjects (two controls, two major depressives, and two early ADs) plotted in a manner similar to Figure 4.3. The top two panels show the performances of two healthy older subjects compared with the average performances of their own peers. Healthy subject #167's mean performances for the various cognitive tasks were exactly the same as the average of his peers, and health subject #158 performed better than the average of his peers. Both regressions could account for more than 90% of the data variance.

The two middle panels show the performances of two depressed subjects compared to the mean of healthy controls. Both subjects seemed to perform well compared to the controls. Depressed subject #179 performed similarly to the controls, and depressed subject #158 was more variable, with some tasks performed at the same level as the controls and others worse than control. The more variable nature of the performances of depressed subject #158 is reflected in the lower variance accounted for by the linear regression.

The lower two panels show the performances of two early AD patients. Visual inspection of the performances easily differentiated these patients from the major depressives and controls. Visual inspection of the performance profiles could also

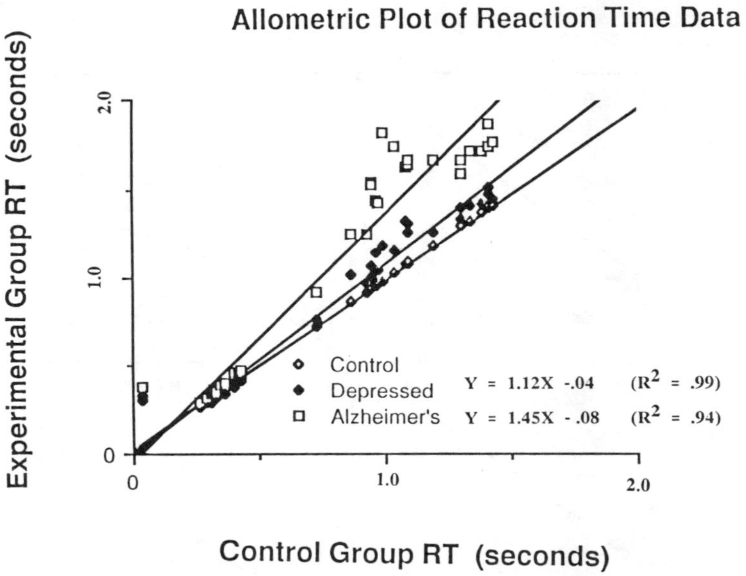

FIGURE 4.3 The mean reaction of the early AD group (□) and the major depressives (◆) for each condition of the five cognitive tasks are plotted against the mean reaction times in the same condition of the control group (◇). The diagonal represents the performance of the control group plotted against itself. Positive departure from the diagonal indicates lower performance of the experimental group compared to the control, and negative departure indicates better performance.

provide an indication of homogeneity of performances as well as strengths and weaknesses of the subjects across the various cognitive performances. All six panels seem to be representative of the characteristics of group performances presented in Figure 4.3.

In summary, the clinical utility of our profile analysis technique remains to be further explored and developed. The above exercise demonstrates one effort to translate laboratory-based findings about age-related effects on the complexity phenomenon to a profile analysis technique to examine cognitive competence for an individual.

In describing the profile analysis technique (Poon et al., 1989), we might say that "a picture is worth a thousand words." These pictures give us information about (1) the homogeneity of performances over a range of cognitive functions for a particular person, (2) strengths and weaknesses within a range of cognitive tasks, and (3) an individual's performance in comparison with an appropriate control group. We propose that this profile analysis could lead to a useful clinical diagnostic tool for cognitive assessment.

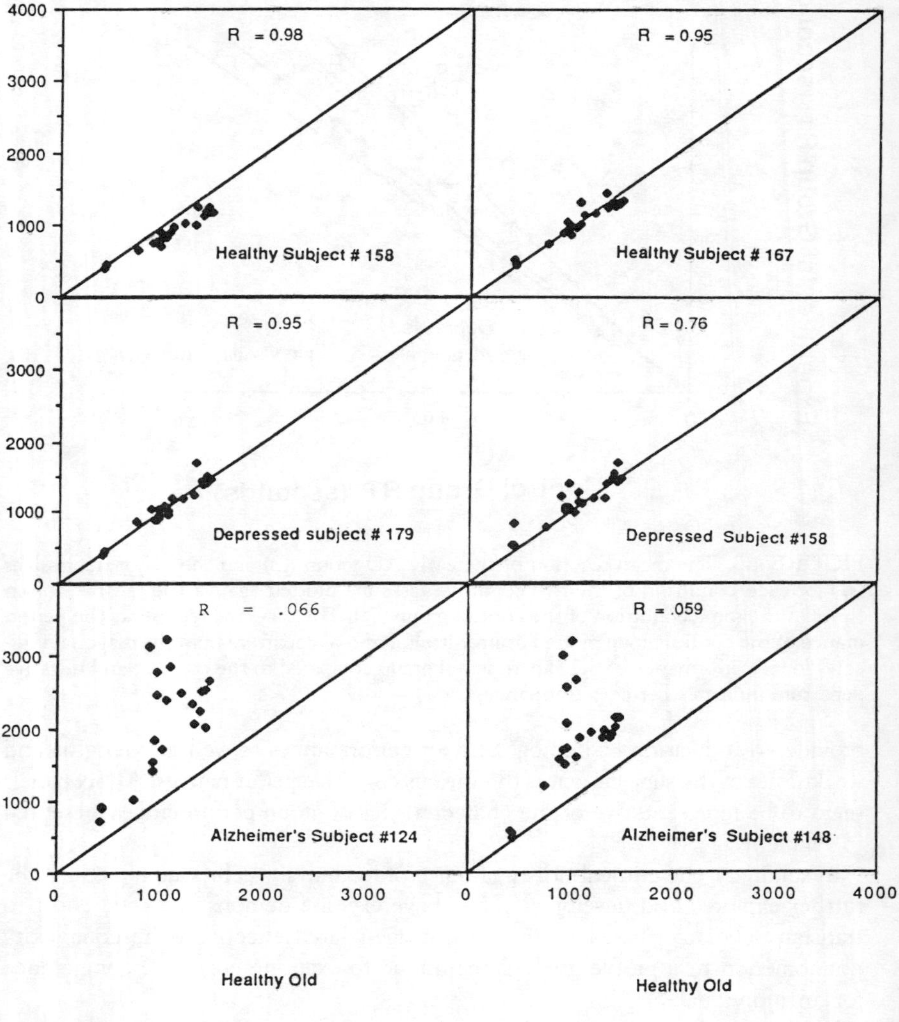

FIGURE 4.4 Profiles of reaction time performances of six subjects plotted against the performances of the controls (diagonals). Each point is the mean performance in one condition of a cognitive task. The top row shows the performances of two control subjects plotted against the mean of their peers. The second row shows the performances of two major depressive patients, and the third row two subjects diagnosed with early AD.

REFERENCES

American Psychiatric Association. (1980). *Diagnostic and statistical manual of mental disorders* (3rd ed.). Washington, DC: American Psychiatric Association.

Birren, J. E. (1965) Age changes in speed of behavior: Its central nature and physiological correlates. In A. T. Welford & J. E. Birren (Eds.), *Behavior, aging and the nervous system* (pp. 191–216). Springfield, IL: Charles C Thomas.

Cerella, J., Poon, L. W., & Williams, D. (1980). Age and the complexity hypothesis. In L. W. Poon (Ed.), *Aging in the 1980's: Psychological issues* (pp. 332–340). Washington, DC: American Psychological Association.

Erickson, R., Poon, L. W., Walsh-Sweeney, L. (1980) Clinical memory testing for the elderly. In L. W. Poon, J. Fozard, L. Cermak, D. Arenberg, & L. Thompson, (Eds.), *New Directions in Memory and Aging* (pp. 379–402). Hillsdale, NJ: Erlbaum Associates.

Erickson, R., & Scott, M. (1977) Clinical memory assessment: A review. *Psychological Bulletin*, 84:1130–1149.

Gilbert, J., & Levee, R. (1971) Patterns of declining memory. *Journal of Gerontology*, 26(1):70–75.

Hale, S., Myerson, J., & Wagstaff, D. (1987) General slowing of nonverbal information processing: Evidence for a power law. *Journal of Gerontology* 42:131–136.

Lowenthal, M. F., Berkman, P. L., Brissette, G. G., et al. (1967). *Aging and Mental Disorder in San Francisco.* San Francisco: Jossey Bass.

Poon, L. W., Gurland, B., Eisdorfer, C., Crook, T., Thompson, L. W., Kaszniak, A., & Davis, K. (1986) *Handbook for Clinical Memory Assessment of Older Adults*. Washington, DC: American Psychological Association.

Poon, L. W., Dudley, W. N., Myerson, J., Hale, S., Prinz, P., & Vitiello, M. (1989). Differentiation of cognitive profiles in early dementia and major depression. Paper to be presented at Pathological Aging: The Case of Alzheimer's disease. the 10th Biennial Meeting of the International Society for the Study of Behavioral Development, July 9, 1989. Jyuäshylä, Finland.

Poon, L. W., Rubin, D., & Wilson, B. (in press). *Everyday cognition in adulthood and late life*. New York: Cambridge University Press.

Randt, C., Brown, R., & Osborne, D. (1980). A memory test for longitudinal measurement of mild to moderate deficits. *Clinical Neuropsychology*, 2, 184-194.

Salthouse, T. (1982). *Adult cognition*. New York: Springer-Verlag.

Welford, A. T. (1965). Performance, biological mechanisms and age. In A. T. Welford & J. E. Birren (Eds.), *Behavior, Aging and the Nervous System* (pp. 3–20). Springfield, IL: Charles C Thomas.

Williams, D. E., Vitiello, M. V., Ries, R. K., Bokan, J., & Prinz, P. N., (1988). Successful recruitment of elderly community-dwelling subjects for Alzheimer's disease research. *Journal of Gerontology* 43:M69–74.

5

Neuropsychological Differentiation of Memory Impairments in Dementia

William C. Heindel, David P. Salmon, and Nelson Butters

The primary goal of our recent research has been to uncover the specific cognitive deficits that underlie the anterograde and retrograde memory deficits of various forms of amnesia and dementia. Actuarial approaches to neuropsychology that rely on standardized quantitative indices of memory and intelligence have seemed to suggest that memory deficiencies of such patient populations are highly similar and have supported the notion that dementia may be conceptualized as a single homogeneous phenomenon. In contrast, investigations applying the concepts and models of cognitive neuropsychology often have demonstrated important differences among these superficially similar memory dysfunctions. Such studies have stressed that a close scrutiny of error patterns is often vital to a full understanding of the cognitive factors involved in the patients' learning impairments (Albert & Kaplan, 1980; Milberg, Hebben, & Kaplan, 1986). Any extension of neuropsychology into the realm of pharmacological therapies for the memory deficiencies associated with either abnormal or normal aging will require extensive knowledge of these underlying processes.

To exemplify the utility of cognitive psychology to the study of impaired memory, Butters (1984) reviewed a series of studies comparing the memory disorders of patients with diencephalic (i.e., alcoholic Korsakoff) patients and basal ganglia (i.e., Huntington's disease) patients damage. It was noted that the anterograde amnesia of alcoholic Korsakoff (AK) patients involved a failure in storage caused by an increased sensitivity to proactive interference and limited encoding, whereas the severe deficit of Huntington's disease (HD) patients on recall measures of learning was related to an inability to initiate systematic retrieval processes. The memory failure of AK paitents, but not those of HD patients, could be attenuated by the introduction of procedures that reduced proactive interference (e.g., distributed rather than massed learning trials). However, only the HD patients performed at almost normal levels when recognition rather than recall measures of learning were employed.

In addition to this distinction between storage and retrieval impairments, AK and HD patients appeared to differ in their ability to acquire a visuomotor skill (Martone et al., 1984). Using the reading of mirror-reflected words as a measure of skill learning, Cohen and Squire (1980) had concluded that AK patients were capable of normal learning and retention of this skill (as measured by reduction in the temporal durations necessary to read mirror-reflected word triads), despite a severe inability to recognize the specific words used to train the skill. When Martone et al. (1984) extended the mirror reading paradigm to HD patients, a double dissociation between recognition memory and skill learning emerged. Although AK patients performed as described by Cohen and Squire (1980), the HD patients were significantly impaired in the acquisition of the visuomotor skill despite normal recognition of the words employed on the test. On the basis of these findings, Martone et al. (1984) suggested that the learning of motor skills and the storage of factual (i.e., data-based) materials might depend on the integrity of the basal ganglia (especially the caudate nucleus) and limbic-diencephalic regions, respectively.

In addition to comparisons between amnesic and HD patients, recent investigations from our laboratory have also focused on the performance of patients with Alzheimer's disease on episodic (Tulving, 1983), semantic (Tulving, 1983) and implicit (Graf & Schacter, 1985; Schacter, 1987) memory tasks. The findings, which will be reviewed in this chapter, have not only demonstrated the heuristic value of these taxonomic concepts but also provided clues as to their neuroanatomical substrate. The relevance for Cummings and Benson's (1984) proposed distinction between "cortical" and "subcortical" dementia will also be discussed.

Tulving (1983) has defined episodic memories as those dependent on temporal and/or spatial cues for their retrieval. For instance, attempts to recall the previous day's breakfast meal or a specific encounter with a colleague requires the use of temporal and spatial contextual cues and, therefore, would represent retrieval from episodic memory. Most of the traditional verbal learning techniques (e.g., paired-associate learning, list learning) employed by experimental psychologists are categorized as episodic memory tasks. In comparison to episodic memories, semantic memories are totally independent of contextual cues for their retrieval. Various numerical (e.g., the number of feet in a yard), historical (e.g., the name of the first president of the United States), and geographical (e.g., the capital of California) facts serve as examples of semantic memories. Because of repetition and overlearning, memories that are initially episodic in nature may become context-free and part of an individual's semantic fund of knowledge.

Implicit memory refers to a class of diverse memory tasks that, unlike traditional tests of recall and recognition, do not require the explicit, conscious recollection of previous experiences (Schacter, 1987) and are usually preserved in severely amnesic patients (Squire, 1987). Classical conditioning, lexical and semantic priming, motor skill learning, and perceptual learning have all been considered forms of implicit memory. It should be stressed that the distinction between explicit memory and implicit memory is intended to be purely descriptive, and it remains to be determined how valid this dichotomy will be when applied to the entire spectrum of learning and memory phenomena. Also, whether various types of implicit memory are mediated by single or different neurologic entities has not been adequately addressed.

The Alzheimer patients who participated in our recent studies were diagnosed using the clinical criteria developed by the National Institute on Neurological and Communicative Disorders and Stroke and the Alzheimer's Disease and Related Disorders Association (NINCDS-ADRDA) (McKhann et al., 1984). All patients scored at or above 104 out of a possible 144 points on the Dementia Rating Scale (DRS), a mental status examination that assesses a broad spectrum of cognitive functions (Mattis, 1976). In addition, the patients averaged 7–10 errors out of a possible 33 errors on Fuld's (1978) adaptation of the Information-Memory-Concentration Test (Blessed, Tomlinson, & Roth, 1968), and they earned 21–24 correct responses out of a possible 30 on the Mini-Mental State examination (Folstein, Folstein, & McHugh, 1975).

The HD patients were similar to those described by Butters (1984). They have a genetically transmitted disorder resulting in a progressive atrophy of the basal ganglia, especially the caudate nucleus. The most common behavioral symptoms included choreiform movements, a progressive dementia, and in most cases marked personality changes (e.g., depression, increased irritability). Although the first onset of symptomatology is difficult to determine, almost all of the patients used in these investigations initially evidenced choreiform movements in the third, fourth, or fifth decades of life. These HD patients had a mean age of 46 years and had been diagnosed 3 months to 19 years prior to testing. Although some of the HD patients had moderate choreiform movements (i.e., many had only mild chorea), none were considered to be in the terminal stages of the disease.

Most of the amnesic patients in these studies were alcoholics with Korsakoff's syndrome. They were male veterans with a mean age of 58 years. They all had 10- to 30-year histories of alcohol addiction accompanied by malnutrition prior to the onset of their Wernicke-Korsakoff syndrome. At the time of testing, all of the Korsakoff patients were residing in a Veterans Administration facility or nursing home. They had severe anterograde and retrograde amnesias, as measured by the Wechsler Memory Scale and on the basis of clinical assessment, but their general intellectual functioning, as measured by the Wechsler Adult Intelligence Scale, was within normal limits. Although it is generally assumed that these patients' severe amnesia is related to hemorrhagic lesions in the medial diencephalon (Victor, Adams, & Collins, 1971), there is some evidence that AK patients, like patients with dementia of the Alzheimer type (DAT), may also have a significant loss of neurons in various structures of the basal forebrain (Arendt et al., 1983).

EPISODIC AND SEMANTIC MEMORY

The dichotomy between *episodic* and *semantic* memory has been used to differentiate the impairments of amnesic and demented patients (Martin & Fedio, 1983; Weingartner et al., 1983). Although both amnesic and demented patients are impaired in the acquisition and recall of materials associated with particular temporal and/or spatial contexts (i.e., episodic memory), only demented patients are severely impaired in recalling general knowledge such as rules of grammar and multiplication tables (i.e., semantic memory). In one study, Weingartner et al. (1983) compared the performances of AK patients with those of patients with progressive dementias (presumably DAT) on both episodic (e.g., verbal list learning) and semantic (e.g., sentence completion, verbal fluency) memory tasks. As anticipated, both the AK and DAT patients were severely impaired in the acquisition of word lists and the immediate recall of short passages, whereas only the demented patients evidenced severe deficits in the completion of highly structured sentences and on a letter fluency task. Other studies utilizing verbal fluency tasks to assess semantic memory have reported significant impairments even during the early stages of DAT and HD (Butters et al., 1978; Ober et al., 1986; Rosen, 1980).

In addition to demonstrating the existence of episodic and/or semantic memory problems in amnesic and demented patients, some investigations have focused on the processes underlying these cognitive deficiencies. Although AK patients encounter more difficulty with episodic than with semantic memory tasks, their performances on both are marked by several indices of increased sensitivity to proactive interference. For example, AK patients are highly prone to prior-item (list, passage) intrusions on short-term memory tasks (Butters & Cermak, 1980), verbal paired-associate learning (Winocur & Weiskrantz, 1976), recall of short passages (Butters et al., 1986) and on verbal fluency tests (Butters et al., 1986). In comparison to AK patients, HD patients appear to be severely impaired on both episodic and semantic memory tasks as a result of a general retrieval problem. On list learning tests and tasks involving memory of prose passages, HD patients perform as poorly as do Korsakoff patients when recall measures are employed, but the HD patients are superior to amnesic patients if recognition tests are introduced (Butters et al., 1985; Butters et al., 1986). On letter fluency tasks, HD patients generate fewer correct responses (as well as perseverative errors) than do AK patients. This double dissociation between HD and Korsakoff patients on verbal recognition and verbal fluency tests has been cited as evidence that HD patients are impaired in the initiation of systematic strategies for searching both episodic and semantic memory (Butters et al., 1986). More specifically, as the retrieval demands are reduced (e.g., the use of recognition rather than recall memory tests) or increased (e.g., letter fluency test), the performances of HD patients change dramatically in comparison to those of amnesic subjects.

Butters et al. (1987) have extended these analyses of episodic and semantic memory to patients with DAT. The performances of DAT, HD, and AK patients were compared to those of young and elderly intact control subjects on memory for passages (i.e., episodic memory) and two (letter, category) verbal fluency tasks (i.e., semantic memory). Based on previous findings (Butters et al., 1985; Butters et al., 1986), it was anticipated that the quantitative and qualitative features of the AK and HD patients' responses would again reflect an increased sensitivity to proactive interference (AK patients) and a general retrieval deficit (HD patients). Since patients with DAT also commit numerous perseverative and intrusion errors on episodic (Butters et al., 1983; Fuld, 1983) and semantic (Ober et al., 1986) memory tasks, some similarities in the memory deficiencies of the AK and Alzheimer patients were anticipated. However, in view of Alzheimer patients' aphasic difficulties, they were expected to demonstrate a distinctive pattern of problems on the letter and category fluency tasks. If searching for exemplars of an abstract concept (i.e., animals) requires that the hierarchical organization of semantic knowledge be relatively intact (Martin, 1987), Alzheimer patients should be more impaired on category than on letter fluency tasks, especially in the very early stages of the disease.

A total of 60 subjects participated in Butters et al.'s (1987) study: 12 HD patients; 13 patients with DAT; nine AK patients; 13 young normal controls age-matched to the HD patients; and 13 elderly normal controls age-matched to the patients with DAT. The three patient groups were matched in terms of overall degree of dementia as assessed with the DRS. Such matching for general cognitive loss helps reduce the confounding of differences caused by disease entity (e.g., HD vs. DAT) with those caused by severity of dementia (e.g., mild vs. severe dementia). As might be expected, only the Alzheimer patients showed a moderate degree of aphasia (i.e., dysnomia).

The episodic memory task involved the recall of four thematically neutral stories similar in format and length to the Logical Memory Passages of the Wechsler

Memory Scale. Following the presentation of each story, the subjects were asked to count backwards from 100 by 3's for 30 seconds, and then were asked to recall as much of the story as they could remember. All stories were scored according to a verbatim scale that gave one point credit for each verbatim informational unit (maximum of 23 units per story) recalled by the subject. In addition to the items correctly recalled, the examiner recorded prior-story intrusion errors (i.e., a correctly recalled item from one story that is recalled as part of a subsequent story) and extra-story intrusion errors (i.e., ideas recalled by the subject that were never presented in any story).

The evaluation of semantic memory was comprised of two parts: a letter fluency task (FAS) developed by Benton (1968) and Borkowski, Benton, and Spreen (1967), and a category fluency task. On the letter fluency task, the subjects were read the letters "F," "A," and "S" sequentially and asked to produce "as many *different* words as they could think of" that began with the given letter. For each of the three letters, the subjects were allowed 60 seconds to orally generate words. On the category fluency task, the subjects were allowed 60 seconds to produce "as many different *animals* as they could think of." The subjects' responses on the two fluency tasks were categorized into four types: (1) correct responses; (2) perseverative errors (i.e., the repetition of a correct word within a given trial); (3) intrusion errors (i.e., responses that did not conform to the criteria established for the given letter or animal category); and (4) variation errors (i.e., words repeated within a given trial with a different or added suffix).

On the episodic memory task (i.e., memory for passages), all three patient groups were found to be severely impaired in comparison to their age-matched controls in the number of phrases they correctly recalled. The major differences among the three patient groups became apparent when the numbers of prior-story and extra-story intrusion errors were examined. Both the AK patients and the patients with DAT made more intrusion errors than did their age-matched controls and the HD patients. When the performances of the patient groups were evaluated in terms of proportions (%) of total responses, the differences among the three patient groups were even more striking. Although the HD patients did not recall many phrases from the four stories, what little they did recall was usually correct (78%). In contrast, less than 50% of the impaired recall of the AK and Alzheimer patients was correct; most of their recall represented some combination of prior- and extra-story intrusion errors.

The results for the fluency tasks revealed four major differences among the patient groups:

1. The HD patients were severely impaired on both letter and category fluency tasks. Of the three patient groups, the HD patients produced the fewest number of correct words on both tests.
2. The AK patients showed a mild-to-moderate impairment on both fluency tests, and like the HD patients, the severity of their fluency problem was

not related to the linguistic constraints (i.e., letter vs. category fluency) of the semantic memory task.

3. The performance of the Alzheimer patients was directly related to the linguistic demands of the two fluency tasks. On the letter fluency test, the patients with DAT generated almost as many correct words as did their age-matched controls and actually produced more correct words than did the HD and AK patients. However, on the category fluency task, the performance of the patients with DAT was severely impaired. They generated significantly fewer correct animal names than did their elderly age-matched controls, and their performance was indistinguishable from that of the severely impaired HD patients.
4. On the letter fluency task, both the DAT and AK patients made significantly more perseveration errors than did the HD patients and the two groups of control subjects.

These findings indicate that patients with DAT have a pattern of deficits on episodic and semantic memory tasks that differentiates them from other dementing (e.g., HD) and amnesic (e.g., AK) disorders. When asked to recall short passages, the patients with DAT remembered few correct facts and made numerous prior-story and extra-story intrusion errors. The ubiquitousness of these intrusions exemplifies the Alzheimer patients' increased sensitivity to proactive interference and confirms other reports that intrusion errors are an important characteristic of these patients' episodic memory disorder (Fuld, 1983; Fuld et al., 1982).

On the two fluency taks (i.e., semantic memory), the Alzheimer patients were adversely affected by their aphasic disorder as well as by their increased sensitivity to interference. Although the patients with DAT generated nearly as many correct responses as did the intact elderly controls on the letter fluency tasks, they emitted significantly more perseveration errors. Of even greater import for the Alzheimer patients' problems with semantic memory was the difference in their performances on the category and letter fluency tests. They were severely impaired in producing names of animals but encountered few problems on the letter fluency task. That is, their deficits in semantic memory were most apparent when they had to search for exemplars of an abstract category (i.e., animals). If, as Martin and Fedio (1983) and Ober et al. (1986) have suggested, the Alzheimer patients' language problems involve a reduction in the number of exemplars comprising an abstract category, scores on the category fluency task should be a highly sensitive measure of deficiencies in semantic memory. Since the letter fluency task can be performed using phonemic cues to search a very extensive set of appropriate exemplars, impairments on this task may not be apparent until the disease has progressed beyond its earliest stages.

The HD patients' performances on the story recall and fluency tasks indicate that their episodic and semantic memory disorders involve processes different from those of Alzheimer patients. The HD patients were impaired on story recall and fluency measures, but their pattern of deficits and errors does not suggest a special role for proactive interference and general language dysfunctions. The HD patients produced relatively few intrusion and perseveration errors in comparison to Alzheimer patients, and yet were severely impaired on *both* letter and category fluency tests. Although Butters et al.'s (1987) study was not designed to evaluate the hypothesis that HD patients' episodic and semantic memory disorders reflect a general retrieval deficit (Butters, 1984; Butters et al., 1986; Caine et al., 1978), the findings are certainly consistent with this notion. Patients who encounter unusual difficulty in retrieving successfully stored information should be impaired on virtually all fluency tasks regardless of their linguistic demands.

The AK subjects performed as anticipated on the episodic memory task. They recalled few verbatim items from the stories and made numerous prior- and extra-story intrusion errors. The prior-story intrusions serve as another indicator of the Korsakoff patients' well-known increased sensitivity to proactive interference (Butters & Cermak, 1980), whereas the extra-story intrusions may be a remnant of these patients' tendency to confabulate during the acute phase of the disorder. The AK patients' propensity for perseverative intrusion errors was also evident on one of the semantic memory tasks (i.e., letter fluency), where they often repeated correct words (e.g., *field*, found, factory, *field*) during the 60-second test period. Apparently, whether episodic or semantic memory is being assessed, those memories dominating a Korsakoff patient's response hierarchy at a given moment will be repeatedly emitted and remain unmonitored by any inhibitory feedback.

The parallels in the performances of the Korsakoff and Alzheimer patients are deserving of some mention. As Butters (1985) reported in a preliminary comparison of these patients' story recall and letter fluency, both Alzheimer and Korsakoff patients are prone to perseveration and intrusion errors. Although such error tendencies are not necessarily indicative of a specific brain dysfunction or etiology (Shindler, Caplan, & Hier, 1984), one recent neuropathological report provides some basis for considering a common neurochemical factor in these two disorders. Arendt et al. (1983) have reported that the number of neurons in basal forebrain structures was reduced by 70% and 47% in the brains of Alzheimer and Korsakoff patients, respectively. Examination of the brains of HD patients revealed a significant loss of neurons in the globus pallidus but not in the basal forebrain. Given that the basal forebrain is the source of cholinergic input to the hippocampus and frontal association cortex, one might speculate that the common error patterns of Alzheimer and AK patients might reflect a similar underlying cholinergic deficiency. Although this suggestion is certainly worthy of further neurochemical and neuropathological investigation, the differences between Alzheimer and AK patients in terms of aphasic and dyspraxic symptoms must not be overlooked. The lack of aphasia and severe constructional apraxia in AK patients may be indications that the noted similarities in the two disorders are coincidental.

Another recent study (Granholm & Butters, 1988) provides further support for some common underlying deficits in Korsakoff and Alzheimer patients. Using an encoding specificity paradigm (Tulving & Thomson, 1973), Cermak, Uhly, and Reale (1980) found that Korsakoff patients were so impaired in their encoding of the semantic relationships between two words that they could not use the product of such encoding to facilitate retrieval. The encoding specificity hypothesis, as developed from verbal memory studies with normal subjects (Thomson & Tulving, 1970), predicts that words present at both encoding and retrieval, whether strong or weak associates, should be the most effective retrieval cues. However, unlike intact subjects, AK patients consistently benefited more from strong associates than from weak associates of the to-be-remembered (TBR) word, regardless of which associate was present during encoding (Cermak, Uhly, & Reale, 1980). Granholm and Butters (1988), using the same stimuli and design employed by Cermak, Uhly, and Reale (1980), examined the associative encoding and retrieval abilities of Alzheimer and HD patients. If, as Martin et al. (1985) have suggested, Alzheimer patients have a limited ability to perform adequate semantic encoding during presentation, they should demonstrate a pattern of performance similar to that of the AK patients. Since HD patients' memory deficits primarily involve retrieval problems (Butters et al., 1986), it was anticipated that these patients should evidence a pattern of performance on the encoding specificity task similar to that of intact controls.

Forty subjects participated in this study: 10 HD patients; 10 patients with DAT; 10 middle-aged normal controls (i.e., age-matched to the HD patients); and 10 elderly normal controls (i.e., age-matched to the patients with DAT). Since the HD and DAT patient groups did not differ in terms of their DRS scores, they appeared to be matched in terms of overall severity of dementia.

The materials and design employed in this study are described in detail elsewhere (Cermak, Uhly, & Reale, 1980; Granholm & Butters, 1988). Briefly, 60 word triads were constructed consisting of a TBR word plus a strong and weak associate of the TBR word (e.g., TBR word = DAY; strong associate = night; weak associate = sun). The 60 TBR words were then divided into five lists of 12 words each and printed on index cards in uppercase letters. Four encoding/retrieval conditions and a free recall condition were created by varying the types of cues (i.e., strong: S; weak: W; or no cues: 0) that were present at presentation and recall. The five experimental conditions were designated by the following abbreviated terms: 0-0, S-S, W-W, W-S, and S-W. For example, condition 0-0 was a standard free recall condition with no associates present at either presentation or recall. In the S-S condition, each TBR word was accompanied by a strong cue at presentation (e.g., DAY–night), and the subjects were cued with the same strong associate at recall. In condition W-S, each TBR word was accompanied by a weak associate (e.g., DAY–sun) at presentation, and subjects were cued with an appropriate strongly associated (but not previously presented) word (e.g., night) at recall, etc.

Subjects were presented a list of 12 word pairs each consisting of a capitalized TBR word and, in the four encoding/retrieval conditions, an associated word printed in lowercase letters and enclosed in parentheses above the TBR word. First, the subject was shown a sample card and told to read aloud and memorize each capitalized word and also to pay attention to the related word as a possible aid in recalling the capitalized one at a later time. Following the presentation of this practice card, each of the 12 word pairs was presented individually for three seconds. After a second presentation of the 12 word pairs, the subject was given a sheet of paper containing a typed column of 12 cue words with a space beside each for the appropriate TBR words. The subject was instructed that each word on the list was a cue or aid to recalling one of the capitalized words that had been read aloud and to write the remembered words in the space next to the cue that helped. Words remembered without the help of a cue were to be written separately on the page. In the 0-0 condition, subjects were shown no cues at recall; rather, they were handed a sheet containing 12 blank spaces and asked to recall as many of the TBR words as possible. A maximum of 5 minutes was allowed for each recall test. The same procedures were followed for each of the five experimental conditions. Subjects were allowed a 2- to 3-minute rest period between lists.

In addition to the number of words correctly recalled, the number of omission errors, prior-list intrusion errors (i.e., words recalled that were present as either TBR words or cues on a previous trial), and extra-list intrusion errors (i.e., words recalled by the subject that were not presented as TBR words or cues in any other list) were also recorded.

Figure 5.1 shows the total number of correctly recalled words for the four subject groups in the free recall condition and each of the four encoding/retrieval conditions. Both the HD and Alzheimer patients were impaired relative to their age-matched controls in total words recalled. Although the two patient groups demonstrated similar overall levels of recall performance, they displayed different patterns of performance across the five experimental conditions. For all four subject groups, recall performance was best in the S-S condition (i.e., strong associates presented both at encoding and retrieval) and worst in the S-W condition. The HD group, like the two control groups, also demonstrated a similar level of recall on the three remaining conditions (i.e., W-W, W-S, 0-0). In contrast, the DAT group performed significantly better in the W-S conditions than in the W-W and 0-0 conditions. These different patterns of performance were still apparent when proportion scores (percentage of total correct responses) were used to correct for group differences in the total number of words recalled (Figure 5.2).

Analyses of prior-list intrusions, extra-list intrusions, and omission errors also revealed different patterns of performance between the HD and DAT groups. Specifically, the Alzheimer patients made a larger proportion (i.e., percentage of total errors) of extra-list intrusions than did the HD patients, while the HD patients produced a larger proportion of omission errors.

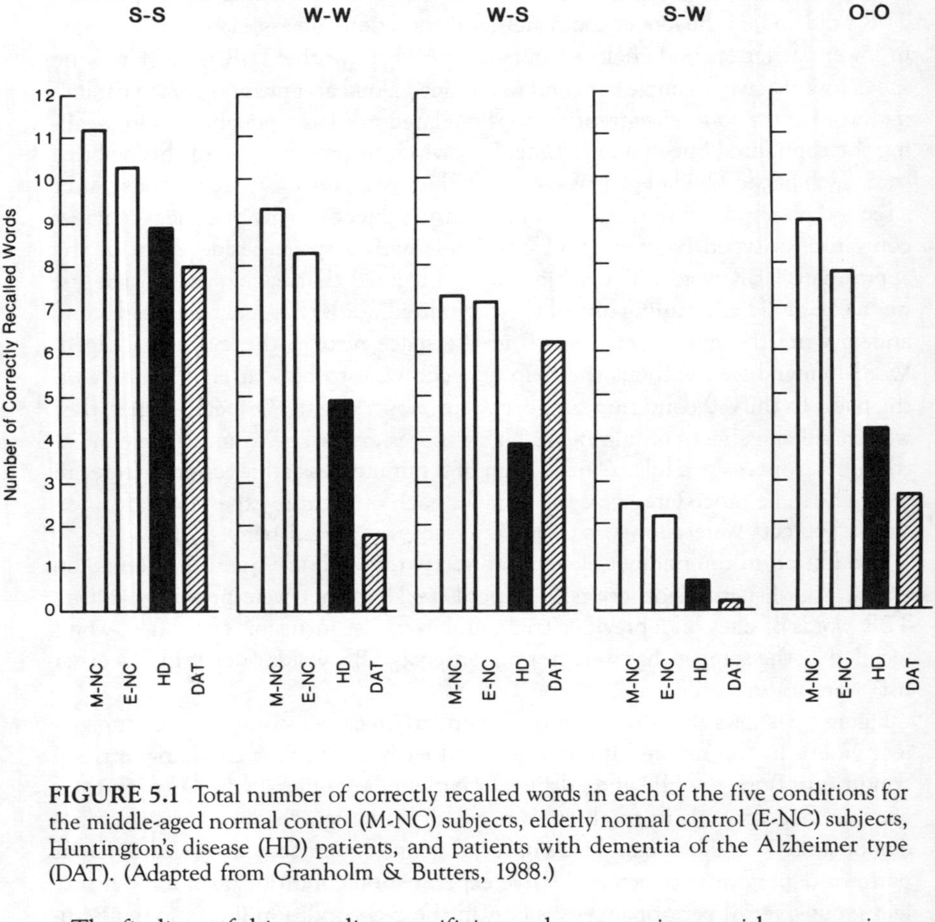

FIGURE 5.1 Total number of correctly recalled words in each of the five conditions for the middle-aged normal control (M-NC) subjects, elderly normal control (E-NC) subjects, Huntington's disease (HD) patients, and patients with dementia of the Alzheimer type (DAT). (Adapted from Granholm & Butters, 1988.)

The findings of this encoding specificity study are consistent with our previous demonstrations that the semantic memory impairments of DAT and HD patients involve different underlying processes. Although both patient groups evidenced poor recall overall, they were clearly distinguished by their ability to utilize strong and weak cues for retrieving TBR words. As anticipated by their general difficulty with initiating systematic retrieval processes (Butters, 1984; Butters et al., 1986; Caine et al., 1978), the HD patients demonstrated the same pattern of performance with the various combinations of weak and strong cues at encoding and retrieval as did the two intact control groups. The HD patients and control subjects were generally most successful recalling words when the strength of the cues were identical during encoding and retrieval, and were least successful when the cue words differed during presentation and recall. It appears, then, that both the HD patients and control subjects successfully encoded the relationships between

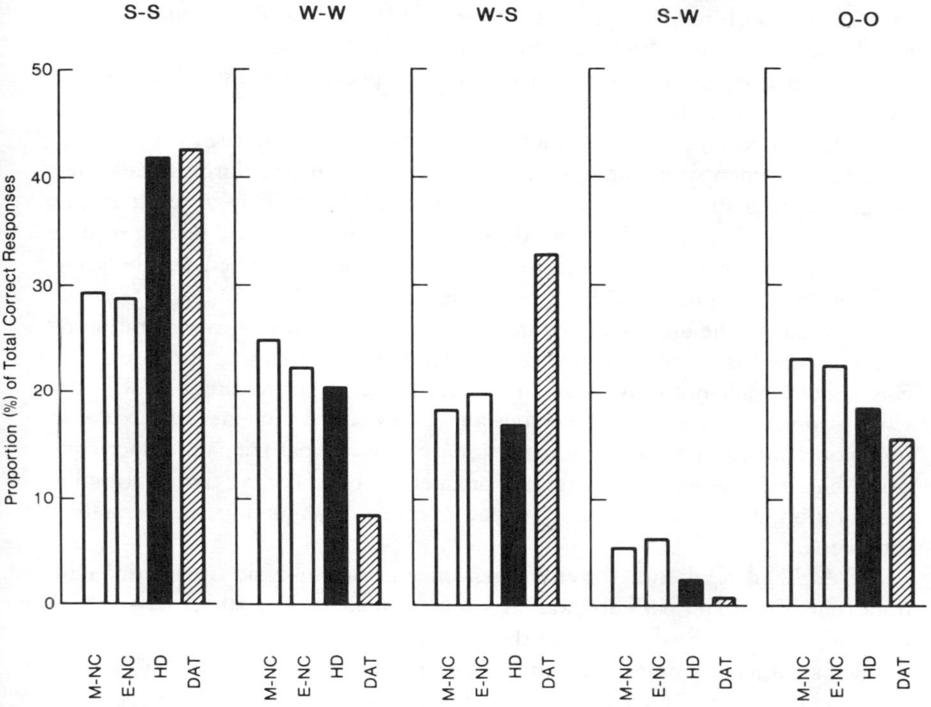

FIGURE 5.2 Recall performance in each of the five conditions is presented as a proportion of total correctly recalled words for the middle-aged normal control (M-NC) subjects, elderly normal control (E-NC) subjects, Huntington's disease (HD) patients, and patients with dementia of the Alzheimer type (DAT). (Adapted from Granholm & Butters, 1988.)

the cue and TBR words and subsequently were able to use the cue word to facilitate retrieval. The HD patients' overall impaired performance probably demonstrates their inability to initiate efficient retrieval strategies despite relatively intact encoding.

The Alzheimer patients' pattern of performance with the various combinations of strong and weak cues indicated that they either did not encode the relationships between cue and TBR words or were unable to utilize the product of encoding at the time of cued recall. In comparison to the HD patients, the Alzheimer patients were severely deficient in recall when the same weak associate was shown at both encoding and retrieval. Also, the Alzheimer patients performed relatively well whenever a strong cue was present at recall, regardless of whether a strong or weak cue was present at encoding. These results suggest that the encoding of specific relationships between associates and TBR words was not responsible for the Alzheimer patients' success in retrieval with strong cues. Instead of relying upon semantic encoding, the patients with DAT appear to have simply generated their most dominant associations to the cue words during recall testing. Such an associative strategy would account for the huge discrepancies in the DAT patients' performance when strong and weak associates were available during recall. Free associating to a strong associate is obviously much more likely to result in the chance production of the TBR word. The other subject groups, relying on the product of their encoding as a retrieval cue, were hindered whenever the same associate was not present at both encoding and retrieval.

The results of the error analyses are also consistent with this interpretation of the Alzheimer patients' performance. Any tendency to free associate to retrieval cues should result not only in an increased probability of recalling TBR words when strong associates are present but also in a marked increment in extra-list intrusion errors regardless of cue conditions. Since HD patients and intact control subjects did rely primarily on the product of the encoding during stimulus presentation, they should not have been prone to generating such extra-list intrusions.

The Alzheimer patients' pattern of performance on this task, though different from that of the HD patients, was strikingly similar to the pattern reported by Cermak, Uhly, and Reale (1980) for the AK patients. Both DAT and AK patients recalled significantly more words in the W-S condition than in the W-W condition, and neither performance differed significantly from that of control subjects in the W-S condition. These results suggest that Alzheimer and Korsakoff patients are both impaired in their ability to utilize semantic information present at encoding to facilitate recall performance. Again, whether such similarities in cognitive mechanisms truly reflect some common neurologic dysfunction (e.g., loss of cells in the basal forebrain) can only be determined by future neuropathological investigations.

Finally, the findings of our recent investigations (Butters et al., 1987; Granholm & Butters, 1988) not only support the notion that episodic and semantic memory are disturbed in the dementias, but also demonstrate that the processes underlying failures in episodic and semantic memory systems may vary from one form of dementia to another. Patients with HD perform poorly on both episodic and semantic memory tasks because of their inability to initiate suitable retrieval strategies, whereas the deficits of patients with DAT on these same memory tasks reflect linguistic aberrations, an increased sensitivity to proactive interference, and reduced semantic encoding ability. It appears then that the notion that all dementias may be characterized as a loss of both episodic and semantic memory seems too simplistic and likely blurs many important distinctions among various degenerative diseases of the central nervous system.

IMPLICIT MEMORY

In addition to the differences between HD and Alzheimer patients on explicit tests of episodic and semantic memory, there is now some evidence that these patient groups may be dissociated by their performance on implicit memory tests as well. Martone et al. (1984) found that HD patients were impaired in their ability to acquire a visuomotor skill (i.e., reading mirror-reversed words), whereas Eslinger and Damasio (1986) have reported that Alzheimer patients could acquire in a normal fashion the motor skills underlying a pursuit rotor task. Together, these results suggest that the neostriatum (damaged in HD but preserved in the early stages of DAT) may be critically involved in the acquisition of visuomotor skills. That is, in addition to the well-known motor dysfunctions (e.g., chorea, bradykinesia, tremor, rigidity) associated with basal ganglia lesions, patients with various forms of the so-called "subcortical" dementias (Cummings & Benson, 1984) may be deficient in forming the motor programs and links so vital to the acquisition of motor skills.

To assess this hypothesis, Heindel, Butters, and Salmon (1988) compared the ability of HD and Alzheimer patients to learn a pursuit rotor task. This classical test of skill learning has a major methodological advantage over mirror-reading, in that patients' initial levels of performance may be equated readily by adjusting the speed of rotation of the disk. Since HD patients' initial level of performance on a mirror-reading task is much slower than that of intact controls and even other neurologic groups (Martone et al., 1984), ceiling and floor effects may cloud any interpretation of significant group differences in rate of learning.

A total of 44 patients participated in Heindel, Butters, and Salmon's (1988) study: 10 HD patients; 10 patients with DAT; four amnesic patients of mixed etiologies; and 20 intact control subjects. As in our other studies (Butters et al., 1987; Granholm & Butters, 1988), the three patient groups were matched for overall degree of dementia with the DRS. The small group of amnesic patients was included to confirm previous findings of spared motor learning in amnesia (Cermak et al., 1973; Corkin, 1968).

Subjects were asked to maintain contact between a stylus held in their preferred hand and a small metallic disk (2 cm in diameter) on a rotating turntable (25 cm in diameter). The turntable could be adjusted to rotate at 15, 30, 45, or 60 rotations per minute (rpm) for a given 20-second trial. All subjects were tested over three sessions of eight trials each, with each session separated by approximately 30 minutes of other psychometric testing. Within each test session, subjects were also allowed a 1-minute rest interval between the fourth and fifth trials, thereby creating six blocks of four trials each. The total time on target was recorded for each 20-second trial.

For each subject the first test session was preceded by a block of practice trials to determine the speed of rotation (i.e., 15, 30, 45, or 60 rpm) of the turntable. On each successive practice trial the speed of the turntable was increased. The turntable was then set for the remainder of the subject's testing to that speed associated with a score (i.e., time on target) closest to 5 seconds (i.e., contact maintained 25% of the time). In this manner, the initial level of performance on the pursuit rotor task was equated for the four subject groups.

The results showed that three of the four groups evidenced systematic skill learning over the six blocks of testing. Specifically, the Alzheimer and amnesic patients and normal control subjects all improved their performance to approximately 52% time on target on block 6, whereas the HD patients maintained contract between the stylus and the disk for only 35% of the time on this last test block. When difference scores (block 6 − block 1) were calculated to measure the amount of skill acquisition, the HD patients demonstrated significantly less learning than did the other three groups. As anticipated, the amnesic and Alzheimer patients did not differ from the intact control subjects on any measure of skill acquisition.

Like previous findings, the results of Heindel, Butters, and Salmon's (1988) study support the notion that the basal ganglia (especially the neostriatum) are involved in the acquisition of motor skills. Since the four subject groups were matched for initial level of performance on the pursuit rotor task, the impairment of the HD patients cannot be attributed to ceiling or floor effects. Furthermore, the HD patients with the least amount of functional disability were found to be as impaired on this task as were those with the greatest disability, indicating that pursuit rotor learning in HD does not appear to be directly related to primary motor deficits. It should also be noted that the matching of the three patient groups in terms of overall level of dementia with the DRS reduces the possibility that the differences in the learning of the motor skill might reflect differences in degree of overall cognitive loss (i.e., dementia).

The proposed linkage between motor skill learning and the basal ganglia is consistent with current understanding of the organization of the motor system. The neostriatum, along with the other subcortical components of the extrapyramidal motor system (i.e., the pallidum, substantia nigra, and subthalamic nucleus), appears to influence voluntary motor behavior in an indirect way through thalamocortical projections to the pyramidal system. In addition, basal ganglia dysfunction has been associated more with an impairment in self-initiated movements than simply with the direct control of movement per se (Evarts & Wise, 1984). Given the massive topographical projection from most of the neocortex to the neostriatum (Kemp & Powell, 1970), the neostriatum may play a role in converting general strategies for motor action formed by the association cortex into purposeful motor behavior (Brooks, 1986; Groves, 1983).

Given the HD patients' impairment in acquiring visuomotor skills, the question arises concerning the general role of the basal ganglia in implicit memory.

Are the basal ganglia critically involved in all forms of implicit memory, or are different forms of implicit memory mediated by their own distinct neural systems? An investigation of verbal priming in amnesic and demented patients (Shimamura et al., 1987) supports the latter hypothesis. Priming, another form of implicit memory, has been defined as the temporary (and unconscious) facilitation of performance via prior exposure to stimuli. Shimamura et al., using a lexical priming paradigm in which subjects were asked to complete three-letter word stems with the first words that came to mind, found that AK patients, HD patients, and normal controls all demonstrated a similar tendency to complete these stems with previously presented stimuli. Alzheimer patients, however, were found to be severely impaired in their lexical priming ability. These results suggest that this form of implicit memory is not dependent on the integrity of the basal ganglia but rather is mediated by a neural system that is selectively disrupted in DAT.

Since patients with DAT show marked pathology in temporal, parietal, and frontal association cortices along with a relative sparing of the primary sensory areas (Brun, 1983), their impaired priming ability may be related to damage to those neocortical association regions that store the lexical representations of semantic memory. This notion that Alzheimer patients are deficient in activating preexisting representations stored in semantic memory is also consistent with the difficulty Alzheimer patients have on explicit tests of semantic memory such as category fluency (Butters et al., 1987; Martin, 1987; Martin & Fedio, 1983; Ober et al., 1986). In both instances, the Alzheimer patients' impairment may be related to a breakdown in the hierarchical organization of their semantic knowledge.

To further explore these possible ties between patients' priming and semantic memory deficits, Salmon et al. (1988) administered a semantic priming task to Alzheimer, HD, and intact control subjects. Subjects were asked to judge categorically or functionally related word pairs (e.g., bird-robin, needle-thread) and later to say the first word that came to mind (i.e., "free-associate") when presented with the first word (e.g., bird, needle) of a pair. Semantic priming, as well as an intact organization of semantic memory, are indicated by the subjects' tendency to produce the second word of the related word pairs. Nine patients with DAT, 10 HD patients, nine elderly control subjects, and 10 middle-aged control subjects participated in this study. The Alzheimer and HD patients were again matched for overall level of dementia with the DRS.

Forty-eight *functional* word pairs were created by pairing 24 stimulus words with both a "strong" associate and a "moderate" associate. The two words in each of these functional pairs were semantically related either by common function (e.g., needle-thread), by tendency to occur in the same context (e.g., doctor-nurse), or by part-whole relationships (e.g., hand-finger). Forty-eight *categorical* pairs (e.g., bird-robin) were also created by pairing 24 different stimulus words with both a "strong" and "moderate" exemplar. Six additional word pairs, three categorical and three functional, were designated as filler pairs and used to control for primacy and recency effects. Another six word pairs with no apparent semantic association were created. These unrelated pairs were used to control for the possibility that subjects might respond with target words during the free association task, not because an existing semantic association had been primed, but simply because the two words had been presented together.

The test was administered in three identical blocks composed of a rating task and a free association task. Subjects were presented pairs of words one pair at a time and were asked to rate how closely the two words were related on a five-point scale. Each group of 12 word pairs (four categorical, four functional, two unrelated, two filler) was presented to each subject twice in succession, in the same order both times. Of the categorical and functional pairs, half of each type were strong associates, the other half moderate associates. Filler pairs were always presented first and last in each group of twelve pairs.

Immediately following the second presentation of word pairs in each block, the free association task was presented. The examiner never mentioned that this task was related to the previous rating task. Subjects were told that single words would be presented visually and they were to say "the first word that came to mind" in response to each stimulus word. Stimuli for the free association task included the first words of the categorical, functional, and unrelated pairs presented during the rating task. In addition, eight distractors (four strong associates and four moderate associates) were presented that were members of categorical and functional stimulus pairs that had not been presented to the subjects at any time. Distractors were included as a measure of the probability of a correct response due simply to chance. The same procedures were followed for the remaining two blocks.

Figure 5.3 shows the percentage of previously presented words produced on the semantic priming task by each group. Since the production of previously presented words from unrelated word pairs was extremely rare and isolated, subjects in all four groups apparently treated the task as one of free association rather than adopting a conscious recall strategy. The HD patients demonstrated normal semantic priming in this task, and performed significantly better than did the Alzheimer patients. The DAT group was significantly impaired compared to the control group and was the only group that did not prime above baseline guessing rates. The priming performance of the four groups was further subdivided into categorical vs. functional items (Figure 5.4) as well as strongly vs. moderately associated items. In all four cases, the Alzheimer patients, but not the HD patients, were severely impaired in their semantic priming ability.

The results of this study support the idea that Alzheimer patients experience a breakdown in the associative structure of their semantic memory. The categorical and functional cues may have failed to activate traces of previously presented stimuli because of the dissolution of the semantic network governing verbal materials. For example, the cue "bird" may not have evoked an unconscious

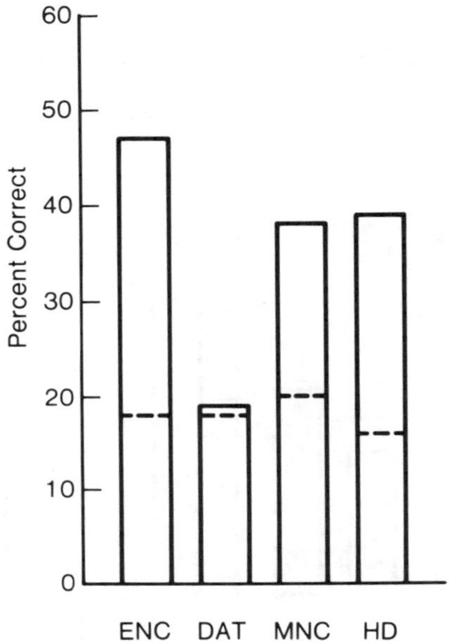

FIGURE 5.3 The percentage of previously presented words correctly produced in the free association task by patients with dementia of the Alzheimer type (DAT), patients with Huntington's disease (HD), elderly normal control subjects (ENC), and middle-aged normal control subjects (MNC). The baseline guessing rate of each group is indicated by the broken line. (Adapted from Salmon et al., 1988.)

activation of the categorical associate "robin" because the association between the two words has been greatly weakened. Such a disruption of the organization of semantic memory would also account for the Alzheimer patients' previously noted impairment on a lexical priming task (Shimamura et al., 1987). That is, the association in semantic memory between a word stem such as "mot" and the word "motel" may be sufficiently disrupted to negate the facilitating effect of the word's presention.

This interpretation of the semantic priming results allows for the integration of the Alzheimer patients' performance on explicit and implicit semantic memory tasks. Like deficits in semantic priming, deficiencies in the effortful retrieval of specific exemplars of an abstract category may also reflect significant changes in the structure and organization of semantic memory. As Martin and Fedio (1983) have noted using a supermarket fluency task, the number of specific exemplars associated with a given category is greatly reduced in DAT. Alzheimer patients can often name many of the general categories of items found in a supermarket (e.g., meats, vegetables, fruits) but are unable to produce specific examples (e.g., veal, beef, tomatoes, lettuce, apples) of these categories.

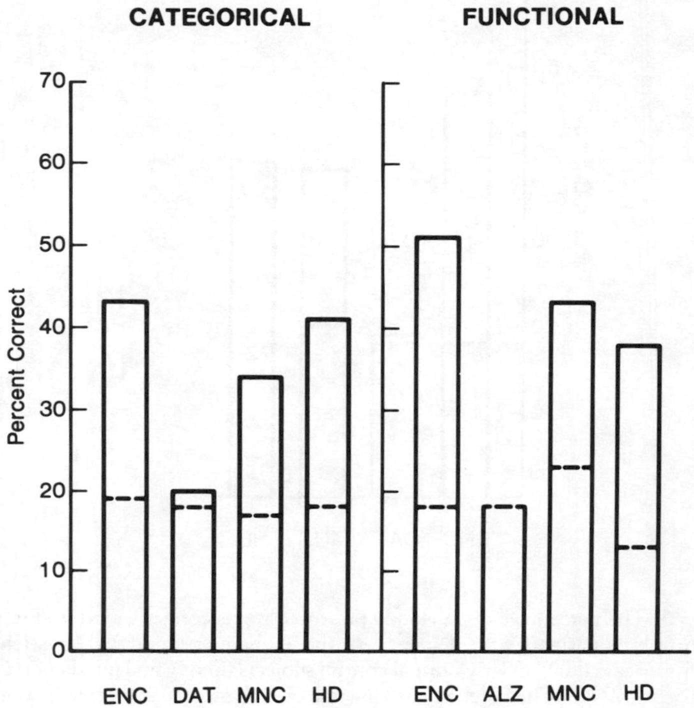

FIGURE 5.4 The percentage of previously presented words correctly produced in response to categorically or functionally related semantic associates in the free association task by patients with dementia of the Alzheimer type (DAT), patients with Huntington's disease (HD), elderly normal control subjects (ENC), and middle-aged normal control subjects (MNC). The baseling guessing rate of each group is indicated by the broken line. (Adapted from Salmon et al., 1988.)

The intact semantic priming of HD patients supports the conclusion drawn from the lexical priming study (Shimamura et al., 1987) that the integrity of the basal ganglia is not critical for the activation of stored representations in semantic memory. These results, in conjunction with those from the skill learning studies (Martone et al., 1984; Eslinger & Damasio, 1986; Heindel, Butters, and Salmon, 1988), suggest that different forms of implicit memory do depend on different anatomical substrates. Specifically, the HD patients' impairments on pursuit rotor and mirror-reading tests are consistent with the critical role of the basal ganglia in skill learning, whereas the Alzheimer patients' deficiencies on lexical and semantic priming tasks may be attributable to the cortical neuropathology reported in DAT (Terry & Katzman, 1983).

The double dissociation between the HD and Alzheimer patients on implicit memory tasks has relevance for Cummings and Benson's (1984) distinction between cortical and subcortical dementias. Patients with subcortical dementias (e.g., HD) usually have much less dysphasia and dyspraxia than do patients with cortical dementias (e.g., Alzheimer's disease) but are also much slower to initiate and complete most cognitive and motor processes than are patients with cortical degenerative diseases. The present results suggest that patients with cortical and subcortical dementias can also be differentiated by their performance on different implicit memory tasks. Patients with cortical dementias may have a preserved capacity to acquire and retain motor skills, but may be severely impaired on other tests of implicit memory that depend on the intactness of the association cortex in the dominant hemisphere. In contrast, patients with some forms of subcortical dementia may appear very limited in their ability to learn motor skills, despite their normal performance on implicit memory tasks mediated by verbal processes (e.g., lexical priming).

In a recently published study, Heindel et al. (1989) evaluated whether this double dissociation between the two implicit memory tasks and the DAT and HD patients would generalize to patients with idiopathic Parkinson's disease (PD). Although not included in James Parkinson's (1817) original description of the disorder, dementia has consistently been found to occur more frequently in PD than would be expected in a general population of the same age (Brown & Marsden, 1984; Lieberman et al., 1979). Although there is now general agreement that dementia can be an integral feature of the disease, considerable disagreement still exists concerning the underlying nature of the dementia. Since the primary lesion in PD appears to be a loss of cells in the substantia nigra pars compacta, several investigators (Albert, 1978; Huber et al., 1986; Mayeux et al., 1981) have stressed the common features (e.g., preserved language) of the dementias of PD, HD, and other subcortical dementias. However, others (Alvord et al., 1974; Boller et al., 1979) have noted that the dementing form of PD shares many enuropathologic features with DAT and may be the result of the superimposition of Alzheimer-type changes on primary subcortical pathology. In view of these uncertainties about the etiology and neurologic basis of the dementia of PD, the performances of demented PD patients on priming and motor skill learning tasks seems of some importance.

Heindel et al. (1989) administered to demented and nondemented PD patients two of the implicit memory tasks (pursuit rotor learning, stem-completion priming) found to differentiate DAT from HD patients. If the dementia of PD is similar to that of DAT, impaired performance on lexical priming combined with intact motor skill learning would be expected. Conversely, if demented PD patients manifest deficient skill learning combined with normal lexical priming, their cognitive impairments would appear similar to those of HD patients.

A total of 68 subjects participated in this study: 16 patients with DAT; 13 HD patients; eight demented PD patients; nine nondemented PD patients; 12 elderly control subjects; and 10 middle-aged control subjects. The demented PD patients all obtained DRS scores that were at least two standard deviations below the mean of the elderly control subjects (i.e., less than 134). The nondemented PD group, in contrast, did not differ significantly on the DRS from either control group. All PD patients were rated from 0 (absence of symptoms) to 4 (greatest severity) on each of the three classic parkinsonian symptoms (i.e., tremor, rigidity, and bradykinesia). Ten of the HD patients were also rated with a five-point scale for the severity of their choreiform movements.

The lexical priming paradigm used in this study was adapted from that used by Shimamura et al. (1987). Briefly, subjects were shown 10 words (e.g., motel, abstain) one at a time and were asked to rate how much they liked each word on a five-point scale. Three additional filler words were placed at the beginning of the list and two at the end in order to reduce primacy and recency effects, respectively. After the subjects completed this initial rating of the entire set of 10 words, the examiner requested that they perform a second rating of the same words presented in the same order. Following the two presentation trials, subjects were shown 20 three-letter word stems (e.g., mot, abs) and were asked to complete each stem with the first word that came to mind. Ten of the stems could be completed using study words, and the other 10 stems were used to assess baseline guessing rates. The entire stem-completion study/test procedure was then repeated in exactly the same manner using a different list of 10 words. In this way, stem completion was assessed twice, using two different lists of 10 words.

The procedure for the pursuit rotor task was identical to that used in the previously described study by Heindel, Butters, and Salmon (1988).

As can be seen in Figure 5.5, all six subject groups began the pursuit rotor task at about the same level of performance (i.e., 25% time on target). Despite these similar initial levels, the HD and demented PD groups both demonstrated significantly less learning over the six test blocks than did their control groups (Figure 5.6). The HD and demented PD groups, though not differing significantly from each other, also demonstrated significantly less motor learning than did both the DAT and nondemented PD groups. In contrast, the Alzheimer and nondemented PD patients did not differ from their controls in the amount they learned on this task.

The motor learning ability of the HD patients was found to be significantly correlated with their scores on the DRS but not with the severity of their choreiform movements. Similarly, the performance of the PD patients (demented and nondemented combined) was significantly correlated with DRS but not with the severity of their tremor, rigidity, or bradykinesia. Thus motor learning in both HD and PD patients appears to be related more to the severity of their dementia than to the severity of their motor dysfunction.

The results of the lexical priming task are shown in Figure 5.7. Baseline guessing rates (dotted lines) did not differ across the groups, indicating that the subject groups were very similar in their ability to perform the basic stem-completion task. Although the HD and nondemented PD groups demonstrated normal priming ability, the DAT and demented PD groups were both severely impaired relative to their control groups. Furthermore, the HD and demented PD groups were both impaired in their

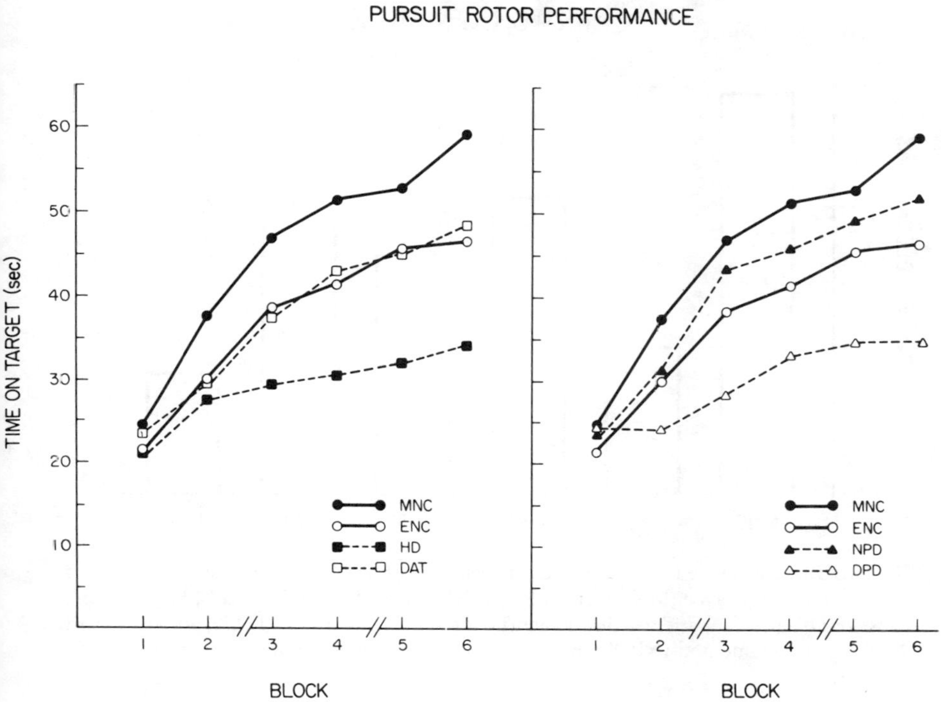

FIGURE 5.5 Performance of middle-aged (MNC) and elderly (ENC) normal control subjects, Huntington's disease (HD) patients, patients with dementia of the Alzheinmer type (DAT), and demented (DPD) and nondemented (NPD) Parkinson's disease patients on the pursuit rotor task. (Adapted from Heindel et al., 1989.)

priming ability compared to the HD and nondemented PD groups, but did not differ significantly from each other.

Besides providing a replication of the previously reported dissociations between HD and DAT patients on the two implicit memory tasks (Heindel, Butters, and Salmon, 1988; Shimamura et al., 1987), these findings suggest that demented PD patients may not fit neatly into Cummings and Benson's (1984) "cortical-subcortical" taxomony of dementia. The impaired performances of the demented PD patients on both pursuit rotor and lexical priming tasks indicate that these patients share some common features with both HD and DAT patients. The demented PD patients' deficiencies in acquiring motor skills may be caused by their basal ganglia dysfunction, whereas their lack of lexical priming may have its origins in neuropathological changes in cortical association areas. It appears likely then that previous attempts to define the dementia of PD may have been hampered by the failure to recognize the coexistence of both "cortical" and "subcortical" features within the same disease.

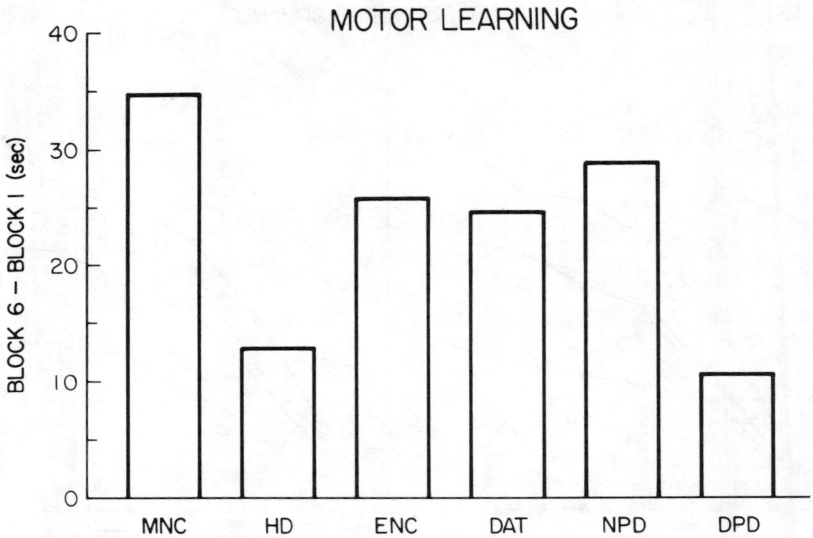

FIGURE 5.6 Difference in performance between the last and first test blocks on the pursuit rotor task for middle-aged (MNC) and elderly (ENC) normal control subjects, Huntington's disease (HD) patients, patients with dementia of the Alzheimer type (DAT), and demented (DPD) and nondemented (NPD) Parkinson's disease patients. (Adapted from Heindel et al., 1989.)

CONCLUSIONS

The neuropsychological studies reviewed in this chapter are consistent with the notion that patients with dementias of different etiologies can be differentiated from each other and from patients with amnesic conditions. Although both DAT and HD patients are impaired on episodic and semantic memory tasks, they seem to fail for quite distinct reasons. The HD patients' capacity to store new verbal information seems relatively preserved, but these patients appear extremely deficient in initiating systematic retrieval strategies when asked to recall information from either episodic or semantic memory. In contrast, patients with DAT encounter unusual difficulty in consolidating new information, and their attempts to recall information from semantic memory are often hindered by their dysphasia. The deleterious effects of proactive interference are also more apparent in the episodic and semantic memory deficits of DAT than of HD patients.

Investigations focusing on the learning of motor skills and other types of implicit memory usually preserved in amnesic patients suggest additional dissociations between cortical and subcortical dementias. Although HD patients appear severely impaired in their attempts to acquire motor skills, they perform normally on stem-completion priming tasks. The opposite relationship is seen in patients with DAT.

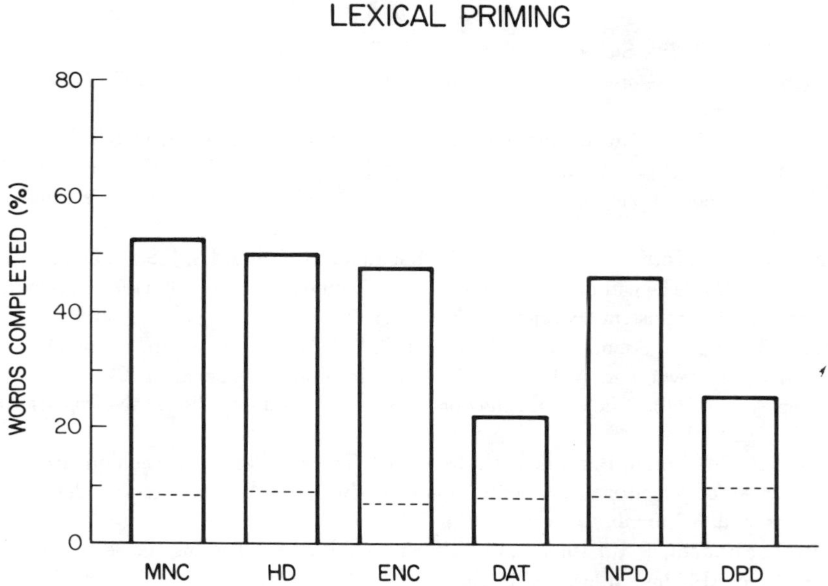

FIGURE 5.7 The percentage of work stems completed with previously presented words on the lexical priming task by middle-aged (MNC) and elderly (ENC) normal control subjects, Huntington's disease (HD) patients, patients with dementia of the Alzheimer type (DAT), and demented (DPD) and nondemented (NPD) Parkinson's disease patients. (Adapted from Heindel et al., 1989.)

Alzheimer patients acquire and retain motor skills with the same facility as intact controls and amnesic patients, but they evidence little tendency to complete three-letter stems with words previously exposed to them. These findings suggest that the learning of motor skills and stem-completion priming depend on different neuroanatomical systems and lend support to the previously proposed distinction between cortical and subcortical dementias. The impaired performances of demented PD patients on both tests of implicit memory suggest the presence of both cortical and subcortical dysfunctions in this disorder.

From a clinical perspective, it is important to stress again that the present findings emanate from the application of concepts borrowed from cognitive psychology and from careful analyses of the processes underlying the patients' achievements and deficits. These demonstrations of the utility of experimental concepts with pathological populations also provide the constructs themselves with a form of validity and legitimacy unavailable through studies limited to normal subjects. In our view, the mutual benefits that have been described represent an ideal model for the interaction between experimental and clinical approaches in neuropsychology.

REFERENCES

Albert, M. L. (1978). Subcortical dementia. In R. Katzman, R. D. Terry, & K. L. Bick (eds.), *Alzheimer's disease: Senile dementia and related disorders* (pp. 173-180). New York: Raven Press.

Albert, M. S., & Kaplan, E. (1980). Organic implications of neuropsychological deficits in the elderly. In L. Poon, J. Fozard, L. Cermak, D. Arenberg, & L. Thompson (Eds.), *New directions in memory and aging* (pp. 403-432). Hillsdale, NJ: Lawrence Erlbaum Associates.

Alvord, E. C. Jr., Forno, L. S., Kusske, J. A., Kauffman, R. J., Rhodes, J. S., & Goetowski, C. R. (1974). The pathology of parkinsonism: A comparison of degeneration in cerebral cortex and brainstem. *Advances in Neurology, 5*, 175-193.

Arendt, T., Bigl, V., Arendt, A., & Tennstedt, A. (1983). Loss of neurons in the nucleus basalis of Meynert in Alzheimer's disease. *Acta Neuropathologica*, 61:101–108.

Benton, A. L. (1968). Differential behavioral effects in frontal lobe disease. *Neuropsychologia*, 6, 53-60.

Blessed, G., Tomlinson, B. E., & Roth, M. (1968). The association between quantitative measures of dementia and of senile change in the cerebral grey matter of elderly subjects. *British Journal of Psychiatry*, 114, 797–811.

Boller, F., Mizutani, T., Roessmann, U., & Gambetti, P. (1980). Parkinson disease, dementia, and Alzheimer disease: Clinicopathological correlations. *Annals of Neurology*, 7, 329–335.

Borkowski, J. G., Benton, A. L., & Spreen, O. (1967). Word fluency and brain damage. *Neuropsychologia*, 5, 135–140.

Brooks, V. B. (1986). *The neural basis of motor control*. New York: Oxford University Press.

Brown, R. G., & Marsden, C. D. (1984). How common is dementia in Parkinson's disease? *Lancet*, 2:1262–1265.

Brun, A. (1983). An overview of light and electron microscopic changes. In B. Reisberg (Ed.), *Alzheimer's disease* (pp. 37-47). New York: Free Press.

Butters, N. (1984). The clinical aspects of memory disorders: Contributions from experimental studies of amnesia and dementia. *Journal of Clinical Neuropsychology,* 6(1):17–36.

Butters, N. (1985). Alcoholic Korsakoff's Syndrome: Some unresolved issues concerning etiology, neuropathology and cognitive deficits. *Journal of Clinical and Experimental Neuropsychology*, 7(2):181–210.

Butters, N., Albert, M. S., Sax, D. S., Miliotis, P., Nagode, P., & Sterste, A. (1983). The effect of verbal mediators on the pictorial memory of brain-damaged patients. *Neuropsychologia, 21*,307–323.

Butters, N., & Cermak, L. S. (1980). *Alcoholic Korsakoff's Syndrome: An Information Processing Approach to Amnesia*. New York: Academic Press.

Butters, N., Granholm, E., Salmon D. P., Grant, I., & Wolfe, J. (1987). Episodic and semantic memory: A comparison of amnesic and demented patients. *Journal of Clinical and Experimental Neuropsychology,* 9, 479–497.

Butters, N., Sax, D., Montgomery, K., & Tarlow, S. (1978). Comparison of the neuropsychological deficits associated with early and advanced Huntington's Disease. *Archives of Neurology, 35*, 585–589.

Butters, N., Wolfe, J., Granholm, E., & Martone, M. (1986). An assessment of verbal recall, recognition and fluency abilities in patients with Huntington's Disease. *Cortex, 22*, 11–32.

Butters, N., Wolfe, J., Martone, M., Granholm, E., & Cermak, L. S. (1985). Memory disorders associated with Huntington's Disease: Verbal recall, verbal recognition and procedural memory. *Neuropsychologia*, 23(6):729–743.

Caine, E. D., Hunt, R. D., Weingartner, H., & Ebert, M. H. (1978). Huntington's dementia: Clinical and neuropsychological features. *Archives of General Psychiatry*, 35, 377–384.

Cermak, L. S., Lewis, R., Butters, N., & Goodglass, H. (1973). Role of verbal mediation in performance of motor tasks by Korsakoff patients. *Perceptual and Motor Skills*, 37, 259–262.

Cermak, L. S., Uhly, B., & Reale, L. (1980). Encoding specificity in the alcoholic Korsakoff patient. *Brain and Language, 11*, 119–127.

Cohen, N. J., & Squire, L. R. (1980). Preserved learning and retention of pattern analyzing skills in amnesia: Dissociation of knowing how and knowing that. *Science, 210*,207–210.

Corkin, S. (1968). Acquisition of motor skill after bilateral medial temporal-lobe excision. *Neuropsychologia*, 6, 255–265.

Cummings, J. L., & Benson, D. F. (1984). Subcortical dementia: Review of an emerging concept. *Archives of Neurology, 41*(8):874–879.

Eslinger, P. J., & Demasio, A. R. (1986). Preserved motor learning in Alzheimer's Disease: Implications for anatomy and behavior. *Journal of Neuroscience,* 6, 3006–3009.

Evarts, E. V., & Wise, S. P. (1984). Basal ganglia outputs and motor control. In D. Evered & M. O'Connor (Eds.), *Functions of the basal ganglia: Ciba foundation symposium 107* (pp. 83-102). London: Pitman Press.

Folstein, M. F., Folstein, S. E., & McHugh, P. R. (1975). "Mini-Mental State": A practical method for grading the cognitive state of patients for the clinician. *Journal of Psychiatric Research, 12*, 189–198.

Fuld, P. (1978). Psychological testing in the differential diagnosis of the dementias. In R. Katzman, R. D. Terry, & K. L. Bick (Eds.), *Alzheimer's disease: Senile dementia and related disorders* (pp. 185-193). New York: Raven Press.

Fuld, P. A. (1983). Word intrusion as a diagnostic sign in Alzheimer's Disease. *Geriatric Medicine Today, 2*, 33–41.

Fuld, P. A., Katzman, R., Davies, P., & Terry, R. D. (1982). Intrusions as a sign of Alzheimer's dementia: Chemical and pathological verification. *Annals of Neurology, 11*, 155–159.

Graf, P., & Schacter, D. L. (1985). Implicit and explicit memory for new associations in normal and amnesic subjects. *Journal of Experimental Psychology [Learning Memory Cognition], 11*(3), 501–518.

Granholm, E., & Butters, N. (1988). Associative encoding and retrieval in Alzheimer's and Huntington's disease. *Brain and Cognition, 7*:335–347.

Groves, P. M. (1983). A theory of the functional organization of the neostriatum and the neostriatal control of voluntary movement. *Brain Research Reviews, 5*: 109–132.

Heindel, W. C., Butters, N., & Salmon, D. P. (1988). Impaired learning of a motor skill in patients with Huntington's disease. *Behavioral Neuroscience*, 102, 141–147.

Heindel, W. C., Salmon, D., Shults, C., Walicke, P., & Butters, N. I. (1989). Neuropsychological evidence of multiple implicit memory systems: A comparison of Alzheimer's, Huntington's, and Parkinson's Disease patients. *Journal of Neuroscience*, 9(2), 582–587.

Huber, S. J., Shuttleworth, E. C., Paulson, G. W., Bellchambers, M. J., & Clapp, L. E. (1986). Cortical vs subcortical dementia: Neuropsychological differences. *Archives of Neurology, 43*(4), 392–394.

Kemp, J. M., & Powell, T. P. S. (1970). The cortico-striate projection in the monkey. *Brain*, 93, 525–546.

Lieberman, A., Dziatolowski, M., Kupersmith, M., Serby, M., Goodgold, A., Korein, J., & Goldstein, M. (1979). Dementia in Parkinson disease. *Annals of Neurology*, 6, 355–359.

Martin, A. (1987). Representation of semantic and spatial knowledge in Alzheimer's patients: Implications for models of preserved learning in amnesia. *Journal of Clinical & Experimental Neuropsychology*, 9, 191–224.

Martin, A., Brouwers, P., Cox, C., & Fedio, P. (1985). On the nature of the verbal memory deficit in Alzheimer's disease. *Brain and Language, 25*, 323–341.

Martin, A., & Fedio, P. (1983). Word production and comprehension in Alzheimer's Disease: The breakdown of semantic knowledge. *Brain and Language, 19*, 124–141.

Martone, M., Butters, N., Payne, M., Becker, J. T., & Sax, D. S. (1984). Dissociations between skill learning and verbal recognition in amnesia and dementia. *Archives of Neurology*, 41(9), 965–970.

Mattis, S. (1976). Mental status examination for organic mental syndrome in the elderly patient. In L. Bellak & T. B. Karasu (Eds.), *Geriatric Psychiatry* (pp. 77–121). New York: Grune & Stratton.

Mayeux, R., Stern, Y., Rosen, J., & Benson, D. F. (1981). Subcortical dementia: A recognizable clincial entity. *Annals of Neurology, 10*, 100–101.

McKhann, G., Drachman, D., Folstein, M., Katzman, R., Price, D., & Stadlan, E. M. (1984). Clinical diagnosis of Alzheimer's Disease: Report of the NINCDS-ADRDA Work Group under the auspices of Department of Health and Human Services Task Force on Alzheimer's Disease. *Neurology, 34*, 939–944.

Milberg, W., Hebben, N., & Kaplan, E. (1986). The Boston process approach to neuropsychological assessment. In I. Grant & K. M. Adams (eds.), *Neuropsychological assessment of neuropsychiatric disorders* (pp. 65-86). New York: Oxford University Press.

Ober, B. A., Dronkers, N. F., Koss, E., Delis, D. C., & Friedland, R. P. (1986). Retrieval from semantic memory in Alzheimer-type dementia. *Journal of Clinical & Experimental Neuropsychology*, 8(1):75–92.

Parkinson, J. (1817). *An essay on the shaking palsy*. London: Sherwood, Neely, & Jones.

Rosen, W. G. (1980). Verbal fluency in aging and dementia. *Journal of Clinical Neuropsychology, 2*, 135–146.

Salmon, D. P., Shimamura, A. P., Butters, N., & Smith, S. (1988). Lexical and semantic priming deficits in patients with Alzheimer's disease. *Journal of Clinical & Experimental Neuropsychology*, 10, 477–494.

Schacter, D. L. (1987). Implicit memory: History and current status. *Journal of Experimental Psychology [Learning Memory Cognition], 13*, 501–517.

Shimamura, A. P., Salmon, D. P., Squire, L. R., & Butters, N. (1987). Memory dysfunction and word priming in dementia and amnesia. *Behavioral Neuroscience, 101*, 347–351.

Shindler, A. G., Caplan, L. R., & Hier, D. B. (1984). Intrusions and perseverations. *Brain and Language, 23*, 148–158.

Squire, L. R. (1987). *Memory and brain*. New York: Oxford University Press.

Terry, R. D., & Katzman, R. (1983). Senile dementia of the Alzheimer type. *Annals of Neurology, 14*:497–506.

Thomson, D. M., & Tulving, E. (1970). Associative encoding and retrieval: Weak and strong cues. *Journal of Experimental Psychology, 86*, 255–262.

Tulving, E. (1983). *Elements of episodic memory*. New York: Oxford University Press.

Tulving, E., & Thomson, D. M. (1973). Encoding specificity and retrieval processes in episodic memory. *Psychology Review, 80*,352–373.

Victor, M., Adams, R. D., & Collins, G. H. (1971). *The Wernicke-Korsakoff syndrome*. Philadelphia: F. A. Davis.

Weingartner, H., Grafman, J., Boutelle, W., Kaye, W., & Martin, P. R. (1983). Forms of memory failure. *Science, 221*,380–382.

Winocur, G., & Weiskrantz, L. (1976). An investigation of paired-associate learning in amnesic patients. *Neuropsychologia*, 14,97–110.

ACKNOWLEDGMENTS

The research reported in this manuscript was supported by funds from the Medical Research Service of the Veterans Administration, by NIAAA grant AA-00187 to Boston University, and by NIA grant AG-05131 to the University of California at San Diego. Portions of this chapter are based on a manuscript, "Processes underlying the memory impairments of demented patients," published in E. Goldberg (Ed.), (1989). *Contemporary neuropsychology and the legacy of Luria* (pp. 99–126). New Jersey: Erlbaum.

6

Assessment of Secondary Memory Function in Dementia

James L. Mack, Marian B. Patterson, and Nancy L. Adams

In preceding chapters, memory has been described as a dynamic, complex process that changes with age in some respects but is stable in others. The concept of memory described in this volume represents a major change from concepts in vogue not too many years ago. Consequently, the manner in which clinicians have traditionally approached memory assessment is outdated. It is no longer appropriate to think of memory as a single process, isolated from other cognitive or conative functions. One must seek assessment techniques capable of distinguishing aspects of memory function relevant to a particular clinical question. Further, one should expect continuing changes in our understanding of memory, changes that will require commensurate changes in assessment approaches. To meet these needs, we have utilized techniques that allow the application of theoretical constructs to the individual assessment of memory in a manner that we hope will be adaptable to future developments.

In this chapter we will first discuss general considerations in the clinical assessment of memory. Second, we will describe some techniques of memory assessment. Third, we will present case material to demonstrate how these techniques can be used in the context of a particular clinical problem.

NEUROPSYCHOLOGICAL EVALUATION IN DEMENTIA

Purpose

There are several reasons that a neuropsychological evaluation of a demented patient may be requested:

Differential Diagnosis

The neuropsychologist may be asked for assistance in providing a differential diagnosis. The evaluation may be used to determine the presence of cognitive impairment; the nature of that impairment (whether it is global or specific and, if specific, what functions are affected); and whether depression or other psychiatric disorders play a role in the patient's illness.

Identifying the Basis of a Complaint

The neuropsychologist may be asked to explain the basis of specific symptoms. While many patients complain of problems in retrieving old information or learning new information, similar complaints may stem from quite different problems. Detailed testing is often required to determine just what cognitive deficits underlie the patient's complaints.

Evaluation of Future Change

A neuropsychological evaluation may be requested to establish a baseline to measure disease progress or response to treatment. Unless the nature of the expected treatment effect or the disease progression is highly specific, a comprehensive evaluation of memory may be important in identifying not only the presence but also the nature of the patient's change in function.

Development of a Treatment Program

Testing may be required to provide a basis for establishing a treatment program for the amelioration of or compensation for the patient's deficits. As memory rehabilitation becomes more sophisticated, it is becoming increasingly important to identify just what aspects of memory are being targeted by a specific treatment program.

Considerations Guiding the Evaluation

Subjects differ with respect to a number of variables that may influence performance on memory tasks. These variables include relatively stable or slowly changing values such as age, intelligence, educational level, vocational and avocational experience, general physical health, and personality type.

The general medical state of the patient may provide critical information to direct the memory assessment. Is there a history of stroke, tumor, encephalitis, head injury, alcohol abuse, or other condition known to be associated with memory deficits? Is the subject taking medications that may influence directly or indirectly cognitive performance? Sensory functioning is also important, especially in assessment of the elderly. Decrements of vision or hearing can interfere with processing test stimuli in ways that may be hard to detect or to separate from cognitive defects.

Other subject variables that influence performance on memory tasks but are less stable in their effects include the specific physical and emotional condition of the subject at the time of testing. Although enduring, disease-related deficits are often relatively obvious, more variable physical factors may be equally important but less obvious influences. Similarly, both the subject's long-standing personality adjustment and his or her present emotional state may be important determiners of performance on memory testing. The presence of acute depression or anxiety and their effects on the subject's memory performance are usually readily observable. It is important, however, not to lose sight of long-standing behavioral patterns that may also influence that performance. A subject's results on memory testing may be greatly affected, for example, by tendencies to be impulsive or make questionable judgments, to be cautious and conservative, or to be overwhelmed by failure or task difficulty.

Performance on tests of memory is particularly susceptible to motivational level, which should be carefully assessed. Does the subject appear to be making a serious effort to remember, or does he or she seem to lack motivation on some or all of the tests? What is behind the lack of effort? Are there rewards for not doing well, such as receiving financial assistance, relief from responsibilities, or satisfaction of a need to be dependent? Is the subject so fatigued, stressed, preoccupied, or depressed that he or she has an overwhelmingly negative self-concept and expects failure?

The clinician is occasionally asked to evaluate a subject who, because of depression, distrust, or disagreement about the need for testing, is uninterested or frankly uncooperative. Before administering any tests, the clinician must spend the time necessary to gain the subject's cooperation. Most subjects eventually accept being tested, though considerable examiner effort may be necessary to achieve such cooperation. If the subject remains resistant and uncooperative, the likelihood of obtaining useful information is small, and testing is probably not worth attempting, even when the reason for referral is critical.

A carefully obtained, detailed history of a subject's complaints is crucial to accurate assessment of memory. When did the problems begin, and what has been their course? Was the onset acute or insidious, and is the deficit static or progressive? Perhaps the most common mistake made by inexperienced examiners is to fail to delineate the precise nature of the subject's memory problem. Does the subject complain of failure to learn new information or to retrieve old, familiar information? When a subject complains of inability to acquire new information, are whole episodes absent from memory, or does the subject simply recall episodes that are lacking in detail? When a retrieval failure occurs, is the subject helped by cuing or reminding (i.e., do more details come to mind or does the target information seem familiar following cuing)? Does the subject experience difficulty in learning information globally, or is the problem specific to the verbal or nonverbal nature of the material?

In seeking answers to these questions regarding the nature of the subject's complaints, it is usually necessary to ask for specific examples, confirmed whenever possible by another person. Examples are important, because most persons have little insight into memory processes and will rarely specify their problems along dimensions useful to the assessment of memory. Indeed, many subjects actually obscure the underlying problem by focusing on an aspect of their problem that is, to the examiner, relatively incidental. A number of memory questionnaires, suitable for use with both subjects and caregivers, are available for clinical use and may help examiners elicit comprehensive information regarding memory function (c.f. Herrmann, 1982, and Gilewski & Zelinski, 1986, for a general review of memory questionnaires).

Determination of the precise nature of the subject's complaints is important for several reasons. To the extent that the complaints suggest a particular basis for the subject's memory problem, the examiner can select the tests maximally useful in delineating the subject's deficits. Further, if the examiner can interpret test findings by demonstrating how a patient's complaints can be explained by the underlying deficits, the results are made meaningful to a subject or subject's family. Consequently, the likelihood that any suggestions regarding therapeutic or ameliorative procedures are followed is increased.

Evaluation of Nonspecifc Cognitive Abilities That Affect Secondary Memory Function

Baddeley (1982) has made an important distinction between types of memory disorder. In an unfortunately confusing, though understandable, choice of terminology, Baddeley identifies what he calls *primary amnesia*, a gross difficulty in learning new material (i.e., secondary memory impairment) characteristic of the classic amnesic syndrome. The classic amnesic syndrome is distinguished from a far more common memory problem that he terms *secondary amnesia*, in which the memory problem is a secondary consequence of some deficit or deficits in the ability of the subject to process information (e.g., a deficit in primary memory). An evaluation of memory disorder should be able to distinguish between these two very different problems.

A good assessment of attention, or primary memory, is essential to assessing secondary memory, because, generally speaking, in order to remember something one must first have registered it adequately. Attentional problems are very common in dementia, and they sometimes account for a good deal of what subjects experience or interpret as memory problems.

Several aspects of attentional ability should be included in a comprehensive assessment. The first is the immediate *span of attention*. This is most frequently assessed by asking the subject to repeat sequences of digits of gradually increasing length. A number of investigators have found the serial recall of digits (Kopelman, 1985), letters (Morris, 1984), and words (Corkin, 1982; Morris, 1984) to be impaired in demented subjects, although others have found the repetition of digits to be relatively spared (Bayles, 1982; Tweedy et al., 1982). Using visually presented, nonverbal, and less familiar stimuli, however, investigators have found substantial deficits in immediate span of attention in demented subjects, even though digit span was relatively less affected (Cantone et al., 1978; Grossi, Orsini, & Ridente, 1977; Winegardner & Mack, 1982). A useful method of evaluating attention span is to use a nonverbal stimulus such as the Knox Cubes (Bornstein, 1983), in which the subject is asked to repeat the exact sequence in which a row of four blocks have been touched. Performance can then be contrasted with that on an analogous span task in which the subject is asked to touch a row of four written digits in the same sequence in which they were presented auditorily (Winegardner & Mack, 1982).

In addition to span, the subject's *breadth of attention*, the ability to divide one's attention between several sources of stimulation, should be tested. This is done by giving a task in which a subject must hold more than one thing in primary memory at a given moment. For example, the subject can be presented a small amount of information, something well within the limitations of attention span such as three letters or words, and then distracted briefly by an interfering task, such as counting backwards or carrying out a serial addition or subtraction task (the Brown-Peterson technique; Brown, 1958). Substantial deficits in Alzheimer disease patients have been reported on the Brown-Peterson task (Corkin, 1982; Kopelman, 1985; Morris, 1986).

There are additional aspects of attention likely to be affected in dementia, which, when impaired, may have debilitating effects on secondary memory. However, these functions are usually not formally tested. *Freedom from distractibility* can be measured by experimental tasks in which an ongoing activity is randomly interrupted by interfering stimulation. *Sustained attention*, or vigilance, is usually evaluated by tasks requiring subjects to continue a relatively simple, repetitive task for periods of a half an hour or more to determine whether error rate increases over time. Typically, however, problems with distractibility and sustained attention have not been formally measured but simply observed in the clinical assessment of subjects. Indeed, examiners have usually attempted to eliminate interference and to switch from one task to another to minimize the effects of distractibility and vigilance deficits on secondary memory task performance. A related issue concerns brief fluctuations in efficiency often noted in the performance of demented subjects. Such fluctuations may not represent an attentionally based deficit but instead may be related to executive disabilities, although they can certainly be considered in the context of Baddeley's concept of a central executive system in working memory (Baddeley, 1983; 1986). A discussion of working memory, however, is beyond the scope of this chapter (c.f. Chapter 1).

Executive abilities (Lezak, 1983) represent another area of cognition that has an important effect on secondary memory function. Executive abilities refer to a subject's ability to organize and carry out a plan of action, and consist of the following aspects: (1) identification of a need state (i.e., that there is a problem to solve); (2) formulation of a goal and a plan to achieve it; (3) initiating the activity necessary to implement the plan and work toward the goal; (4) monitoring of goal-directed activity, including appropriate modification of that activity; and (5) cessation of the activity once the goal is accomplished.

There is no single task that reflects all aspects of executive abilities. Failure to identify need states is often indicated by gross passivity, which may be overcome by providing a subject with direction (Lezak, 1983). Subjects who lack spontaneity, appear apathetic, and fail to initiate activity may appear depressed because they no longer seem to become involved in their former activities. However, careful evaluation can usually demonstrate that they show none of the cognitive, conative, or vegetative signs of depression and that they respond to the immediate directing and organizing efforts of the examiner, i.e., that the underlying problem is an executive deficit.

A test like the Porteus Maze Test (Porteus, 1965) is useful for assessing a subject's capacity for mental planning and organization. The Tinker Toy test, described by Lezak (1983), may be better at tapping the initiation of goal-directed activity. The Cognitive Estimation Test (Shallice & Evans, 1978), which we use in a form modified for U.S. residents, appears sensitive to deficits in monitoring ongoing behavior and is often quite useful in identifying defective judgment. Especially important in assessing executive abilities is the process by which the subject goes about solving the problems presented by the tasks. Careful observation will usually reveal a failure to initiate, monitor and correct, or appropriately terminate the activity.

Subjects with defective ability to organize their thinking and behavior will have great difficulty getting material into memory in a form that can be easily retrieved. They may also use ineffective strategies for learning and be quite unsystematic in attempting to retrieve information at recall. For example, one nonverbal memory test requires a subject to copy a complicated geometric figure and then, after a delay interval, reproduce it from memory. Subjects whose initial copying was unsystematic and disorganized have a much more difficult task in recalling the figure than subjects whose original copy was organized in such a way that they can retrieve major structural elements of the design and then fill in the details.

The Value of Various Approaches

There are a number of tests and procedures available for the assessment of memory (Erickson & Scott, 1977; Erickson, Poon, & Walsh-Sweeney, 1980). They vary with respect to such factors as the means by which the stimuli are presented, the nature of the stimuli to be remembered, and the way in which what the subject has remembered is evaluated. Each of these factors may affect the way in which a specific memory impairment is revealed. Therefore, to determine the nature of the underlying deficit and what can be done about it, it is useful to work with a set of tests that include a number of procedures to reveal the full nature of a particular memory deficit.

Presentation of the Stimuli to be Remembered

Tests vary with respect to the number of times that information is presented and the amount of information presented in a single trial. When material is presented only once, the task is often referred to as a memory test, while tasks with more than one presentation are called learning tests. The effect of multiple presentations of the stimuli, however, is primarily a reduction in the attentional demands of the task.

A popular *one-trial memory* task is a recall of a prose paragraph, such as the Logical Memory subtest from the Wechsler Memory Scale-Revised (Wechsler, 1987).* Prose recall tasks are usually presented aloud, and subjects are asked to recall the story both immediately after its presentation and following a delay interval. The stories typically consist of an amount of information that far exceeds a subject's span of attention. Subjects must be able not only to register long strings of information but to hold what they have just heard in their mind while they are attending to the following sentences. Because of the heavy information load, subjects with limited attention span or difficulty in dividing their attention are likely to perform quite poorly, even though they may have a perfectly intact secondary memory. Their poor performance on what is nominally a secondary memory task is thus a consequence of a more general problem.

Some one-trial memory tasks, however, such as complex visual design copying (e.g., the Rey-Osterrieth Figure; Lezak, 1983), minimize attentional demands, because the subect is allowed unlimited time to copy the design and typically spends considerable time examining it in order to organize the copying task. Thus, adequate recall of a complex design copying task suggests that secondary memory is not globally deficient, even if a subject's prose recall performance is quite

*For an extensive description of the Wechsler Memory Scale-Revised see *The Clinical Neuropsychologist* 2:(2), March, 1988.

impaired. Obviously there are other important differences between prose and design recall tasks, differences that will be discussed subsequently.

If attentional deficits are thought to be interfering with the evaluation of secondary memory, memory tests that involve *multi-trial stimulus presentations* should be used. List learning tests (Rey, 1964; Buschke & Fuld, 1974; Delis et al., 1987) are probably the most common type of multi-trial memory test, although the Wechsler Memory Scale-Revised (Wechsler, 1987) includes a brief multi-trial paired associate learning test. On list learning tests, subjects with attentional deficits typically demonstrate slow acquisition; normal subjects can usually repeat six to seven words per trial, while attentionally impaired subjects may register only two or three and thus take longer to learn the list. If a subject's deficits are limited to attentional problems, however, with additional trials he or she should be able to master the list at a normal level and retain what has been learned over a delay interval.

List learning tests do present some practical difficulties. Elderly subjects frequently find list learning and other "laboratory" techniques artificial and not representative of everyday learning situations. Consequently, they may be poorly motivated to perform. Some test developers have attempted to minimize this problem by using items on the list that represent a practical memory task, for example, remembering a list of items to be purchased at the grocery store. The actual importance of making the memory task a "practical" one remains to be determined. A further problem with list learning tasks is that they take a long time to administer. The number of learning trials may be limited, but then the advantage of a list learning test is reduced, since there is less opportunity for a subject to compensate for attentional deficits. We believe that the effect of attentional problems on the memory performance of demented subjects is so great and the compensatory techniques needed to deal with "primary" and "secondary" amnesia (Baddeley, 1982) so different that the time required for more trials is more than justified.

In some cases it is relevant to consider the *sensory modality of the stimulus*. In evaluating demented subjects, the sensory modality of the test stimuli is usually only critical when sensory loss prevents the presentation of a test in the usual manner. Usually verbal stimuli are presented auditorily, although with subjects who have normal reading skills, they may be presented visually. Because of the spatial aspects involved in nonverbal processing tasks, nonverbal material is usually presented visually. However, some spatially demanding tests use tactual presentation (c.f. Lezak, 1983), and there are tests of nonverbal auditory stimuli using, for example, tunes or tonal patterns, which have been used experimentally. In practice, most memory tests confound sensory modality and the nature of the stimulus and are either auditory-verbal or visual-nonverbal.

It is worth noting that the *rate of stimulus presentation* can have an important impact on how well subjects are able to process it, whether they have the time to elaborate on it to help them remember it, and whether the memory will be interfered with by subsequent incoming information. In elderly and demented subjects, a presentation rate as slow as one item every five seconds can often demonstrate retained learning ability when faster presentation rates produce apparent deficits.

A final consideration is whether the learning is *intentional or incidental* (also referred to as "rehearsal-independent" in Chapter 2). On many tests subjects are specifically instructed to remember. On other tests, however, the subject is asked to recall without warning, a situation that often arises in everyday life. The strength of incidental learning is clearly related to the depth at which a subject processes information. On some tasks depth of processing is implicitly controlled. When, for example, a subject is asked to recall a complex design that was previously copied, it is reasonable to assume that the design must have been processed deeply in order to have been copied. On relatively effortless tasks such as object naming, however, an unexpected recall may reflect the depth at which subjects spontaneously process material and thus measure a relevant aspect of a subject's memory function.

Nature of the Stimuli to be Remembered

The nature of the material to be remembered is a critical influence on memory test performance. One factor that must be considered is the *complexity* of the stimulus, which must be distinguished from the information load. Stimuli that consists of a number of elements with complex interrelationships are easier to remember when they are processed in an organized, systematic fashion. To the extent that a subject cannot or does not use appropriate organizing strategies during the acquisition phase of a memory task, his or her recall is apt to be deficient. Indeed, many age-related memory deficits appear to be the result of failures of elderly subjects to avail themselves of organizing strategies when storing material for subsequent recall (cf., Chapter 2).

Many commonly used memory tests include complex stimuli that clearly require extensive organization if they are to be remembered efficiently. Story recall is perhaps minimally affected by organizational deficits since the basic gist of the story is evident to all but the most demented subjects; when subjects fail to grasp the gist of a brief story, it is usually because their attentional deficits have prevented them from registering crucial elements. Complex design copying and recall, however, demands considerable organizing ability. Subjects with impaired planning and organizational abilities have great difficulty recalling the design because copying is carried out in a disorganized, unsystematic fashion that does not facilitate identification of the basic elements of the design, which are usually easier to recall and on which additional details may be "mapped."

Most list learning tasks are also sensitive to organizational deficits. Subjects typically group recalled items in a consistent order, although the basis for that order may be quite subjective. The material to be remembered can be varied with respect to what cues are available for encoding, since material that is capable of being organized should be easier to remember if the subject is able to take advantage of that organization. It is much harder to remember twelve unrelated words than three distinct categories containing four words each. Some tests have not provided any obvious categories to promote intralist organization (Rey, 1964), others have lists of items all drawn from a single category (Buschke & Fuld, 1974), while others include items from several categories so that grouping within a category can be evaluated (Delis et al., 1987). The categories may be explicit, when the subject is told that there are categories to be remembered; or unmentioned, so that the examiner may see if the subject can discover and use organizational strategies to help his or her memory. If a list includes several categories of items, subjects with executive deficits or conceptual impairments (which hinder their ability to identify categories of items) may do poorly, though they may improve relative to normal subjects on tests whose items are not related. When evaluating subjects with executive or conceptual impairments, it would be ideal to see performance on lists with and without categorizable items under instructions that do and do not draw a subject's attention to the categories.

Another important aspect of the stimuli to be remembered is its *verbal or nonverbal* nature. Verbal memory tasks typically ask the subject to learn and/or recall factual information, past experience, brief stories, lists of words, or arbitrary pairs of words. Nonverbal memory tests include such tasks as complex design recall and maze learning. Often tests that are nominally verbal or nonverbal allow subjects to use more than one method of processing the stimulus information. "Verbal" material, for example, may be visualized, while "nonverbal" material may be named or otherwise verbally mediated. It is not always possible to determine how an individual subject is processing a given stimulus nor, consequently, whether that stimulus is functioning as intended. In general, nonverbal memory tests are more difficult to construct than verbal tests. Because people are by nature verbal beings, they tend to verbally mediate when possible. Tests that show the subject familiar objects to remember are readily verbally mediated. To avoid the use of verbal mediation, designers of nonverbal memory tests have used as stimuli complex geometric designs, abstract shapes or pictures, nonmeaningful spatial arrays or dot patterns, or abstract sound patterns (c.f. Lezak, 1983).

In patients with focal lesions, it is not uncommon to see material-specific memory deficits (e.g., a verbal memory deficit with intact nonverbal memory). Demented patients usually have global memory deficits, so that both verbal and nonverbal memory are affected. However, because demented patients often have additional cognitive deficits such as language or visual-spatial disabilities, a knowledge of the relative strengths of verbal and nonverbal memory is useful in designing treatment strategies.

Manner in Which Memory Is to be Tested

Memory tests vary with respect to how the quality and quantity of what the subject has remembered is evaluated. To evaluate what a subject remembers of a particular stimulus or episode, he or she may be asked to recall freely all that can be remembered, to respond to questions concerning specific aspects of the stimulus, to recall the stimulus in response to a cue, or to recognize the stimulus among several alternatives.

Free recall is one of the most commonly used techniques for assessing memory. Recall quality may be evaluated in terms of gross accuracy alone or with regard to its order (as in serial list learning techniques). An advantage of free recall testing is that it is usually quickly administered. Because ordering of the material to be remembered tends to facilitate recall, free recall testing is quite vulnerable to executive deficits. Furthermore, free recall is highly dependent on a subject's motivation, the extent to which he or she is willing to make an effort to retrieve the material. Free recall testing is therefore affected to a considerable degree in both primary and secondary amnesia (Baddeley, 1982). It is a sensitive measure of memory problems but is not particularly discriminating.

Some subjects may have actually stored information successfully but do poorly on free recall tasks, either because their retrieval strategies are inefficient or because they lack the motivation to search effortfully. Such subjects may be helped by direct questions concerning the stimulus content. In a story recall task, for example, the subject might be asked the identity of the main character, what happened first, or the point of the story. In a list learning test, the examiner might provide the name of a category in which some or all of the items fall. The next step in helping a subject overcome difficulties in organizing or mounting an effortful search is to provide partial information. Sometimes simply reading the first phrase or two of a story is sufficient to elicit good detail for its remainder.

When cued by questions or partial information, nearly all subjects will show some improvement over free recall. In the absence of normative data regarding the expected degree of improvement under conditions of cued recall, one must be conservative in concluding that a subject's memory is intact despite poor free recall performance. Nevertheless, some subjects are so strikingly accurate following cuing that the examiner can be confident that the poor free recall performance did not reflect defective secondary memory.

The end point of cuing is a recognition testing procedure. Among techniques of evaluating the quality of memory, recognition testing has generally been considered the least effortful and least sensitive to executive deficits (c.f. Chapter 2). Recognition testing is often used to demonstrate that learning has taken place in spite of little or no free recall, but this interpretation is subject to the same qualifications that apply to the use of partial cues to promote recall. One way to avoid this dilemma is to use a test that is standardized as a recognition memory test, such as Warrington's Recognition Memory Test (Warrington, 1984).

There are, however, potential misconceptions regarding the demands made by recognition memory testing. While it is true that recognition testing minimizes the role of organization and effortfulness when memory is tested, it is potentially susceptible to the effect of those factors at acquisition. If the stimulus to be recognized is highly complex or if a subject expends little effort in initially processing it, recognition accuracy will suffer. If, on the other hand, the stimuli are not amenable to organizational strategies (as in a long list of unrelated words), or they are presented very quickly or with instructions that do not lead to deep processing, then motivational or executive deficits are not likely to diminish recognition accuracy.

Recognition testing paradigms have several possible disadvantages. The subject may respond correctly by guessing. On a test with 50 two-choice items, for example, purely random responses would produce, on average, 25 correct answers, so that the effective range of the test is 25, not 50. Consequently, many alternatives or many test items must be included, so that testing takes longer than with recall procedures.

Recognition testing is often carried out by presenting one stimulus to be recognized at a time, so that the subject must identify whether it has been previously presented. When the subject is free to answer yes or no, bias can be an important influence on response accuracy. Some subjects may be quite conservative, hesitant to recognize a stimulus unless they are quite certain, while others may "recognize" nearly every stimulus, previously presented or not.

There are two ways of dealing with response bias. By changing the recognition procedure to a forced choice response in which a target and distractor are presented simultaneously and the subject must choose which of the two was previously presented, gross response bias may be avoided. This procedure is used in the Warrington Recognition Memory Test (1984). A problem with the forced choice procedure, however, is that by eliminating a subject's opportunity to demonstrate response bias, the examiner is prevented from observing a feature that may be quite significant clinically. A consistent response bias is likely to affect a subject's memory performance in real life as much as in the laboratory. Thus it may be preferable to use a single-item recognition procedure but to correct for response bias by using a mathematical technique such as signal detection analysis, which distinguishes the particular operating characteristics of the subject, bias, from his or her accuracy (Hannay, 1986).

A further way of testing for memory is to use a savings paradigm. The examiner presents a series of learning trials until the subject reaches a particular response criterion and then subsequently repeats the procedure to see if learning occurred at a faster rate. Using this procedure, some form of memory can at times be demonstrated, sometimes even if the subject has no explicit memory of the test at all (see Chapter 5).

From the foregoing considerations, it should be evident that secondary memory cannot be evaluated in isolation. No single method of presention of stimuli, type of stimulus, or testing of memory can provide a comprehensive picture of secondary memory.

Influence of Emotional Factors on Secondary Memory Function

It is well known that emotional factors have an impact on secondary memory. The differentiation of the effects of depression and dementia in aged subjects is a frequent diagnostic problem. Anxiety can have a profound impact on memory function. One occasionally sees selective memory loss as a result of emotional factors quite distinct from depression and anxiety, such as repression and denial. Further, emotional or characterological problems that can produce lack of cooperation, indifference, preoccupation, or withdrawal can have a major impact on secondary memory function. Consequently, the impact of emotional factors on memory must be an important consideration in any evaluation. In fact, there are times when a subject's emotional impediments to cooperation make it necessary to abandon testing until the basis for the subject's lack of cooperation can be dealt with. *The effects of depression on memory function* represent, perhaps, the most prevalent subject of investigation and have been recently reviewed (Poon, 1986; Caine, 1986; Kaszniak, Sadeh, & Stern, 1985). Experimental comparisons of the memory performance of depressed and nondepressed subjects vary widely in methodology, including both the selection of depressed subjects and the procedures used to assess memory. Furthermore, the application of experimental observations to individual cases can be hazardous, since clinical situations rarely replicate conditions in the original research. Even when significant effects of depression are found, there may be considerable overlap between depressed and nondepressed subjects. Also, many of the studies have been made on relatively young populations, and it is not certain to what extent their results can be generalized to the elderly. For the purposes of this discussion, we will briefly survey the effects of depression on memory in the elderly and present some guidelines for assessing these effects.

The first step in *differentiating the emotional and cognitive bases of memory problems* is to identify the nature of the patient's emotional problems. This step is not as simple as it may seem. Frequently, a subject's cognitive deficits may mimic the symptoms of emotional disturbance. Patients with executive deficits sometimes present a picture of limited initiative and inertia that can be confused with depression, or they may demonstrate an absence of reflection and self-monitoring that may suggest hysteria. Before considering the possible emotional bases of cognitive problems, it is important to evaluate the subject's emotional adjustment.

Many investigators in the studies of depression and memory have relied on the *DSM III-R* (American Psychiatric Association, 1987) or earlier diagnostic systems for the diagnosis of such conditions as major depressive disorder and dysthymic disorder. Frequently, however, when working with mildly affected subjects, diagnostic classification is not as useful as directly measuring the degree of emotional maladjustment. There are specific scales, for example, for measuring depression on the basis of examiner judgment (Gallagher, 1986) or self-rating (Yesavage, 1986).

Using specific scales for measuring a particular emotional difficulty is appealingly simple but poses some difficulties. In the first place, most scales have been developed and validated on relatively young subjects and may not be appropriate for the elderly. Recently, scales for rating depression in elderly subjects have become available (Alexopoulos et al., 1988; Yesavage, 1986), although their psychometric properties and validity are unclear simply because of their newness. Even with reliable scales that have been shown to be sensitive to a particular set of symptoms such as depression, another problem remains. Other significant psychological problems may be present in addition to the particular symptoms measured by the scale. As Caine (1986) reminds us in his discussion of "pseudodementia," emotional disorders other than depression can affect intellectual functioning. Measuring a single aspect of emotional adjustment, such as depression, may be appropriate for certain types of research, but in the clinical evaluation of a patient, a subject's overall personality adjustment should be evaluated to identify emotional problems that might affect performance on cognitive tasks.

Once the presence of emotional problems that may be affecting memory function has been established, the examiner must then determine the manner in which a subject's memory is actually affected. As we have discussed earlier in this chapter, memory is multifactorial. Research regarding the effects of, for example, depression on memory is useful in determining how these effects can be differentiated from the effects of both normal aging and dementia.

Although there is considerable divergence among the findings of existing studies, some findings are particularly relevant to the clincial evaluation of memory (cf., Niederehe, 1986). With depressive subjects in particular, subjective reports of memory problems may not be related to memory test performance (e.g., Kahn et al., 1975). Some investigators have found depressives to show a conservative response bias (i.e., a tendency to deny remembering information unless they are quite certain). Depressed subjects have also been noted to show decrements on tasks that require rapid processing of information or sustained effort. Many of these same findings have been reported in studies of normal elderly subjects. In both depressed and elderly subjects, decrements on memory testing have often been attributed to such factors as response bias, diminished processing speed, and reduction of effortful processing (Niederehe, 1986; Weingartner, 1986). It is not surprising, therefore, that both depressives and elderly subjects have been reported to show deficits on tests of arousal and attention. In contrast, both depressed and elderly subjects have performed relatively adequately on untimed tests and on tests that require relatively non-effortful processing.

Findings from the studies of elderly normal and depressed subjects suggest that before evaluating memory function in all of its varied aspects, the examiner might first look at performance on cognitive tasks with fewer sources of variance. Experimentally and clinically, depressed subjects and the elderly have been observed to perform relatively well on many tests of verbal and nonverbal abilities, as long as those tests did not require speed or sustained, effortful processing (including, for example, such tasks as picture naming and the Porteus Maze Test). In contrast, while demented subjects may do well on some relatively automatic, low-effort tasks they do poorly on tests of executive ability, not only with respect to working memory (Baddeley et al., 1986) but also on tests of general planning ability such as the Porteus Maze Test.

An important guideline in determining the source of a subject's impairment on a given task is, clearly, the extent to which effort is demanded by the task, and how much effort the subject has extended. The subject's reduced effort or motivation may be observable in the form of slowness, apathy, verbal and nonverbal indications of discouragement and futility, or an inability to be diverted from preoccupations or worries. As the case example that follows will illustrate, it is often possible to elicit improved performance by inducing a depressed subject temporarily to exert a greater effort. The subject is unlikely to sustain this effort over several tasks without enormous support and encouragement from the examiner, but without this time and effort, the evaluation may not be worth undertaking.

Once the subject has been evaluated on relatively automatic, untimed, low–effort demanding tasks and considerable effort has been expended to maximize his or her motivation, the examiner is ready to begin testing memory. Performance on primary memory tasks is not likely to help in the differentiation of depression and dementia, since not only depressed and demented subjects but the normal elderly as well have been found to show primary memory deficits (Niederehe, 1986). It is possible, however, to differentiate the performance of demented subjects from that of normal elderly and depressive on some secondary memory tasks. Acquisition of new information is reduced in normal aging, depression, and dementia. All three groups have been reported to fail to elaborate information spontaneously or to use deep encoding strategies such as organization, semantic association, or imagery. However, providing instructions to promote the use of appropriate strategies has been shown to improve the memory performance of elderly (Craik & Simon, 1980) and depressed (Niederehe, 1986) subjects but not that of demented subjects (Corkin, 1982).

Studies have also suggested that while normal elderly and depressed subjects may perform better in comparison to younger controls on recognition rather than recall testing, demented subjects do not (Niederehe, 1986). This last finding, however, illustrates one of the hazards in applying research results to clinical situations. One might presume that a good way to differentiate depression from dementia would be to contrast the subject's performance on free recall versus recognition memory tests; a demented subject would do poorly on both, while a depressed subject would be aided by the recognition procedure. Unfortunately, recognition performance will be accurate only if the subject has successfully encoded the information in memory. If the depression has interfered with the subject's ability to attend to the information as it is presented or reduced the effort he or she made to encode the information in some organized way, recognition performance is likely to be as poor as recall. The findings of research studies do not necessarily apply to the evaluation of individual subjects.

In the next section we will illustrate how the ideas presented in this chapter can be put into practice. It must be emphasized that we are interested in characterizing the nature of a subject's deficits rather than looking for tests to measure a particular dysfunction. Trying to differentiate between clinical syndromes by using specific tests with cutting scores does not seem to us to be a clinically useful endeavor. Performance on most tests is multi-determined; it is the result of more than one cognitive ability. Defects with respect to one ability may be compensated by utilization of another and the underlying cognitive deficit obscured. Or, alternatively, problems with respect to one of the factors underlying test performance could obscure relatively normal ability on another. In essence, neither high nor low scores on a single test necessarily reveal the nature of the problem underlying the test score. In a group of subjects as heterogeneous as we find in the study of dementia, it is likely that subjects receiving the same score on the same test might well have very different problems. Therefore it seems unlikely to us that performance on any specific test will provide a basis for the useful differentiation of subjects according to the etiology of their problem. Furthermore, research studies that evaluate the performance of two distinct groups on a cognitive task provide little help in dealing with patients who may very well have the problems of both groups.

Perhaps the more relevant criticism of the use of single tests to discriminate groups of subjects, however, is related to our interest in dealing with the specific complaints of each patient. Even if a test score correctly categorizes a subject and establishes that the basis of the memory problem is emotional or neurological, we would still know little about the nature of the subject's deficit. Consequently we would have difficulty making specific recommendations about what could be done to ameliorate the memory problems.

In summary, when beginning a clinical evaluation, the first consideration is a subject's background and presenting complaints and what is known about the disorder under investigation. In assessing the secondary memory of subjects who are possibly demented and/or emotionally disturbed, we are especially concerned with the subject's ability to handle complexity, to expend effort, to work under time constraints, to attend to incoming information, and to hold material briefly in primary memory while processing additional information.

Case Studies

Case 1

The first case is that of patient RE, a retired 55-year-old woman. She was referred for evaluation by a neurologist, who noticed that she was tearful at times and seemed depressed and questioned whether depression was causing her problems with attention, concentration, and memory.

RE completed high school with average grades and worked in a very demanding secretarial position for a large corporation until she stopped work to raise a family. Her hobbies included golf, flower arranging, and gardening. She lived with her husband and teen-age daughter and had two grown sons. RE complained that she felt overprotected by her family.

Her medical history included surgery in her thirties to remove breast cysts, a hysterectomy in her forties (following which she was treated with estrogen replacement therapy), and at about age 45, surgery to remove polyps from her throat. About 6 or 7 years before her neuropsychological evaluation, her husband thought she had become forgetful, and within the previous 2 or 3 years friends noticed lapses in her speech. Two years before testing, Alzheimer's disease was diagnosed, and RE dated the onset of her dysphoria from that time. There had been little change in her behavior during the 2 years prior to our evaluation, and consequently her neurologist had begun to question the diagnosis of dementia and to consider that her problems might simply be the result of depression.

Her problems included difficulty in remembering things she had done, such as where she put things or whether she had turned off the gas. Clearly such problems may be the result of impairment of attention rather than secondary memory. She also had difficulty independently carrying out familiar tasks, such as cooking meals, setting the table, and doing housework. In dressing she occasionally put on her clothing incorrectly. These latter tasks are often presented by patients and families as a memory disturbance ("She doesn't remember how to prepare a meal"), but they are frequently a consequence of executive deficits, problems in organizing and integrating familiar tasks.

RE had an extensive neuropsychological evaluation that included assessment of language, conceptual, and nonverbal abilities, attention, and executive functioning.* She demonstrated many deficits, although this discussion will focus on those tests that relate most directly to her memory function.

A useful way to begin the assessment of memory is to present a task that is sensitive to a wide variety of factors that influence memory in order to get a general index of the extent of the subject's problems. Recall of a brief story is sensitive

*The tests administered included the National Adult Reading Test, Wide Range Achievement Test—Revised (Arithmetic), Woodcock Reading Mastery Test (Passage Comprehension), Wisconsin Card Sorting Test, Weigl Color-Form Test, Cognitive Estimation Test, Oldfield-Wingfield Picture Naming Test with Recall, Controlled Word Search, Token Test (short form), Auditory Comprehension Test for Sentences, Dot Centering Test, Dot Cancellation Task, Benton Visual Retention Test (copy), Form Assembly Test, Finger Tapping, Grip Strength, Stereognosis Test with Recall, Auditory Verbal Sequencing Span, Nonverbal Sequencing Span, Verbal Divided Attention Task, Prose Recall Test, Visual Design Copying Test with Recall, Verbal Recognition Memory Test, Nonverbal Recognition Memory Test, Verbal List Learning Test, Minnesota Multiphasic Personality Inventory.

to most of the variables that influence memory, and subjects usually find it an acceptable, valid task. The following prose passage was read to RE:

> On a holiday trip to Boston a Texas cowboy left his dog with a friend and went out to purchase a new suit. Upon returning in fancy dress, the proud fellow whistled to his dog and attempted to pat him on the head. Instead of greeting his master, the confused pet failed to recognize him and fearfully backed away. The odd looking stranger took off the new hat and coat and put on his old clothes, and the happy dog jumped up eagerly and licked his face. Most animals are likely to act peculiar in unusual situations.

Her immediate recall of the story was as follows:

> "This is a story of a man and his dog, uh, going to, uh Texas. And uh . . . □ . . . it just seemed like it was going fine and then all of a sudden there were so many words it didn't come out."

Considerable encouragement produced no additional recollections. She recalled so little that it wasn't surprising that, when asked to recall the story 36 minutes later, she also did poorly:

> "This is the story of the dog and his master took him for a walk? and uh, I'm not, uh the master took the dog for a walk and there was a scramble or uh, that's it."

Again, extra time and encouragement availed her naught. To see if she retained more of the story than she could express on free recall, she was presented questions about the story and asked to select her answer from among five multiple choice alternatives. Although she had failed to recall substantial elements of the original story and had not grasped its basic gist, she did correctly recognize three items that she had failed to recall. Her overall performance was, nevertheless, well below average.

What are we to make of RE's performance? Clearly, her recall was quite poor, but why? Examination of her responses suggests some tentative hypotheses. The fact that she initially retained three elements from the first sentence of the story (man, dog, Texas) and nothing else, along with her comment that she was overwhelmed by the amount of detail, leads one to speculate that much of her problem may have been the result of an overwhelmed attentional system. On delayed recall she retained one item from her immediate recall, dog, and improved her recall of a second item (man → master) but dropped the third item, Texas. One could argue that her ability to retain information in secondary memory was essentially intact, since she lost little information during the 36 minutes following her immediate recall, but her immediate recall was so sparse that its retention scarcely constituted a challenging test of long-term storage. Having determined that she was having a major problem in retaining complex information presented on a single trial, we were now ready to tease out the basis of her problem.

First, we needed to determine if she was able to attend well enough to get the story into memory in the first place. Although RE could repeat a series of six digits on a standard digit span task, on the Nonverbal Sequencing Span Test (a modified version of the Knox Cubes Test) she could repeat a sequence of touching no more than three blocks, and then only on two of four trials. Most people her age can repeat a sequence of at least five or six blocks. Clearly, RE could not adequately register information presented in the form of long sentences.

Even with a limited span of attention, however, subjects can retain more than a few words from a prose paragraph if they are able to hold what they have just heard in their primary memory while they attend to the next section being presented. If a subject has difficulties in dividing attention, however, he or she encounters an additional problem in registering supra-span information. To assess RE's ability to hold information in mind in the face of the distraction provided by a competing task, we presented the Verbal Divided Attention Test, using a Brown-Peterson procedure. On this task, RE was also grossly impaired. The distractor test had to be changed to counting forward rather than backward, since she could not perform the latter task. She retained a total of only three of 15 letters on five trials, at which point the test was discontinued because of the great difficulty she was experiencing.

Given RE's attentional deficits, it was not surprising that she seemed to retain very little information. It's quite difficult to remember something that is not registered. The next question was whether RE's memory would be better in a situation where attentional demands were minimized. To assess this, she was given a verbal list learning test. Twelve concrete words were read to her with the instruction that she was to recall them in any order. The words fall into three categories, with four words in each category. She remembered only one word the first time the list was read. [We use a restricted reminding technique (Buschke & Fuld, 1974): whenever the subject has correctly remembered a word twice in a row, that word is no longer presented, although the subject is still asked to recall it every trial.] Most people readily notice the categories and group the words to help them remember. After 12 trials, RE had recalled only six of the 12 words without reminders. She showed a slight tendency to recall the words of a particular category in association, but this tendency was not marked, and she verbalized no awareness of the categories when subsequently questioned. After a 45-minute delay from among the six words she had recalled without reminders, she only remembered four.

RE did no better on recognition testing. When the 12 original words were combined with 12 words from the same categories that had not been on the list, she correctly identified all 12 of the words on the list but also "remembered" eight of the 12 distractors. Her "liberal" response bias thus colored her results, but even when her score was corrected for response bias, it was still low. Clearly her severe attentional problems that interfered with her ability to register information did not fully account for her memory problems. Before we could draw any firm conclusions about the nature of her memory problem, however, we had to examine her executive abilities. Her relatively limited use of categorization and her gross liberal response bias suggested the possibility of problems in planning, organization, and self-monitoring.

On the Porteus Maze Test she could not get beyond the 5-year level. On this and other executive ability tasks, it was apparent that her organizational skills were quite deficient. On the Plan of Search, where she had to show how she would go about searching for a set of keys that had been lost in a field, she drew a line that meandered seemingly at random. There appeared to be no coherent plan directing her search. She was unable to use simple conceptual principles in matching stimuli on either the Wisconsin Card Sorting Test or the Weigl Color-Form Test. Her performance on the Cognitive Estimation Test was very severely impaired. She estimated, for example, that the average American woman was six feet tall.

It is clear, therefore, that RE's performance on memory testing was affected by both severe attentional and executive deficits. Indeed, the only problem was in trying to determine whether her secondary memory was impaired beyond the effect of those deficits. She was not grossly amnesic, because she was able to retain some information over significant delay intervals. On the other hand, her overall performance on all secondary memory tasks was so poor that it seems quite likely that her deficit could not be attributed solely to the effect of her more generalized deficits. Further testing seemed unwarranted in view of the overall severity of her problems.

RE seemed fairly unconcerned about her deficits, showing a lack of insight that was striking in view of the extent of her impairment. Also, her MMPI (which had to be read to her) showed no scales elevated above a T score of 66. Her score on the Depression scale was only 55. Overall her profile suggested a rather denying, repressive, hysteroid style of adjustment.

As to the role depression plays in this patient's dementia, RE's test results leave little doubt. Her performance was globally impaired. She performed best on tasks that demanded little speed, effort, or organization, and no amount of encouragement enabled her to improve her performance. Finally, she showed no signs of depression either clinically or on personality testing, although her lack of initiative and involvement may initially have appeared to be depression.

Case 2

Like RE, 59-year-old TI was referred by his neurologist to differentiate between dementia and depression. He had an essentially normal medical history, though he had had classic migraine headaches from age 18 to 53. Nine months prior to the neuropsychological evaluation, TI had an aortic valve replaced and an aortic aneurysm repaired. In the hospital he experienced a transient episode of numbness, disorientation, and blurred vision, and 3 months later he had a transient episode of disorientation and loss of memory for the day's events.

Following his hospitalization, TI experienced continuing problems with memory and concentration. For example, he couldn't remember how many golf strokes he played on a particular hole, and he forgot where he put things. He had a new computer, and working with it had become increasingly difficult for him. His wife said that he would become confused about when things had happened and would think that an event occurring a few days ago happened several weeks earlier. TI also complained that he had difficulty completing his work. He said he couldn't get things together right or do things on time. He delayed tax preparation until the last minute and had postponed writing reports.

TI had completed high school, attended some college, and obtained an engineering certificate. He worked as an industrial engineer in a supervisory position. At age 56, he bought his own business, which he ran with his sons. His hobbies were golfing and boating, but he spent most of his time working, 60–70 hours per week. He lived with his wife.

As with RE, TI was administered an extensive set of tests.* When asked to repeat the prose story, his immediate recall was:

> "There was this person, man, in Boston who went to Texas. The guy, oh, I don't know, that's all I can remember. [Tell me as much as you can remember.] Something about a dog and he got some new clothes while he was in Texas. [Good] No, it's not good, because I can't remember. [Keep going.] That's all I remember. I wasn't concentrating on it. [Anything else?] I don't remember anything."

Like RE, TI remembered very little and failed to get the gist of the story. Fifty-three minutes later, he recalled all of what he had initially learned:

> "Seems like there was a man from Boston that went to Texas. Seems like he got some new clothes, and somewhere in there he also came across a dog. That's about all I remember. [Anything else?] I didn't remember it when you gave it to me."

On multiple-choice recognition testing, he recognized three elements he had not recalled, but his overall recognition performance was well below normal. On two

*The following tests were administered: Wisconsin Card Sorting Test, Columbia Mental Maturity Scale, Cognitive Estimation Test, Porteus Maze Test, Plan of Search, Controlled Word Search, Oldfield-Wingfield Picture Naming Test with Recall, Cookie Theft Description, Fairy Tale Recitation, Stereognosis Test with Recall, Nonverbal Sequencing Span Test, Auditory Verbal Sequencing Span Test, Visual Verbal Sequencing Span Test, Verbal Divided Attention Task, Nonverbal Divided Attention Task, Paced Auditory Serial Addition Test, Prose Recall, Segmented Prose Recall, Design Copying with Recall, Verbal Recognition Memory Test, Nonverbal Recognition Memory Test, Verbal List Learning Test, Nonverbal List Learning Test, Minnesota Multiphasic Personality Inventory.

specific tests of recognition memory, his performance was mildly to moderately impaired, even when corrected for response bias.

In an attempt to increase the depth of his processing of story material, he was subsequently given a story construction task in which he was required to place five disordered sentences in a sequence to make a sensible story. He assembled the story correctly. When he was asked without prior warning to recall the story after a delay interval, his memory, though still somewhat sparse, was considerably superior to his performance on the original story recall task.

Although his presenting complaints suggested deficits of attention and organization, no deficit emerged on testing. TI was able to reproduce a sequence of seven digits and six blocks, and on a Brown-Peterson interference task he was above average.

Unlike the demented patient, TI was able to organize and plan systematically, to solve problems, and to reason normally. For example, he had no difficulty copying a complex geometric figure, and he did it quite systematically. Forty-three minutes later his recall was quite adequate.

The most consistent observation that emerged in TI's testing was that he did best when he had to process the stimulus actively rather than by passively listening or watching. The best example of this was seen when he was asked to tell the fairy tale, *Cinderella*. His initial attempt was quite inadequate. He mixed up the story with *Snow White*, produced very few details, and was sure that he could not do it. However, when he was provided a great deal of encouragement to try again, to pretend that he was telling the story to a child, he finally seemed to get into the proper spirit of the task and gave a full and accurate account of the story. At the end he even corrected an inconsistency that he remembered making during the early part of the story.

This patient shows several of the features that are typical of depressives. He did not show difficulties on testing consistent with either the nature or the extent of his complaints. The difficulties he did show on testing did not seem to be related to the memory demands of the tasks. By looking at TI's performance on both memory and non-memory tasks, it became apparent that his difficulties were associated with the amount of effort the task required. Given the opportunity to process information quite passively, he would do so and fail to remember it, even with recognition testing. When the task required him to process the stimulus actively or when he was provided with a great deal of encouragement and support, he performed quite normally. The MMPI in this case confirmed the presence of a significant amount of depression and anxiety, combined with a tendency to repress and deny emotional concerns. Consistent with these denying tendencies, TI's presenting complaints had included only irritability.

REFERENCES

Alexopoulos, G. S., Abrams, R. C., Young, R. C., & Shamoian, C. A. (1988). Cornell scale for depression in dementia. *Biological Psychiatry, 23*, 271–284.

American Psychiatric Association. (1987). *Diagnostic and statistical manual of mental disorders* (3rd ed.—revised). Washington, D.C.: American Psychiatric Association.

Baddeley, A. D. (1982). Amnesia: A minimal model and an interpretation. In L. S. Cermak (ed.), *Human memory and amnesia* (pp. 305–336). Hillsdale, NJ: Lawrence Erlbaum.

Baddeley, A. D. (1983). Working memory. *Philosophical Transactions of the Royal Society of London*, B302: 311–324.

Baddeley, A. D. (1986). *Working memory*. Oxford: Clarendon Press.

Baddeley, A. D., Logie, R., Bressi, S., Della Sala, S., & Spinnler, H. (1986). Dementia and working memory. *The Quarterly Journal of Experimental Psychology, 38A*, 603–618.

Bayles, K. A. (1982). The use of language tasks in identifying etiologically different dementias. Paper presented at the International Neuropsychological Society, Pittsburgh.

Bornstein, R. A. (1983). Construct validity of the Knox Cube Test as a neuropsychological measure. *Journal of Clinical Neuropsychology, 5*, 105–114.

Brown, J. (1958). Some tests of the decay theory of immediate memory. *Quarterly Journal of Experimental Psychology, 10*, 12–21.

Buschke, H., & Fuld, P. A. (1974). Evaluating storage, retention, and retrieval in disordered memory and learning. *Neurology*, 24(11):1019–1025.

Caine, E. D. (1986). The neuropsychology of depression: Pseudodementia syndrome. In I. Grant & K. M. Adams (Eds.), *Neuropsychological assessment of neuropsychiatric disorders* (pp. 221–243). New York: Oxford University Press.

Cantone, G., Orsini, A., Grossi, D., & De Michele, G. (1978). Verbal and spatial memory span in dementia. *Acta Neurologica (Napoli), 33*, 175–183.

Corkin, S. (1982). Some relationships between global amnesias and the memory impairments in Alzheimer's disease. In S. Corkin, K. L. Davis, J. H. Growdon, E. Usdin, & R. J. Wurtman (Eds.), *Alzheimer's disease: A report of research in progress*. New York: Raven Press.

Craik, F. I. M., & Simon, E. (1980). Age differences in memory: The roles of attention and depth of processing. In L. W. Poon, J. L. Fozard, L. S. Cermak, D. Arenberg, & L. W. Thompson (Eds.), *New directions in memory and aging* (pp. 95-112). Hillsdale, NJ: Lawrence Erlbaum Associates.

Delis, D. C., Kramer, J. H., Kaplan, E., & Ober, B. A. (1987). *The California verbal learning test-research edition*. New York: The Psychological Corporation.

Erickson, R. C., Poon, L. W., & Walsh-Sweeney, L. (1980). Clinical memory testing of the elderly. In L. W. Poon, J. L. Fozard, L. S. Cermak, D. Arenberg, & L. W. Thompson (Eds.), *New directions in memory and aging* (pp. 379-402). Hillsdale, NJ: Lawrence Erlbaum Associates.

Erickson, R. C., & Scott, M. L. (1977). Clinical memory testing: A review. *Psychological Bulletin, 84*, 1130–1149.

Gallagher, D. (1986). Assessment of depression by interview methods and psychiatric rating scales. In L. W. Poon (Ed.), *Handbook for clinical memory assessment of older adults* (pp. 202-212). Washington, DC: American Psychological Association.

Gilewski, M. J., & Zelinski, E. M. (1986). Questionnaire assessment of memory complaints. In L. W. Poon (Ed.), *Handbook for clinical memory assessment of older adults*. (pp. 93-107). Washington, DC: American Psychological Association.

Grossi, D., Orsini, A., & Ridente, G. (1977). Osservazioni introduttive allo studio neuropsicologica delle demenze organiche. *Acta Neurologica (Napoli), 32*, 682–696.

Hannay, H. J. (1986). Psychophysical measurement techniques and their application to neuropsychology. In H. J. Hannay (Ed.), *Experiemental techniques in human neuropsychology* (pp. 45-94). New York: Oxford University Press.

Herrmann, D. J. (1982). Know thy memory: The use of questionnaires to assess and study memory. *Psychological Bulletin, 92*, 434–452.

Initial Validity Studies of the New Wechsler Memory Scale—Revised [Special Issue]. (1988). *The Clinical Neuropsychologist, 2*(2).

Kahn, R. L., Zarit, S. H., Hilbert, N. M., & Niederehe, G. (1975). Memory complaint and impairment in the aged: The effect of depression and altered brain function. *Archives of General Psychiatry, 32*, 1569–1573.

Kaszniak, A. W., Sadeh, M., & Stern, L. Z. (1985). Differentiating depression from Organic Brain Syndromes in older age. In G. M. Chaisson-Stewart (Ed.), *Depression in the elderly: An interdisciplinary approach* (pp. 161–189). New York: Wiley.

Kopelman, M. D. (1985). Rates of forgetting in Alzheimer-type dementia and Korsakoff's syndrome. *Neuropsychologia, 23*, 623–638.

Lezak, M. D. (1983). *Neuropsychological assessment*. (2nd ed.). New York: Oxford University Press.

Morris, R. G. (1984). Dementia and the functioning of the Articulatory Loop System. *Cognitive Neuropsychology, 1*, 143–157.

Morris, R.G. (1986). Short-term forgetting in senile dementia of the Alzheimer's type. *Cognitive Neuropsychology, 3*, 77–97.

Niederehe, G. (1986). Depression and memory impairment in the aged. In L. W. Poon (ed.), *Handbook of clinical memory assessment of older adults* (pp. 226-237). Washington, DC: American Psychological Association.

Poon, L. W. (ed). (1986). *Handbook for clinical memory assessment of older adults*. Washington, DC: American Psychological Association.

Porteus, S. D. (1965). *Porteus Maze Test: Fifty years' application*. Palo Alto, CA: Pacific Books.

Rey, A. (1964). *L'examen clinique en psychologie*. Paris: Presses Universitaires de France.

Shallice, T., & Evans, M. E. (1978). The involvement of the frontal lobes in cognitive estimation. *Cortex, 14*, 294-303.

Tweedy, J. R., Lapinski, R. H., Hines, T., Reding, M., & Deutsch, G. (1982). Cognitive correlates of arteriosclerotic and depressive symptoms in a series of suspected Alzheimer patients. Paper presented at the International Neuropsychological Society, Pittsburgh.

Warrington, E. K. (1984). *Recognition Memory Test*. Windsor, Berkshire, UK: NFER-Nelson Publishing Co.

Wechsler, D. (1987). *Wechsler Memory Scale—Revised*. New York: The Psychological Corporation.

Weingartner, H. (1986). Automatic and effort-demanding cognitive processes in depression. In L. W. Poon (Ed.), *Handbook for clinical memory assessment of older adults* (pp. 218-225). Washington, DC: American Psychological Association.

Winegardner, J., & Mack, J. L. (1982). Sequencing span deficits in dementia. Paper presented at the International Neuropsychological Society European Conference, Deauville, France.

Yesavage, J. (1986). The use of self-rating depression scales in the elderly. In L. W. Poon (Ed.), *Handbook for clinical memory assessment of older adults* (pp. 213-217). Washington, DC: American Psychological Association.

PART II
Alzheimer's Disease: From Gene to Mind

Affecting 5% to 10% of people over the age of 65, dementia is the most common cause of memory impairment in the elderly. Alzheimer's disease (AD) accounts for at least 50% to 70% of all cases of dementia. The chance of suffering from AD increases as one ages; individuals over the age of 85 have a one in three chance of suffering from clinically significant cognitive impairment. Since those over the age of 85 are the most rapidly growing segment of our population, and the number of elderly is expected to triple by the middle of the next century, clinicians will be dealing with more dementia, particularly the degenerative disorders such as AD, in the future.

The first half of this book focused on general issues of memory impairment in the elderly. A number of investigators referred to AD and compared the memory abnormalities present in this condition to other disorders, particularly the more selective amnesias, such as Korsakoff's disease. It is encouraging that more neuropsychologists have become interested in the cognitive problems in dementia. Previously many neuropsychologists believed that the role of dementia in helping us understand brain–behavior interactions was small, because dementia seemed uninterestingly homogeneous, affecting many different cognitive abilities and brain structures all at one time. It has now become clear that AD is a clinically and biologically heterogeneous disorder and that our neurochemical understanding of the basis of memory is probably greater in this disorder than in other conditions.

In the second half of this book we will focus more specifically on AD. We will try to put the psychological problems in a broader biological and sociological context. Some of the most exciting research in AD relates to genetics and molecular biology. This work will be summarized by Peter St. George-Hyslop and colleagues. Shortly after Alois Alzheimer described his first case in 1906, it became apparent that Alzheimer's disease occasionally clustered in families. Pedigrees suggestive of autosomal dominant inheritance were described, but other cases in which the mechanism of transmission was less clear suggested polygenetic models or autosomal dominant models with incomplete penetrance. In the 1950s, individuals with Down's syndrome (also called Trisomy 21 and caused by the presence of an extra third copy of the 21st chromosome) were noted to have a much greater risk of suffering from AD, both pathologically and clinically, than the population at large. The dementia also occurred at early ages (35–40 years). Recently, the DNA that forms the precursor for one of the amyloid proteins found in senile plaques has been found to be located on chromosome 21. St. George-Hyslop's work has also demonstrated that, in some rare families with the young age of onset, autosomal dominant form of AD, the gene that actually causes the disease appears to be located on chromosome 21. The Alzheimer gene and the amyloid gene are not the same, however. Nevertheless, this work allows, for the first time, the possibility of actually defining the abnormality that causes AD in the rare autosomal dominant form. In addition, these studies have implications for clinicians trying to develop diagnostic tests. For example, in Huntington's disease, the gene has been linked to markers on chromosome 4, and as a result, pre-symptomatic testing is now available at certain research centers. At these selected sites, family members can ask the clinician and geneticist to assess the pattern of genetic markers in their white blood cells. It is now possible to change the 50/50 odds suffered by all at-risk, first-degree relatives of a subject affected by an autosomal dominant condition, such as HD, to approximately 95-99% that the individual either does or does not have the disease. Such tests are not available in AD currently, but the research described in the first chapter of this section sets the stage for this to be accomplished. For psychologists, the additional implication of this presymptomatic testing is that we can identify family members who will, if they live long enough, get the disease, allowing us to study the onset and longitudinal progression of cognitive impairments.

Much of this book has focused on the neuropsychological assessment of memory disturbances. In the second chapter in this section, certain aspects of the clinical diagnosis of AD and related disorders are discussed. AD is a disorder for which we have no specific diagnostic tests in life, as well as no effective biologic therapies to reverse the progression of the disease. These authors review the diagnosis of dementia and attempts to develop more effective in vivo diagnostic tests and treatment.

In the last section of the book, we will turn attention to the psychological and sociological aspects of AD. Recognizing that a biological breakthrough is not on the immediate horizon, our society has to address the problem of meeting the care needs of the individual and the family. The assessment and ongoing care of the AD patient is appropriately interdisciplinary. We will hear, therefore, from several representatives of different disciplines as they outline their approaches to managing caregiving problems in dementia. Finally, AD is not only a disorder that impacts on individual patients and families but on our entire society as well. Our last section will address health care policy issues as well as needed reforms in our health care delivery system.

P. J. WHITEHOUSE

7

Biochemical and Molecular Genetic Investigation of Inherited Alzheimer's Disease

P. H. St. George-Hyslop, J. F. Gusella, and D. R. Crapper McLachlan

Alzheimer's Disease (AD) has recently become a major public health problem in many Western societies, where age-dependent incidence rates (up to 127 cases per 100,000 population per year) and age-dependent incidence rates (up to 5.8 cases per 100 population per year) have made the disorder and its associated medical complications the fourth leading cause of death in North America (Rocca, Amaducci, & Schoenberg, 1986; Katzman, 1986). In view of the anticipated increase in the proportion of the elderly in Western societies, AD is likely to assume even greater importance in the future. Indeed, it has been estimated that $25 billion per year are currently spent on the institutional care of demented patients in the United States alone (Katzman, 1986).

The primary cause of AD remains unknown. However, several epidemiological studies have reported that first-degree relatives of patients with AD have an increased risk of this disorder (Breitner, Silverman, Mons, & Davis, 1988; Fitch, Becker, & Heller, 1988; Heston, Mastri, Anderson, & White, 1981). While familial clustering of AD does not necessarily imply a genetic etiology, several extended pedigrees have been described in which the disease phenotype can be clearly followed through multiple generations (Nee, Polinsky, Eldridge, Weingartner,

Smallberg, & Ebert, 1983; Goudsmit, White, Weitkamp, Keats, Morrow, & Gajdusek, 1981; Foncin et al., 1985). In these pedigrees at least, the familial form of Alzheimer's disease (FAD) clearly results from a dominantly inherited defect in an autosomal gene. Apart from the obvious pattern of inheritance and a somewhat younger age of onset, the clinical, biochemical, and pathological features of FAD are indistinguishable from those of "sporadic" cases of AD (Davies, 1986). Consequently, identification of the primary defect in FAD could provide powerful insights not only into the biochemical pathophysiology of familial AD, but also possibly into that of the non-familial form of the disease.

The existence of large pedigrees with FAD has raised the prospect that the chromosomal location of the causative gene defect could be discovered by identifying a polymorphic genetic marker co-segregating with the disorder. Since the chromosomal location of the "linked" genetic marker is already known, the observation of co-segregation infers that the disease gene is located close to the marker locus on the same chromosome. The discovery of the chromosomal location of the FAD gene will permit subsequent attempts to clone the disease gene based simply on a knowledge of its chromosomal location. In the absence of unambiguous clues as to the likely identity of the FAD gene, this approach avoides the necessity of making any a priori assumptions as to the nature of the FAD gene defect.

Classical genetic linkage studies using polymorphic expressed protein markers such as the blood group antigens, have been previously attempted in FAD without success (Spence, Heyman, Marazita, Sparkes, & Weinberg, 1986; Feldman, Chandler, Levy, & Glaser, 1963). However, in recent years the power of this genetic linkage strategy has been dramatically increased by the discovery of large numbers of DNA markers that detectRestriction Fragment Length Polymorphisms (RFLPs) (see glossary at end of chapter for definition of this and other technical terms) in human genomic DNA (Gusella, 1986). Linkage studies using DNA markers have already identified the chromosomal loci for the gene defects causing such inherited neurological diseases as Huntington's chorea, manic depressive illness, and von Recklinghausen's peripheral neurofibromatosis (Gusella, 1986; Gusella et al., 1983; England et al., 1987; Baron et al., 1987; Seizinger et al., 1987). We have applied the strategy of genetic linkage analysis with DNA markers to four large kindreds with pathologically proven FAD.

A priori, the FAD gene could have been located on any of the 22 autosomal chromosomes. However, it has been known for several years that the brains of elderly individuals with Trisomy 21 [Down's syndrome (DS)] almost invariably harbor the neuropathological changes of AD (Wisniewski, Dalton, McLachlan, Wen, & Wisniewski, 1985; Oliver & Holland, 1986). Furthermore, it seems clear that at least some elderly DS individuals also develop cognitive impairment in late life consistent with AD (Wisniewski et al., 1985; Oliver & Holland, 1986). These observations suggested that genes on chromosome 21 may have a special role in the pathogenesis of AD and prompted an intensive investigation of the molecular genetics of this autosome. We report results that provide strong evidence that chromosome

21 does indeed carry a gene causally related to the familial form of AD. However, contrary to initial expectations, our results indicate that although the FAD gene does map to chromosome 21, it is not located in the 21q22-qter region of chromosome 21 associated with DS. Instead, our data suggest that the FAD gene is located close to two DNA markers on the proximal long arm of chromosome 21 above the DS region. We provide evidence using both recombinant DNA and classical biochemical techniques that three candidate genes on chromosome 21 (the *B-Amyloid Precursor* gene, the *Liver-Type-Phosphofructokinase* gene, and the *Superoxide Dismutase* gene) are not the site of the FAD mutation. Finally, although a gene dose effect may explain the pathophysiology of AD in Trisomy 21, we provide evidence that triplication of at least moderate to large segments of chromosome 21 is not the pathogenetic mechanism in the familial and sporadic forms of Alzheimer's disease.

METHODS

The methods employed in these analyses are described in detail in the original articles reporting these studies (St. George-Hyslop et al., 1987). The interested reader is referred to these articles for further information. The pedigrees of families studied by our group are shown in Figure 7.1.

RESULTS

Molecular Genetic Studies

Several DNA markers from the obligate Down's syndrome region of chromosome 21 were tested for linkage to FAD (Table 7.1). Contrary to initial expectations, all markers from this region gave negative lod scores, allowing this region of chromosome 21 to be excluded as the site of the FAD mutation (Table 7.2). However, the DNA markers D21S1/D21S11 and D21S16, from the more proximal regions of chromosome 21, gave positive lod scores (Table 7.3). It should be noted that the lod scores generated at both of these loci were less than +3 conventionally required to prove linkage. Empirical and theoretical observations, however, suggest that lod scores between +2 and +3 are proven incorrect with the subsequent addition of new data in less than 10% of occasions (Ott, 1985). The probability of finding two genetic markers from the same region of the same chromosome, both giving lod scores in this range and both being in error, is therefore quite small. Consequently, although the two-point analysis was unable to prove the presence of the FAD gene in this region, the results with these markers were considered to be highly suggestive.

The difficulty in proving linkage to this region of the genome using two-point methods of analysis could be explained by the poor pedigree structure typical of

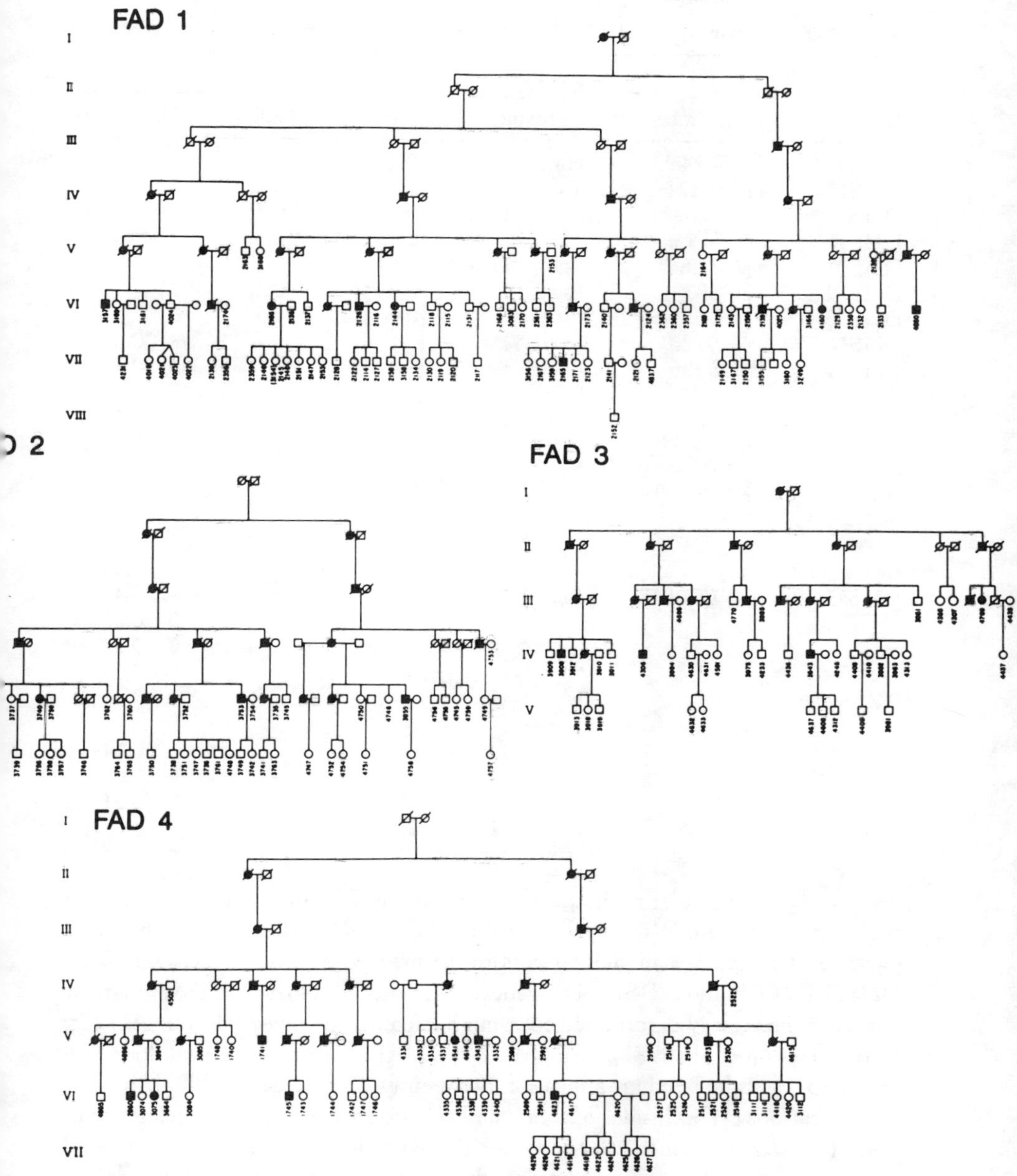

FIGURE 7.1 Pedigree diagrams for four pedigrees with autopsy proven Familial Alzheimer's disease, showing an autosomal dominant pattern of inheritance. Symbols include (○) female; (□) male; (■) affected male; (∅) deceased male. Four digit numbers beneath these symbols indicate individuals who have been examined for evidence of FAD and for whom cell lines have been established.

TABLE 7.1 Polymorphic DNA Markers From Chromosome 21

Locus	Probe	Restriction enzyme	Frequency −Allele	Frequency +Allele	Haplotype
D21S8	pPW245D	Hind 111	0.31	0.69	
D21S13	pGSM21	Taq 1	0.29	0.71	
D21S15	pGSE8	Msp 1	0.54	0.46	
D21S16	pGSE9	Xba 1	0.20	0.80	
D21S17	pGSH8	Bgl 11	0.57	0.43	
D21S19	pGSB3	Pst 1	0.80	0.20	
D21S58	pPW524-5P	Pst 1	0.46	0.54	
D21S1/	pPW228	Msp 1			A 0.26
D21S11	pPW236	BamH 1			B 0.40
		EcoR 1			C 0.25
		Taq 1			D 0.09
D21S53	pPW512-16P	Bcl 1			A 0.26
	pPW512-6B	Sac 1			B 0.20
	pPW512-18P	Apa 1			C 0.59
					D 0.08
					E 0.04
					F 0.03
D21S55	pPW518-1R	Xba 1			A 0.47
					B 0.28
					C 0.22
					D 0.03
B-Amyloid	FB6L	EcoR 1			A 0.36
	HL124	EcoR 1			B 0.40
		Ban 1			C 0.14
					D 0.06
					E 0.01
SOD1	SOD4A	Bgl 11	0.80	0.20	

FAD pedigrees. In order to discover whether the FAD gene was really located in the vicinity of these DNA markers, we utilized LINKMAP from the LINKAGE package of programs (ver 3.5) to perform a three point analysis between FAD, D21S21/D21S11, and D21S16. The genetic relationships of the two DNA markers had been previously determined in a large reference pedigree without AD (St. George-Hyslop et al., 1987). Using the LINKMAP subprogram, a peak lod score of +4.25 was calculated for a location between D21S1/D21S11 and D21S16 (Fig. 7.2). Locations on both sides of these markers also gave lod scores of greater than +4.0 (Fig. 7.2). Since the lod score for the possible locations above, between, or below these markers are not significantly different, it is not yet possible to definitively place the FAD gene relative to D21S1/D21S11 and D21S16. Nevertheless, these results provide strong evidence to suggest that there is a gene located on the proximal long arm of chromosome 21, which when defective is capable of causing FAD.

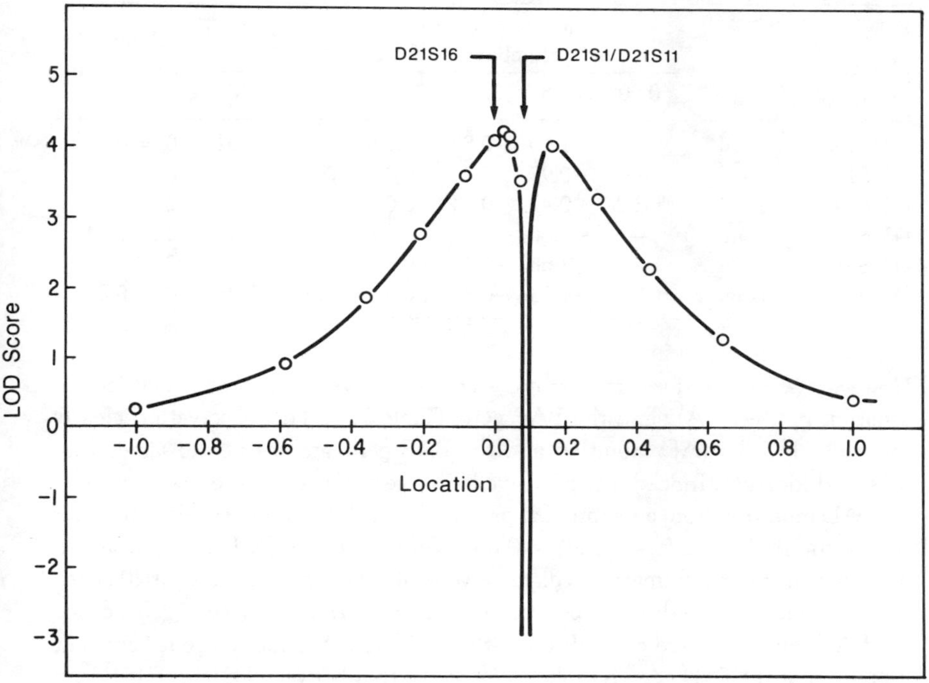

FIGURE 7.2 The multipoint linkage analysis program LINKMAP was used to calculate the relative likelihood of linkage between the FAD gene and various locations above, between, or below the DNA marker loci D21S1/D21S11 and D21S16. A peak lod score of +4.25 was calculated for locations between these markers. Lod scores for locations above and below D21S1/D21S11 and D21S16, however, were also significantly positive ($z > 4.0$).

Candidate Genes

B-Amyloid Gene

The gene coding for the B-Amyloid precursor protein (BAP) has been isolated and mapped to the 21q21-22 region of chromosome 21 (Tanzi et al., 1987; Goldgaber et al., 1987; Robakis et al., 1987). The chromosomal location of this gene, together with preliminary reports of duplication of the BAP gene in genomic DNA from cases of sporadic AD has led to the proposal that this gene may be the start of the FAD mutation. We have tested this hypothesis in several ways. First, we have examined the inheritance of RFLPs in the BAP gene in the four FAD pedigrees. If the FAD mutation did reside in the BAP gene, RFLPs in the BAP gene should show tight genetic linkage with the inheritance of the FAD phenotype.

TABLE 7.2 Lod Scores for Linkage of Markers in 21q22 to FAD.

Marker locus	Pedigree	Recombination fraction (0)						Limit of exclusion (z < −2)
		0.00	0.05	0.10	0.20	0.30	0.40	
D21S15	Total	—	−1.90	−0.88	−0.19	−0.04	−0.02	0 = 0.04
D21S17	Total	—	−0.97	−0.41	−0.03	0.02	0.01	0 = 0.02
D21S19	Total	−3.2	−0.49	−0.24	−0.09	−0.03	−0.02	0 = 0.01
D21S53	Total	—	−3.86	−2.70	−1.49	−0.90	−0.47	0 = 0.14
D21S55	Total	—	−2.68	−1.33	−0.21	0.10	0.10	0 = 0.07
D21S58	Total	—	−1.33	−0.82	−0.30	0.05	0.05	0 = 0.02

However, we observed several meiotic events that revealed chromosomal recombination between FAD and the BAP gene (Table 7.4). This observation clearly indicates that the FAD mutation and the BAP gene are not at the same chromosomal location. Indeed, the negative lod scores at this locus serves to exclude the FAD mutation from a region of approximately 8 million nucleotides on either side of the BAP gene (z <−2, 0 = 0.08) (Tanzi et al., 1987). It is important to note that the most informative pedigree gave weakly positive lod scores at 20 centi-Margan—a measure of distance between two genes (cM) from the BAP gene. Since the BAP gene is located 8 cM distal to the D21S1/D21S11 locus, the latter result suggests that the FAD gene is probably located either between D21S1/D21S11 and D21S16 or, more likely, above D21S16. Further evidence against the presence of

TABLE 7.3 Lod Scores for Linkage of Markers Above 21q22 to FAD.

Marker locus	Pedigree	Recombination fraction (0)						Peak lod score (z)
		0.00	0.05	0.10	0.20	0.30	0.40	
D21S8	Total	—	−1.33	−0.52	0.03	0.10	0.03	
D21S13	Total	−4.2	−0.64	−0.33	0.11	−0.04	0.00	
D21S16	FAD1	0.15	0.10	0.06	0.02	0.01	0.01	
	FAD2	0.13	0.10	0.08	0.04	0.02	0.01	
	FAD3	−0.42	−0.29	−0.20	−0.10	−0.04	0.01	
	FAD4	2.46	2.19	1.91	1.34	0.76	0.23	
	Total	2.32	2.10	1.85	1.30	0.75	0.26	2.32 (O = 0.00)
D21S1/ D21S11	FAD1	—	0.59	0.61	0.41	0.18	0.03	
	FAD2	−0.2	0.04	0.12	0.12	0.07	0.02	
	FAD3	0.6	0.63	0.61	0.49	0.33	0.16	
	FAD4	—	1.00	1.01	0.79	0.47	0.16	
	Total	—	2.26	2.35	1.81	1.05	0.37	2.37 (O = 0.08)

TABLE 7.4 Lod Scores for Linkage of the BAP Gene to FAD*

	Recombination fraction (0)						
Pedigree	0.00	0.01	0.05	0.10	0.20	0.30	0.40
FAD1	—	−2.00	−0.78	−0.39	−0.15	−0.07	−0.04
FAD2	—	−1.92	−0.71	−0.26	0.05	0.05	0.10
FAD3	—	−3.83	−2.28	−1.58	−0.91	−0.53	−0.38
FAD4	—	−0.86	0.40	0.80	0.87	0.60	0.41
Total	—	−8.61	−3.37	−1.43	−0.14	0.10	0.09

* Exclusion (z < −2 at O = 0.08 cM)

a defect in the BAP gene is furnished by the absence of changes in size or quantity of mRNA on Northern blots from FAD cerebral cortex and cultured lymphoblasts (St. George-Hyslop and C. A. Marrotta, unpublished observations).

Although the BAP gene is not the site of the FAD gene, it could be argued that inherited variations in this gene may play an important, permissive role in the familial susceptibility to sporadic AD noted in the epidemiologic surveys (Breitner et al., 1988; Fitch, Becker, & Heller, 1988; Heston et al., 1981). To test this hypothesis, we examined the frequency of particular RFLPs in the BAP gene in patients with AD and compared these frequencies with those expected in the general population. The presence of a significant allelic association between RFLPs in the BAP gene and the occurrence of sporadic AD would provide strong evidence to support a causal role for this gene in "sporadic" AD. However, the allele frequencies at the three RFLP sites in this gene were not different in 63 Caucasian subjects with AD, compared to the general Caucasian population (P >0.10). This observation thus does not support the contention that inherited abnormalities in the BAP gene are causally related to sporadic AD. This conclusion is consistent with the absence of changes in either the quantity or size of mRNA in Northern blots of sporadic AD brain (C. A. Marrotta, personal communication), and with the absence of changes in the nucleotide sequence of cDNAs from AD brain (D. Goldgaber, personal communication).

Superoxide Dismutase 1

The location of the *SOD 1* gene on chromosome 21, the role of this gene in the metabolism of derivatives of oxygen metabolism, and preliminary evidence of duplication of this gene in AD, have led to similar arguments that the *SOD 1* gene may be involved in AD (Schweber et al., 1987; Sinet, 1982). Contrary to these speculations, however, we have determined that the *SOD 1* gene is not linked to the FAD mutation, there is no evidence of an allelic association with "sporadic" AD, and we have been unable to replicate the preliminary observations of duplication at this locus (Table 7.5; Fig. 7.6, Fig. 7.7). The critical role of *SOD 1*

TABLE 7.5 Lod Scores for Linkage of the *SOD 1* Gene to FAD*

	Recombination fraction (0)					
Pedegree	0.00	0.05	0.10	0.20	0.30	0.40
FAD1	0.25	0.20	0.16	0.10	0.06	0.02
FAD2	0.05	0.04	0.03	0.04	0.01	0.00
FAD3	−0.24	−0.18	−0.14	−0.06	−0.06	−0.04
FAD4	—	0.10	0.07	0.04	0.01	0.00
Total	—	0.16	0.12	0.08	0.02	−0.02

in oxygen metabolism suggests that inherited defects in this gene would more likely either be lethal or manifest at an earlier age.

Phosphofructokinase

Positron emission tomography (PET) studies have revealed significant reductions in the rates of glucose metabolism in the cerebral cortex of patients with AD when compared to normal subjects (Alvi, Ferris, & Wolf, 1981; Benson, et al., 1983; Freidland et al., 1983). The degree of reduction of local cortical glucose metabolism rates (LCGMR) correlates closely with the severity of the underlying clinical dementia (Alvi, Ferris, & Wolf, 1981; Benson et al., 1983; Freidland et al., 1983). This suggests that the glycolytic pathway may be abnormal in cerebral cortex afflicted with AD. The major regulatory enzyme of the glycolytic pathway is phosphofructokinase (PFK) (Hoffman, 1970). The liver isoenzyme of PFK, which is expressed in brain and liver, is encoded on the long arm of chromosome 21 (Cox & Epstein, 1985). Preliminary biochemical studies directed toward elucidating the mechanism of reduced LCGMR in AD cortex have reported marked (90%) reductions in PFK activity in AD neocortex, along with lesser reductions (30%) in the activities of other enzymes involved in energy metabolism (Iwangoff, Meier-Ruge, & Reichmeier, 1984; Bowen et al., 1979).

To clarify whether the changes in LCGMR reflect a primary defect in PFK or merely a secondary change consequent to neuronal death, we measured PFK activity and enzyme kinetics in cerebral cortex from sporadic AD, Down's syndrome with AD, non-AD dementia controls, and normal elderly controls. We report that PFK activities from neocortex from AD patients were significantly lower than those in either matched normal controls ($p < 0.001$) or matched non-AD controls ($p < 0.01$) (Fig. 7.3). There was some overlap, however, in the PFK levels observed in the AD and non-AD control groups. It is significant that despite the presence of an extra gene copy, the PFK activities in DS brain were reduced to the same magnitude as those seen in AD cortex (approximately 0.2 Units/gram wet weight of cortex). Michaelis-Menten constants for both ATP (Km) and Fructose-6-phosphate (Km) did not differ between the AD and control groups ($p > 0.05$) (Fig. 7.4).

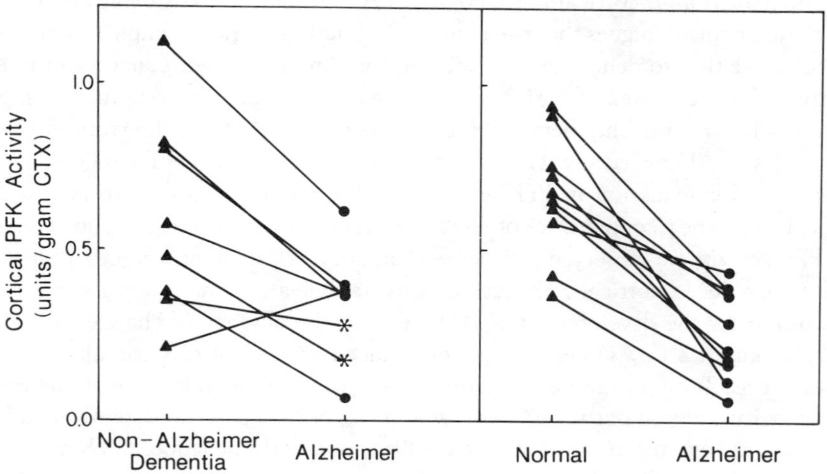

FIGURE 7.3 Phosphofructokinase activity was measured in post-mortem cerebral cortex using a coupled enzyme assay system. The results were expressed as Units/gram wet weight of cortex. PFK activity was significantly reduced in AD and in DS with AD cortices, compared to paired, age-matched normal and non-AD dementia control tissues ($p < 0.001$ and < 0.01 respectively).

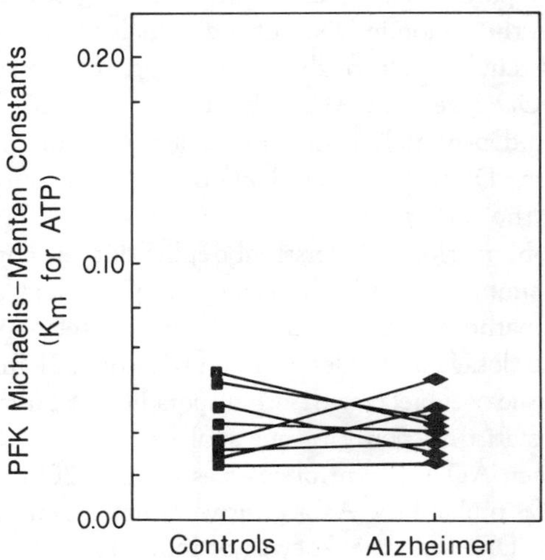

FIGURE 7.4 Michaelis-Menten constants of PFK for Fructose-6-phosphate (Km) (data not shown) and for ATP (Km) (data shown) were not different between AD and controls ($p > 0.05$).

The reduction in cortical PFK activity in AD neocortex compared to non-AD dementia controls argues that the reduced PFK activity is not a simple functional accommodation to dementia. In addition, the similar marked reduction in PFK activities in neocortex of patients with Down's syndrome plus AD further supports a close relationship between the pathogenesis of AD and the reduced PFK activities in AD neocortex. However, for several reasons, our results suggest that although this reduction in PFK activity may be relatively specific to AD, it is more likely to be a consequence of AD rather than a primary cause. First, an overlap in PFK activity was observed between AD and non-AD dementia groups, indicating that reduced cortical PFK activity was neither a necessary nor a sufficient condition for the development of AD. Second, the absence of changes in PFK enzyme kinetics in AD argues that the reduced activity of this enzyme in AD does not result from inherited abnormalities in the PFK peptide, from alterations in relative expression of the PFK isoenzyme genes, or from post-translational modification of the enzyme. It would seem more likely that both the reduced PFK activity and the reduced LCGMR observed in PET scan reflect specific loss of large metabolically active neurons in AD. A similar explanation underlies the specific reductions in Choline Acetyl Transferase and selected neurotransmitters in AD brain (Rossor & Mountjoy, 1986).

Gene Dosage Studies

Delabar et al. (1987) reported preliminary evidence to suggest that the BAP gene may be duplicated in the genomic DNA of individuals with sporadic AD. This observation received tentative although indirect support from similar reports of duplication of the *SOD 1* gene in AD (Schweber et al., 1987). These observations prompted an in-depth analysis of gene dosage not only at these loci but also at other loci in the DS region and at loci on the proximal long arm of chromosome 21 close to the FAD gene.

If confirmed, the observation of interstitial duplication on chromosome 21 in AD would provide a simple answer both to the pathophysiology of AD itself and to the AD-like neuropathology in Trisomy 21. Unfortunately, we were unable to detect abnormal gene dosage at any locus on chromosome 21 in genomic DNA extracted from any tissue of subjects with either sporadic or familial AD ($p < 0.05$) (Figs. 7.5–7.7). The statistical power of our analysis was such that a difference in gene dosage between AD and control cases as small as 20% could have been detected with an 80% probability. As a positive control, gene dosage was also measured in genomic DNA from leukocytes of individuals with DS. As would be predicted, DS DNA consistently showed evidence of an extra copy at each locus on chromosome 21 ($p < 0.0001$, compared to AD and to controls) (Figs. 7.5–7.7). These results indicate that interstitial duplication of moderate or large regions of chromosome 21 is not likely to be a common pathogenetic mechanism

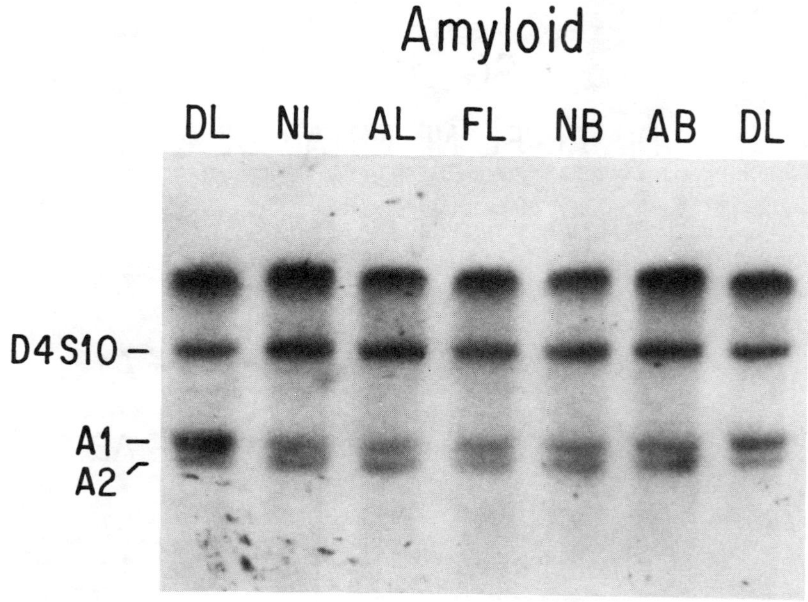

FIGURE 7.5 Gene dosage at the BAP gene was estimated from the intensity of autoradiographic bands produced by hybridizing (^{32}P)-ATP labeled BAP probe (FB6L) to Southern blot filters containing genomic DNA from individuals heterozygous for the EcoR1 RFLP in the BAP gene. The ratio of the signal intensities of the different allelic RFLP bands (A1 and A2) carried on each chromosome did not differ in genomic DNA derived from sporadic AD leukocytes and brain (AL) (AB); FAD leukocytes (FL); and non-AD dementia and normal control leukocytes (NL) and brain (NB) ($p > 0.05$). One allelic band in genomic DNA from Down's syndrome leukocytes (DL) has a significant increase in intensity, reflecting an extra copy of this gene as a result of Trisomy 21 ($p < 0.0001$ compared to AD, FAD, and controls).

in either sporadic or familial AD. Triplication of genes on chromosome 21, however, is the probable mechanism underlying the neuropathologic abnormalities in elderly DS patients.

CONCLUSIONS

The results presented above indicate that the autosomal dominant form of Alzheimer's disease, at least in the four pedigrees examined, is caused by a defective gene on the proximal long arm of chromosome 21. The location of the FAD gene outside the obligate Down's syndrome region of chromosome 21 does not contradict earlier work suggesting a relationship between AD and DS, since the

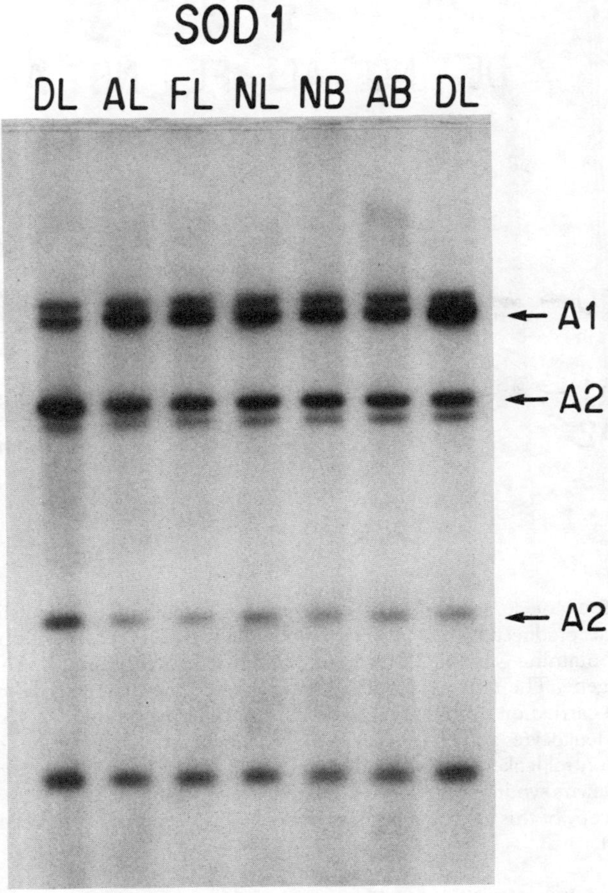

FIGURE 7.6 Gene dosage at the *SOD 1* gene was estimated from the intensity of autoradiographic bands produced by hybridizing (^{32}P)-ATP labeled *SOD 1* probe (SOD4A) to Southern blot filters containing genomic DNA from individuals heterozygous for the Msp1 RFLP in the *SOD 1* gene. The ratio of the signal intensities of the different allelic RFLP bands (A1 and A2) carried on each chromosome did not differ in genomic DNA derived from sporadic AD leukocytes and brain (AL) (AB); FAD leukocytes (FL); and non-AD dementia and normal control leukocytes (NL) and brain (NB) ($p > 0.05$). One allelic band in genomic DNA from Down's syndrome leukocytes (DL) has a significant increase in intensity reflecting an extra copy of this gene as a result of Trisomy 21 ($p < 0.0001$ compared to AD, FAD, and controls).

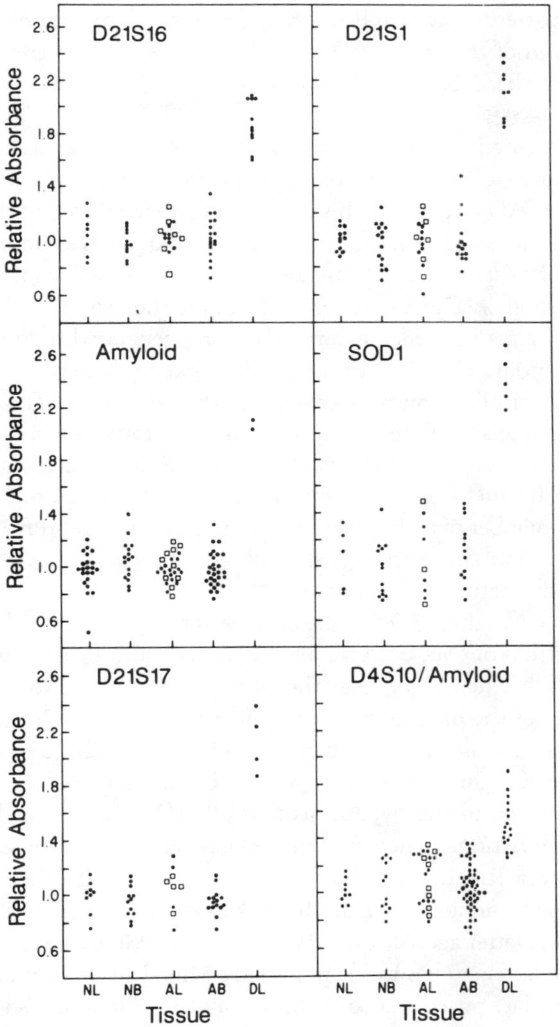

FIGURE 7.7 A laser densitometer was used to accurately measure the density of the allelic bands on the autoradiograms for each chromosome 21 locus as in Figures 7.5 and 7.6. The ratio of the signal intensities of the two allelic RFLP bands was computed and normalized to an arbitrary value of 1.00 (i.e., gene copy number per chromosome). No difference in relative signal intensity, and thus no evidence of alteration in gene copy number, was observed in genomic DNA from normal elderly and non-AD leukocytes (NL); normal elderly and non-AD dementia brain (NB); sporadic AD leukocytes (AL); sporadic AD brain (AB); and FAD leukocytes (FL) ($p > 0.05$). A 100% increase in signal intensity (yielding an abnormal ratio of 2:1) was observed on one allelic band in lanes containing genomic DNA from DS leukocytes (DL), indicating the known presence of an extra copy of chromosome 21 ($p < 0.0001$).

majority of DS patients have triplication of the entire long arm of chromosome 21. Little is known of the fate of the rare DS patients who are trisomic only for 21q22. However, these patients are generally thought to have a milder DS phenotype.

Several genes located on chromosome 21 have been proposed as potential sites for the FAD mutation. We provide compelling evidence that none of these genes are the site of the FAD mutation. This result therefore requires that the FAD gene be isolated using the same molecular genetic techniques that are being applied to the analysis of other inherited diseases, including chromosome walking and differential screening of cDNA libraries. To facilitate the search for the FAD gene, additional anonymous markers are currently being generated from the proximal regions of chromosome 21. It is anticipated that some of these new DNA markers will provide a set of closer markers that flank the FAD gene. The discovery of such "flanking markers" will be a starting point for efforts to clone all the chromosomal DNA between these markers. Since the FAD mutation must reside in one of the DNA fragments cloned from this region, each DNA fragment will be investigated by a number of techniques, including pulse field gel (PFG) electrophoresis, crude restriction site mapping, and, ultimately, nucleotide sequencing in order to detect the actual FAD mutation.

The question of whether AD is a disorder of heterogeneous etiology has long been debated but has not yet been resolved unequivocally. It has been suggested, and contested with equal vigor, that the presenile and senile forms of AD are different subtypes of the disease (Hansen, DeTeresa, Davies, & Terry, 1988; Bondareff et al., 1987). Similarly, some epidemiological surveys have reported a 50% risk of AD by age 90 in first-degree relatives of AD patients (Breitner et al., 1988). These results have led to the hypothesis that all AD results from the effects of an autosomal dominant gene defect with age-dependent penetrance (Breitner et al., 1988). However, this hypothesis is in disagreement with other surveys that have failed to observe an increased familial risk of AD among relatives of patients with late onset AD (after age 70 years) (Heston et al., 1981; Chandra et al., 1987). The results of the latter studies would imply that while young onset AD may have a genetic etiology, late onset AD could have a multifactorial (mixed genetic and non-genetic) or even a purely non-genetic etiology.

At first glance the availability of DNA markers linked to the defective gene responsible for one form of FAD suggests that these markers could be used to test for linkage in other kindreds with multiple affected members. Clearly, a positive result showing linkage of the current markers to all other AD pedigrees would strongly support not only the hypothesis of a unitary disease but also that of a genetic etiology for AD in general. However, for reasons to be discussed, the absence of linkage to these markers does not necessarily prove the contention of heterogeneity.

Two observations dictate cautious interpretation of heterogeneity tests using the current set of markers, especially when small pedigrees are examined. First, in any given small pedigree, it may not be possible to decide whether the presence of several relatives affected with AD reflects a truly genetic disorder rather than merely chance concurrence of a common disease. Second, the more informative marker D21S1/D21S11 is clearly distant from the FAD gene. Consequently, at least 10% of meioses are expected to reveal a recombination event between FAD and this locus. In large pedigrees like those reported here, the significance of an occasional recombination event among many co-segregating events will be obvious—the marker is not located precisely at the site of the FAD gene. In small pedigrees with few matings, the significance of a single recombination event, which will result in a negative lod score for that pedigree, will be difficult to interpret. As noted above, such a recombination could simply reflect the known separation between the marker and the FAD gene. However, a recombination event could equally well indicate that the disease in that pedigree is caused by a gene at another locus (non-allelic heterogeneity), or by a non-genetic but familially clustered disease (e.g., caused by a shared environmental agent). Finally, a recombination event could result from an error in diagnosis. While erroneous recombination events will have some effect in large pedigrees, their effect will be much more profound in small pedigrees where such errors will consume a greater proportion of the available information. Unfortunately, it is often not possible to discriminate between each of these explanations when small pedigrees are investigated. Consequently, in small pedigrees, the absence of linkage to genetic markers that are distant from the actual disease gene does not provide an incontestable argument in favor of heterogeneity.

In general the majority of kindreds with multiple affected members having onset of symptoms after 65 years are typically very small nuclear pedigrees. We have examined the above markers in several small pedigrees in which the age of onset spans the range 60–80 years. The small size and limited informativeness of the majority of these pedigrees results in uniformative lod scores (minimally negative to zero). A few pedigrees show clear co-segregation, while a few show obligate recombination events. The net result is that the cumulative lod scores for these pedigrees is negative. However, bearing in mind the caveats noted above, together with the fact that in many of these small pedigrees the mode of inheritance cannot be unequivocally established, it would seem premature to over-interpret these data.

A conclusive answer to the question of non-allelic heterogeneity in FAD, and to the related question of the true extent of a genetic basis for AD in general, will likely have to await either the positive identification of additional linked loci or the identification of close, flanking markers for the current locus. A more convincing argument for heterogeneity could be made if close flanking markers can be found for the current locus, and if it can be subsequently shown that the genetic defect in some kindreds can be excluded from this "flanked" region. This "negative" proof is not totally satisfying because failure to detect linkage could result from diagnostic errors or from the inclusion of non-genetic cases within a predominantly genetic pedigree, and because the etiology of AD in kindreds with no evidence of linkage within the "flanked zone" could still be either genetic or non-genetic. The most convincing argument in favor of non-allelic heterogeneity would be the demonstration that the genetic defect in some kindreds can be shown to be at a different locus.

Whether AD is eventually proven or disproven to be a single illness, the location of the gene defect causing FAD in at least some pedigrees provides the basis for attempts to clone the defective gene responsible for AD in these families. It would seem likely that an understanding of the function of the normal and disease alleles of this gene that will be gained from this endeavor could provide insights into the pathogenesis of AD in general. Further, in view of certain similarities between AD and normal aging, it is possible that an understanding of the function of this gene may uncover some of the mechanisms responsible for normal neuronal aging.

GLOSSARY

cDNA Cloned DNA fragment with a sequence complementary to that of messenger RNA of a gene.

chromosome walking Technique for cloning DNA in an ordered fashion in order to get close to a desired gene.

chromosome A physical structure made of DNA with a protein scaffolding that contains many genes.

DNA Deoxyribonucleic acid. A molecule composed of a series of nucleotide bases arranged in an ordered sequence to carry the genetic code.

DNA marker/probe A piece of recombinant or cloned DNA that can be tagged with a radioactive label and used to investigate a genetic locus (e.g., a gene or RFLP site).

gene Inheritable substrate that carries certain genetic information (e.g., eye color). Chemically the gene is composed of DNA, the nucleotide sequence of which carries the genetic code of the gene.

genetic locus Site of a gene or RFLP.

genomic DNA DNA extracted from the nucleus of a cell, which carries the complement of genetic information in that cell. Mitochondria in the cytoplasm of the cell contain a small amount of DNA of their own that codes for some of the mitochondrial enzymes (mitochondrial DNA).

library A series of cloned pieces of DNA often carried in a bacterial host cell. The library represents the entire subset of DNA from the original source, each separate cloned piece representing a volume from the library. Libraries can be made from genomic DNA (genomic libraries) representing nuclear DNA, or from cDNA (cDNA libraries) representing only those genes that are functionally active in the tissue from which the cDNA fragments were derived.

linkage analysis A statistical procedure to measure whether two genetic loci are close together on the same chromosome. Tests may be between an unknown test locus and a second site whose chromosomal location is already known (two-point analysis) or between a single unknown locus and a cluster of sites whose location relative to each other are already known (multi-point analysis).

lod score A statistical measure indicating that two genetic loci are close together on the same chromosome (lod score greater than +3) or are unlikely to be close together (lod score less than −2).

Michaelis-Menten constant A biochemical measure of the activity of an enzyme. Altered activity might reflect an inherited defect in the gene coding for this enzyme.

mutation An alteration in the nucleotide sequence of DNA. Mutations may be innocent, causing benign variations in a genetic trait (e.g., eye color or RFLP fragment size), or malevolent, causing disease.

mRNA Messenger RNA. A nucleic acid sequence that carries the genetic code from the gene in the nucleus and is translated into a protein in the cytoplasm of the cell.

recombination event During meiosis (gametogenesis) members of each pair of chromosomes exchange genetic material (recombine). As a result of this genetic recombination, genetic material that was originally on one chromosome (which may have carried a certain marker or disease gene) subsequently appears on the other sister chromosome. Thus, whereas two loci on the same chromosome may have initially been co-inherited, after the recombination event they no longer co-segregate because they are now on different sister chromosomes. The frequency of recombination events between two loci on the same chromosome is roughly related to their physical separation on that chromosome (more possibility for recombination with distant markers). Consequently the frequency of recombination can be used as a measure of the distance (amount of DNA) separating two loci on the same chromosome.

polymorphism An inherited naturally occurring variation in some genetic trait observed in a population (e.g., eye color or blood group).

restriction enzyme An enzyme that cleaves DNA at a specific site.

RFLP Restriction Fragment Length Polymorphism. A naturally occurring inheritable polymorphism in the nucleotide sequence of genomic DNA that leads to variable fragment sizes when genomic DNA is cleaved with a restriction enzyme. Like other inheritable polymorphisms, RFLPs can be used as a genetic marker to follow the inheritance of the chromosomal region that includes the RFLP site.

REFERENCES

Alvi, A., Ferris, J., & Wolf, A. (1981). Determination of cerebral metabolism in senile dementia using F18-deoxy glucose. *Journal of Nuclear Medicine* 21: 22–28.

Baron, M., Risch, N., Hamburger, R., Mandel, B., Kushner, S., Newman, M., Drummer, D., & Belmaker, R. H. (1987). Genetic linkage between X-chromosome markers and bipolar affective illness. *Nature 326*: 289–292.

Benson, D. F., Kuhl, D. E., Hawkins, R. A., Phelps, M. E., Cummings, J. C., & Tsai, S. Y. (1983). The fluordeoxyglucose 18-F scan in AD and MID. *Archives of Neurology 40*: 711–714.

Bondareff, W., Mountjoy, C. Q., Roth, M., Rossor, M. N., Iversen, L. L., & Reynolds, G. P. (1987). *Archives of General Psychiatry 44*: 412–417.

Bowen, D. M., White, O., Spillane, T. A., Goodhardt, M. J., Curzon, G., Iwangoff, P., Meier-Ruge, W., & Davison, A. N. (1979). Accelerated aging, or selective neuronal loss as an important cause of dementia? *Lancet 1*: 11–14.

Breitner, J. C. S., Silverman, J. M., Mohs, R. C., & Davis, K. C. (1988). Familial aggregation of Alzheimer's Disease: Comparison of risk among relatives of early and late onset causes, and among male & female relatives in successive generations. *Neurology 38*: 207–12.

Chandra, V., Philipose, V., Bell, P. A., Lazaroff, A., & Schoenberg, B. S. (1987). Case control study of late onset "probably Alzheimer's Disease." *Neurology 37*: 1295–1300.

Cox, D. R., & Epstein, C. J. (1985). Comparative gene mapping of human chromosome 21 and mouse chromosome 16. *Annals of the New York Academy of Sciences 450*: 169–177.

Davies, P. (1986). The genetics of Alzheimer's Disease: A review and a discussion of implications. *Neurobiology of Aging 7*: 459–466.

Delabar, J. M., Goldgaber, D., Lamour, Y., Nicole, A., Huret, J. L., DeGrouchy, J., Brown, P., Gajdusek, D. C., & Sinet, P. (1987). Beta-amyloid gene duplication in Alzheimer's disease and karyotypically normal Down syndrome. *Science* 235: 1390–1392.

England, J. A., Gerhard, D. S., Pauls, D. L., Sussex, J..N., Kidd, K. K., Allen, C. R., Hostetter, A. M., & Housman, D. L. (1987). Bipolar affective disorder linked to DNA Markers on chromosome 11. *Nature 325*: 783–787.

Feldman, R. G., Chandler, K. A., Levy, L. L., & Glaser, G. H. (1963). Familial Alzheimer's disease. *Neurology 13*: 811–823.

Fitch, N., Becker, R., & Heller, A. (1988) The inheritance of Alzheimer's disease: A new interpretation. *Annals of Neurology 23*: 14–19.

Foncin, J. F., Salmon, D., Supino-Viterbo, V., Feldman, R. G., Macchi, G., Marriotti, P., Scoppetta, C., Caruso, G., & Bruni, A. C. (1985). Demence presenile D'Alzheimer transmise dans une famille etendue. *Revue Neurologique (Paris) 141*: 194–202.

Freidland, R. P., Budinger, T. F., Ganz, E., Yano, Y., Mathis, C. A., Koss, B., Ober, B. A., Huesman, R. H., & Derenzo, S. E. (1983). Regional cerebral metabolic alterations in dementia of the Alzheimer type: Positron emission tomography with (F18)-fluorodeoxyglucose. *Journal of Computer Assisted Tomography 7*: 590–598.

Goldgaber, D., Lerman, M. I., McBride, O. W., Saffiotti, U., & Gajdusek, D. C. (1987). Characterization and chromosomal localization of a cDNA encoding brain amyloid of Alzheimer's disease. *Science 235*: 877–880.

Goudsmit, J., White, B. J., Weitkamp, L. R., Keats, J. B., Morrow, C. H., & Gajdusek, D. C. (1981). Familial Alzheimer's disease in two kindreds of the same geographic and ethnic origin. *Journal of the Neurological Sciences 49*: 79–89.

Gusella, J. F. (1986). DNA polymorphisms and human disease. *Annual Review of Biochemistry 55*: 831–854.

Gusella, J. F., Wexler, N. S., Conneally, P. M., Naylor, S. L., Anderson, M. A., Tanzi, R. E., Watkins, P. C., Ottina, K., & Wallace, M. R. (1983). A polymorphic DNA marker genetically linked to Huntington's Disease. *Nature 306*: 234–238.

Hansen, L. A., DeTeresa, R., Davies, P., & Terry, R. D. (1988). Neocortical morphometry lesion counts, and choline acetyltransferase levels in the age spectrum of Alzheimer's disease. *Neurology 38*: 48–54.

Heston, L. L., Mastri, A. R., Anderson, V. E., & White, J. (1981). Dementia of the Alzheimer type. Clinical genetics, natural history, and associated conditions. *Archives of General Psychiatry 38*: 1085–1090.

Hodge, S. E., Morton, L., Tideman, S., Kidd, K. K., & Spence, M. A. (1979). Estimating Age of onset distributions for disorders with variable onset. *American Journal of Human Genetics 31*: 761–762.

Hoffman, E. (1970). The significance of PFK to the regulation of carbohydrate metabolism. In R. H. Adrian & A. Weber (eds.), *Reviews of Physiology, Biochemistry and Pharmacology*, (p. 1). Berlin: Springer-Verlag.

Iwangoff, P., Meier-Ruge, W., & Reichmeier, K. (1984). Neurochemical enzyme changes in Alzheimer's & Pick's Diseases. *Archives of Gerontology and Geriatrics 3*: 101–165.

Kang, J., Lemaire, H. G., Unterbeck, A., Saulbaum, J. M., Masters, C. L., Grzeschik, K., Multhaup, G., Beyreuther, K., & Muller-Hill, B. (1987). The precursor of the Alzheimer's Disease amyloid A4 protein resembles a cell surface receptor. *Nature 325*: 733–736.

Katzman, R. (1986). Alzheimer's Disease. *New England Journal of Medicine 314*: 964–973.

Nee, L. E., Polinsky, R. J., Eldridge, R., Weingartner, H., Smallberg, S., & Ebert, M. (1983). A family with histologically confirmed Alzheimer's disease. *Archives of Neurology 40*: 203–208.

Oliver, C., & Holland, A. J. (1986). Down's Syndrome and Alzheimer's Disease: A review. *Psychological Medicine 16*: 307–322.

Ott, J. (1985). *Analysis of human genetic linkage*. Baltimore & London: Johns Hopkins University Press.

Robakis, N. K., Wisniewski, H. M., Jenkins, E. C., Devine-Gage, E. A., Houk, G. E., Yao, X. L., Ramakrishna, N., Wolf, G., Silverman, W. P., & Brown, W. T. (1987). Chromosome 21q21 sublocalization of gene encoding B-amyloid peptide in cerebral vessels and neuritic (senile) plaques of people with Alzheimer's disease and Down syndrome. *Lancet 1*: 384–385.

Rocca, W. A., Amaducci, L. A., & Schoenberg, B. S. (1986). Epidemiology of clinically diagnosed Alzheimer's Disease. *Annals of Neurology 19*: 415–424.

Rossor, M., & Mountjoy, C. Q. (1986). Postmortem neurochemical changes in Alzheimer's Disease compared with normal aging. *Canadian Journal of Neurological Science 13*: 499–502.

Schweber, M., Tuson, C., Shiloh, R., & Ben-Neriah, Z. (1987). Triplication of chromosome 21 material in Alzheimer's Disease. *Neurology 37*:222.

Seizinger, B. R., Rouleau, G. A., Ozelius, L. J., Lane, A. H., Faryniarz, A. G., Chao, M. V., Huson, S., Korf, B. R., Parry, D. M., Paricak-Vance, M. A., et al. (1987). Genetic linkage of von Recklinghausen Neurofibromatosis to the nerve growth receptor gene. *Cell 49*: 589–594.

Sinet, P. M. (1982). Metabolism of oxygen derivatives in Down Syndrome. In F. Marott

Sinex & C. Merril (Eds.), *Alzheimer's Disease, Down's Syndrome & Aging* 396 (pp. 83-94). New York: New York Academy of Sciences.

Spence, M. A., Heyman, A., Marazita, M. L., Sparkes, R. S., & Weinberg, T. (1986). Genetic linkage studies in Alzheimer's Disease. *Neurology 36*: 581–583.

St. George-Hyslop, P. H., Tanzi, R., Polinsky, R., Haines, J. L., Nee, L., Watkins, P. C., Myers, R. H., Feldman, R. G., Pollen, D., Drachman, D., Growdon, J., Bruni, A., Foncin, J. F., Salmon, D., Frommelt, P., Amaducci, L., Sorbi, S., Piacentini, S., Stewart, G. D., Hobbs, W. J., Conneally, P. M., & Gusella, J. F. (1987). The genetic defect causing familial Alzheimer's disease maps on chromosome 21. *Science 235*: 885–890.

Tanzi, R. E., Gusella, J. F., Watkins, P. C., Bruns, G. A. P., St. George-Hyslop, P. H., Van Keuren, M. L., Patterson, D., Pagan, S., Kurnit, D. M., & Neve, R. L. (1987). Amyloid B protein gene: cDNA, mRNA Distribution, and genetic linkage near the Alzheimer's Locus. *Science 235*: 880–884.

Tanzi, R. E., St. George-Hyslop, P. H., Haines, J. L., Polinsky, R. J., Nee, L., Foncin, J. F., Neve, R. L., McClatchey, A. L., Conneally, P. M., & Gusella, J. F. (1987). The genetic defect in familial Alzheimer's Disease is not tightly linked to the amyloid B-protein gene. *Nature 329*, 156–157.

Wisniewski, K. E., Dalton, A. J., McLachlan, C., Wn, G. Y., & Wisniewski, H. M. (1985). Alzheimer's Disease in Down's Syndrome: Clinicopathologic studies. *Neurology 35*, 957–961.

8

Diagnosis and Treatment of Alzheimer's Disease and Related Disorders: Issues for the Future

Peter J. Whitehouse, Richard Mayeux, and John Herbert Growdon

The most common causes of memory impairment in the elderly are Alzheimer's disease (AD) and related disorders (Civil & Whitehouse, 1988). AD is a clinical pathological entity defined by progressive dementia and a characteristic pattern of biological alterations, including senile plaques and neurofibrillary tangles. The term "related disorders" is used in several contexts to refer to different groups of disorders. Occasionally, it is used to refer to any non-Alzheimer condition that causes dementia. In this chapter, we will use the term to apply to the degenerative dementias and specifically focus on Parkinson's disease (PD) as an example.

Degenerative dementias are disorders characterized clinically by progressive loss of cognitive abilities and biologically by neuronal loss in specific populations in the brain frequently associated with distinctive pathological hallmarks. Other characteristic features include a lack of clearly defined cause and specific therapeutic agents to reverse the disease progression. These disorders occur more frequently in the elderly, and their clinical and biological features overlap with changes that occur in normal aging.

Like AD, PD is characterized by specific loss of nerve cells, although in a different pattern from that found in AD. The reduction in dopaminergic cells of the substantia nigra in association with intracellular inclusions called Lewy bodies is the primary feature in AD. In approximately 30% of cases, patients with PD also develop dementia, although many more may have cognitive impairment without frank dementia (Mayeux, Stern, Rosen, & Leventhal, 1981; Whitehouse, Struble, Hedreen, Clark, & Price, 1985; Price, Whitehouse, & Struble, 1986).

In this review, we will examine current issues concerning the diagnosis and management of the cognitive and behavioral impairment in AD and PD and identify problems requiring additional research. Ideally, the understanding of diagnosis and treatment should be based on the pathophysiology of a disease condition; therefore, we will start with a review of current understanding of the neurobiology of AD and PD.

NEUROBIOLOGY

As degenerative disorders, both AD and PD are characterized by dysfunction in specific populations in the brain. The mechanisms of cell death in different dementias may be quite different, however (Price et al., 1986). In the previous chapter, Dr. St. George-Hyslop and colleagues demonstrated that in some cases of AD, genetic abnormalities lead to programmed cell death. In some early onset cases, the gene appears to be located on chromosome 21. In Trisomy 21 (Down syndrome), Alzheimer type pathological changes apparently occur in all individuals over the age of 40. The genetic factors in other forms of AD (e.g., late onset) are unclear.

In AD, neuronal loss occurs consistently in cortex, hippocampus, amygdala, cholinergic basal forebrain, noradrenergic locus coeruleus, and serotonergic raphe nucleii (Price et al., 1986). Some of these cell populations express increased amounts of mRNA for the protein that is the precursor of the amyloid found in plaques (Palmert et al., 1988). Current research is also identifying other areas of pathology not previously thought affected, such as retina and white matter.

The role of genes in PD is more limited; most recent attention to pathophysiology has focused on the role of environmental toxins. This work was stimulated by the discovery that 1-methyl-4-phenyl-1,2,3,6-tetrahydropyridine (MPTP), a contaminant in the elicit production of meperidine (Demerol) analogues, causes loss of cells in the substantia nigra and development of parkinsonism in young drug abusers (Kalaria, Mitchell, & Harik, 1987). Some have argued that PD itself may be related to exposure to an environmental toxin. Drug trials are under way to try to slow the progression of PD by blocking the formation of these postulated toxins.

Although neuronal loss in the substantia nigra is characteristic of PD, cell loss also occurs in cortex, cholinergic basal forebrain, locus coeruleus, and raphe nuclei, particularly in those individuals who suffer from cognitive and behavioral abnormalities (Whitehouse et al., 1985).

The challenges for the future will be to define not only *why* nerve cells die in these different conditions, but also to determine *which* nerve cells are at risk. Although the pattern of neuronal loss is obviously different in specific degenerative disorders, certain populations of cells are affected in more than one disease and also tend to be those lost as a part of normal aging. For example, the density of cells in the substantia nigra may be reduced in approximately 30% of cases of AD and to a lesser extent in all of us as we age. Cortical interneurons using somatostatin and corticotropin releasing factor and perhaps neuropeptide Y, glutamate, and GABA are affected in both AD and PD.

The development of more comprehensive pathophysiological models will also allow the development of diagnostic tests based on disease-specific markers and therapies based on a rational understanding of how the disease affects different systems in the brain.

NEUROPSYCHOLOGY

Both AD and the dementia of PD are characterized by the progressive loss of several cognitive abilities (memory, attention, executive systems, visuospatial abilities, praxis, language). The major question for neruopsychological studies is how the dementias that occur in AD and PD vary in their pattern of cognitive loss and how this variability relates to their different biologies. Some patients with PD suffer from coexisting AD as autopsy reveals plaques and tangles (Boller, Mizutani, Roessman, & Gambetti, 1980). However, dementia can occur in PD without plaques and tangles (e.g., Lewy body dementia or simple atrophy). In both AD and PD, neuronal dysfunction in the cholinergic basal forebrain has been correlated with the severity of dementia, although the neurobiological basis of memory undoubtedly involves many other systems as well (Whitehouse et al., 1985; Price et al., 1986). Some authors have suggested that AD and PD belong to fundamentally different neuropsychological classes of dementia. For example, the term "subcortical dementia" has been used to refer to the cognitive impairment found in PD whereas critical dementia has been used to refer AD. Whether all dementias can be classified into these two superordinate categories is uncertain (Whitehouse, 1986). Fruitless argument can be wasted on the semantics of the terms employed to characterize the different types of dementia. Nevertheless, nosology is important, since appropriate classification of dementias may lead to identification of different causes and, eventually, therapies.

The important question is how the cognitive profile at a similar point in the illness in patients with PD differs from that in AD and whether the cognitive disabilities can be related to the biological changes. For example, patients with PD have been characterized as having bradyphrenia (i.e., slowness of mentation) even in the absence of fully developed dementia. Is this a result of pathology in the cholinergic basal forebrain or, perhaps, of dysfunction in dopaminergic neurons such as those in the mesolimbic and mesocortical systems? Since intellectual impairments have been found in drug addicts exposed to MPTP and who have a relatively selective loss of dopaminergic neurons, a role for dopamine in cognition is supported (Mayeux et al., 1981).

Studies have shown neuropsychological differences between the dementia in AD and PD. There may be less language impairment and more visuospatial abnormalities in PD than in AD (Mayeux et al., 1981; Whitehouse et al., 1985). Renewed attention is also being paid to the heterogeneity of the dementias found in AD and PD themselves. There may be subtypes of dementia included in what we currently call AD. For example, some patients with AD have earlier language impairment than others. This clinical variability, such as the relative predominance of language or visuospatial impairment, may be related to the biological substrates (i.e., more pathology found in left vs. right hemisphere). Other subtypes of AD have been proposed, including familial, early onset, benign, myoclonic, and psychotic forms.

NEUROPSYCHIATRY

Psychiatric symptoms occur in both AD and PD and may be major determinants of caregiver burden. Notably, demented patients can suffer from hallucinations, delusions, illusions, paranoia, and affective symptoms as well as other less well defined behavioral symptoms such as agitation and wandering. The phenomenology of the behavioral abnormalities that occur in dementia is poorly understood; it is not clear whether standard diagnostic categories for psychiatric conditions effectively capture well the behavioral disturbances seen in the dementias.

The biological substrate of these psychiatric symptoms occurring in AD and PD also need to be more fully explored. Bioaminergic theories of depression and psychosis have been proposed in cognitively intact patients, primarily supported by evidence that drugs affecting these systems can either cause or alleviate these conditions. For example, drugs that block noradrenergic function (alpha methyl dopa, propranolol) can produce depression, whereas drugs that enhance function (tricyclic antidepressants and monoamine oxidase inhibitors) can alleviate depression. Direct evidence of impairment in bioaminergic systems in brain in depression and psychosis not associated with dementia is weak. In AD and PD, where pathology occurs in the noradrenergic locus coeruleus and serotonergic raphe nuclei, we may be able to establish specific links between the loss of neurons in these systems and the presence of specific psychiatric symptoms (D'Amato et al., 1987; Zweig et al., 1988).

DIAGNOSIS

The diagnosis of AD is currently made by excluding other forms of dementia. History, physical examination, blood tests, and brain imaging allow the exclusion of other common and occasionally treatable forms of dementia, including systemic illness, endocrine disease, vitamin deficiencies, stroke, and brain tumors. The PD patient with cognitive impairment also requires such an evaluation to ensure that the dementia is not caused by a superimposed medically treatable condition before presuming that this is a dementia syndrome that accompanies PD.

No diagnostic test specific for either AD or PD is available in life. Three major lines of research are proceeding to develop an in vivo diagnostic test. Brain imaging, particularly functional imaging with PET or SPECT, may lead to a diagnostic test based either on the pattern of metabolic abnormalities (i.e., decreased parietal metabolism in AD [Johnson et al., 1988]) or by labeling specific markers for the disease (i.e., neurotransmitter receptors). CSF studies are focusing on the presence of abnormal proteins associated with AD, such as the A-68 identified by Peter Davies, or a particular pattern of neurotransmitter abnormalities that reflects the loss of chemical systems in the brain (Beal & Growdon, 1986). As yet, no such pattern of neurochemical abnormalities specific for a particular disorder has been identified. As mentioned, loss of cortical acetylcholine, somatostatin, and corticotropin releasing factor occurs in both AD and PD, whether or not plaques and tangles are found.

The third line of research to develop a diagnostic test is based on the possibility that AD has manifestations outside the central nervous system. Abnormalities in lymphocytes, red blood cells, fibroblasts, and platelets have been described, although consistent patterns of changes in AD or any of the related disorders have not yet been described.

A major diagnostic problem is to separate early dementia from normal age-associated memory impairment (Crook et al., 1986). Nearly all individuals show some minimal changes in speed of cognitive processing and memory performance as they age. Some of the neurochemical systems affected in AD and PD show mild neuronal loss as people age, without major intellectual changes. No specific neurotransmitter or other neurochemical marker change currently allows the discrimination of normal aging from AD *qualitatively*. Even diagnosis at autopsy is based on finding quantitatively greater changes in AD than in normal aging.

TREATMENT

A treatment program for AD or patients with PD who are demented may include both behavioral and biological aspects. Attention to functional abilities (activities of daily living), safety issues, caregiver stress, access to resources, and family education are essential in the management of patients with dementia. Nurses, social workers, physicians and other health care provides all play an important role in management of the patient. Recent attention is also being paid to psychological approaches to maintaining or enhancing memory function, particularly in patients with early AD. AD patients can learn new material, albeit with difficulty. The challenge is to design techniques to permit cognitively impaired patients to enhance their ability to remember even relatively simple information such as the names of caregivers. Attempts are being made to describe the pattern of cognitive impairment and tailor therapeutic approaches based on an understanding of individual differences. This movement to develop what might be called rehabilitative techniques is perhaps most important, because it creates a sense of optimism about care of AD patients, which has for so long been dominated by nihilism.

No consistently effective drugs are available to treat dementia in either AD or PD. Experimental studies based on an understanding of the neurotransmitter abnormalities in both conditions are under way. To date, treatments with agents to enhance cholinergic function have been the most promising, although results have been modest (Civil & Whitehouse, 1988). Studies with noradrenergic and serotonergic drugs are also in progress based on animal studies that suggest a role for bioamines in cognition and on autopsy studies that demonstrate these systems are affected in AD and PD. Nootropics ("toward mind"), such as piracetam, promise much, yet so far have delivered little (Growdon, Corkin, Huff, & Rosen, 1986). For the most part, clinicians should focus more on how the avoidance of medicine can prevent excess cognitive disability than on trying to ameliorate cognitive symptoms with currently available drugs.

Treatment of the co-existing psychiatric and behavioral abnormalities in these conditions can be more successful. Once again, the clinician must attend to the side-effect profiles of medications, particularly anticholinergic properties, which can contribute to the worsening of cognitive symptoms. However, the judicious use of antidepressants and major tranquilizers can be useful in amelioration of depressive and psychotic symptoms, respectively. Even small reductions in the level of anxiety or agitation can make a tremendous difference in terms of caregiver burden to either the family member or professional involved in the care of the patient.

The future for drug treatment of the psychiatric symptoms in AD looks particularly bright. Anti-anxiety agents are being developed that reportedly have less sedation and to which tolerance does not develop. Neuroleptics that seem to have fewer cognitive and extrapyramidal side effects are on the horizon. Antidepressants are being developed that are more selective in their action and appear to have fewer side effects.

CONCLUSION

AD and related disorders such as the dementia in PD will become increasingly common problems for health care professionals in the future as our population ages. A new understanding of the genetics of AD and how environment interacts with the genes to produce the clinical phenotype will ultimately contribute to better models of the mechanism. Comparing the biological and clinical differences between AD and PD and the heterogeneity among the different forms of these diseases will contribute to identifying the roles of specific chemical systems in producing specific behavioral abnormalities. A more precise understanding of the pathophysiology of these disorders may lead to the development of specific markers for the disease process and, subsequently, to diagnostic tests. As we continue to develop new agents that may be more helpful in treating the cognitive impairments present in this condition, we must also recognize that it is the psychiatric and behavioral manifestations that are often painful to the patient and stressful to the caregivers.

REFERENCES

Beal, M. F., & Growdon, J. H. (1986). CFS neurotransmitter markers in Alzheimer's disease. *Progress in Neuro-psychopharmacology and Biological Psychiatry, 10*,259-270.

Boller, F., Mizutani, T., Roessman, U., & Gambetti, P. (1980). Parkinson disease, dementia, and Alzheimer disease: Clinicopathological correlations. *Annals of Neurology, 7*(4),329-335.

Civil, R. C., & Whitehouse, P. J. (1988). Alzheimer's disease. In S. Appel (Ed.), *Current Neurology* (pp. 227-250). Chicago: Yearbook Publisher.

Crook, T., Bartus, R. T., Ferris, S. H., Whitehouse, P. J., Cohen, G. D., & Gershon, S. (1986). Age-associated memory impairment: Proposed diagnostic criteria and measures of clinical change—Report of a National Institute of Mental Health Work Group. *Developmental Neuropsychology, 2*,261-276.

D'Amato, R. J., Zweig, R. M., Whitehouse, P. J., Wenk, G. L., Singer, H. S., Mayeux, R., Price, D. L., & Snyder, S. H. (1987). Aminergic systems in Alzheimer's and Parkinson's disease. *Annals of Neurology, 22*(2),299-336.

Growdon, J. H., & Corkin, S. (1986). Cognitive impairments in Parkinson's disease. In M. D. Yahr & R. C. Duvoisin (Eds.), *Advances in Neurology, Volume 45* (pp. 392-396). New York: Raven Press.

Johnson, K. A., Holman, B. L., Mueller, S. P., Rosen, T. J., English, R., Nagel, J. S., & Growdon, J. H. (1988). SPECT in Alzheimer's Disease: Abnormal IMP uptake reflects dementia severity. *Archives of Neurology, 45*,392-296.

Kalaria, J. N., Mitchell, M. J., & Harik, S. I. (1987). Correlation of 1-methyl-4-phenyl-1,2,3,6-tetrahydropyridine neurotoxicity with blood-brain barrier monoamine oxidase activity. *Proceedings of the National Academy of Sciences of the United States of America, 84*, 3521-3525.

Mayeux, R., Stern, Y., Rosen, J., & Leventhal, J. (1981). Depression, intellectual impairment, and Parkinson disease. *Neurology, 31*,645-650.

Palmert, M. R., Golde, T. E., Cohen, M. L., Kovacs, D. M., Tanzi, R. E., Gusella, J. F., Usiak, M. K., Younkin, L. H., & Younkin, S. G. (1988). Amyloid protein precursor messenger RNAs: Differential expression in Alzheimer's disease. *Science, 241*,1080-1084.

Price, D. L., Whitehouse, P. J., & Struble, R. G. (1986). Cellular pathology in Alzheimer's and Parkinson's diseases. *TINS,* 9,29-33.

Whitehouse, P. J. (1986). The concept of cortical and subcortical dementia: Another look. *Annals of Neurology, 19*(1),1-6.

Whitehouse, P. J., Struble, R. G., Hedreen, J. C., Clark, A. W., & Price, D. L. (1985). Alzheimer's disease and related dementias: Selective involvement of specific neuronal systems. *Critical Reviews in Clinical Neurobiology, 1*,319-339.

Zweig, R. M., Ross, C. A., Hedreen, J. C., Steele, C., Cordillo, J. E., Whitehouse, P. J., Folstein, M. F., & Price, D. L. (1988). The neuropathology of aminergic nuclei in Alzheimer's disease. *Annals of Neurology, 24*(2),233-242.

PART III
Memory, Alzheimer's, and Related Dementias: Intervention and Care

Using an interdisciplinary approach, Part III examines the complicated task of supporting and caring for those individuals affected by the dementia of Alzheimer's disease. Recognizing that a biological breakthrough is not on the immediate horizon, health care professionals have to learn how to deal with the care needs of Alzheimer's patients, their families, and their social units. Insightful and practical perspectives and suggestions from the involved professions of medicine, nursing, social service, and clinical psychology address concerns of the Alzheimer's victim and the enormous burden that often affects the family caregivers. Although the approach to this section is interdisciplinary, the disciplines do not share the same viewpoints of treatment and management issues. In Chapter 9, Kathryn Riley defines and describes the treatment needs of Alzheimer's patients in light of the related cognitive, emotional, and behavioral changes. She emphasizes that the first phase of psychological intervention begins by sharing the diagnoses with the patient and family. Specific psychosocial interventions and therapies are described along with directions for future research and clinical care.

Cameron Camp in Chapter 10 introduces a memory intervention that is effective in teaching the names of people and subjects. The technique was developed to help individuals suffering from Alzheimer's disease. A description of the most recent research involving this technique for facilitating memory is presented. While the amount of information learned by the intervention may be little, on the other hand it could be of significant value for interpersonal relationships between the caregiver and the patient.

Next, Kathleen Buckwalter offers a nursing perspective on the care of Alzheimer's patients. She highlights a few of the many roles nurses embrace in the care and support of Alzheimer's victims, such as management of behavioral problems, environmental change, and evaluation and implementation of relevant research findings. Buckwalter, contrary to Camp's position of using a memory intervention technique that is intensive, supports the introduction of less stressful activities and the progressive reduction of environmental stimulation for Alzheimer's patients. There is also some controversy as to what information is important for the Alzheimer's patient to know. However, it is generally agreed that although success for the Alzheimer's victim may be limited, these various learning techniques give hope, particularly when interventions are started in early stages of the disease. A balance must be found between the interventions and the stress placed on the AD victim and their families.

In Chapter 12, Lisa Gwyther outlines her approach to caregiver problems in dementia. Through vignettes she demonstrates that good care for the person with Alzheimer's disease is family centered. She reminds us that the core responsibility of the professional caregiver is to assist the family with care and provide support for the Alzheimer's victim, both at home and in formal care facilities. Gwyther challenges professionals to look more critically at the type of help offered and what is expected of caregivers.

In Chapter 13, Robert Kane continues the focus on meeting health care delivery service needs of Alzheimer patients and their families. He calls for services that are both rational and compassionate. Alternatives to institutions, client preference, quality assurance, innovative technologies for caregiving, and policy and service issues are explored with sensitive concern. Both health professionals and policy experts must come to grips with social policy and treatment issues surrounding dementia. Examination of health care policy issues and health care delivery system for aged persons will continue to be a major concern as the aged population increases.

MAY L. WYKLE

9

Psychological Interventions in Alzheimer's Disease

Kathryn Perez Riley

During the past 10 to 20 years, Alzheimer's disease (AD) has gone from being considered a fairly rare form of presenile dementia to having the status of a household word. The Alzheimer's Disease and Related Disorders Association (ADRDA), a self-help group founded in 1980, had originally pledged to bring the disease "out of the darkness." Scientific publications, research funding, and clinical care settings have increased dramatically in recent years in response to the great needs of Alzheimer's patients and their families. Most of this work has focused on one of three areas: accurate differential diagnoses of Alzheimer's disease from other dementing illnesses or reversible conditions; biomedical research into the causes and possible cures for the illness; and programs designed to assist the family caregivers of Alzheimer's victims. Each of these areas is tremendously important—yet even taken together, a major gap exists in this growing body of interest and knowledge related to Alzheimer's disease. That gap is consideration of the Alzheimer's patient as an individual. In our zeal to detect the presence of the disease with greater specificity and to discover its biological markers and etiology, as well as to provide care and aid to stressed and burdened caregivers, we have often given short shrift to the needs of the Alzheimer's victim. The aim of this chapter is to bring attention to and document the value of identifying the AD patient as the primary target of psychological interventions. These interventions will be defined broadly to include individual, family, and group psychotherapy, as well as environmental and psychosocial approaches. The small body of available literature in this area will be reviewed, and the author will provide information on treatment methods from her work, along with clinical examples. The much larger literature on interventions with caregivers, while related to the topic at hand, will not be reviewed here. Family caregivers will be discussed as co-participants or adjuncts to the therapeutic procedures designed with the AD patient in mind.

A recent review of literature on Alzheimer's disease revealed that even when the topic at hand was "care," "management," or "interventions" in AD or other dementing diseases, the identified patient generally has been the family caregiver (Rabins, 1981; Zarit & Zarit, 1982; Barnes & Raskind, 1984). When the focus is on the patient, most of the writing has to do with his or her behavioral disturbances that are distressing to the caregiver, with interventions consisting of drug or behavioral management designed to ease the caregiver's stress (Carstensen & Edelstein, 1987; Kerzner, 1984; Hollister, 1985). While caregivers are certainly in need of attention from clinicians and researchers, and issues of burn-out, decreased well-being, and declining physical health of the often frail elderly caregiver are of great importance, we may be doing a disservice to both the AD victim and family by focusing only on the caregiver's stress or the accurate diagnosis of the patient. If we mechanistically prescribe medications or behavioral management of behaviors such as paranoia, hallucinations, or agitation in the AD patient, we are in danger of ignoring the phenomenology of the afflicted individual, for whom these behavioral disturbances may reflect an underlying need that will not be met by even the most judicious and well-titrated dose of haloperidol. Instead, we must re-focus our energies on the individual needs, reactions, and feelings of the AD victim. We must increase our awareness of and sensitivity to these issues, beginning when the patient and family begin the assessment process, continuing during their reactions to the diagnosis of Alzheimer's disease, and remaining available throughout the often long and always painful course of the disease.

INTERVENTIONS WITH THE ALZHEIMER'S PATIENT

While the bulk of the current literature has focused on the caregiver, there are a few recent articles that describe therapeutic interventions for the patient (Byrne, 1984; Akerlund & Norberg, 1986; Solomon, 1980; Zarit, Zarit, & Reever, 1982; Yesavage & Karasu, 1982) as well as the benefits of day care and other psychosocial programs for the demented elderly (Sands & Suzuki, 1983; Panella, Lilliston, Brush, & McDowell, 1984; NIA, 1980; Godber, 1977). A major exception to this focus on either caregivers or medications has been the work in group therapy with cognitively impaired older adults. However, as can be seen in a literature review conducted by Gilewski (1986), almost all of these published efforts have dealt with supportive, remotivation, or socialization therapy for mixed groups of "organically" impaired persons within institutional settings. The applicability of these studies to outpatient psychotherapy with Alzheimer's disease patients is limited, although this does not detract from the usefulness of their results. In addition, most of the articles cited previously present case reports, anecdotal data, or descriptions of programs that do not yet involve the systematic evaluation of interventions. However, as with any new area of clinical work, these kinds of reports are necessary to stimulate more formalized research projects, and it is encouraging to see the AD victim as the primary target of some innovative programs. A problem that remains, however, is the tendency of clinicians and researchers alike to limit their interventions in depth and in scope, presuming perhaps that the AD patient has seemingly, by virtue of a diagnosis alone, already lost the capacity for insight, self-behavior change, and self-initiated symptom relief. Thus, remotivation groups, reality orientation, and day care programs are the most commonly described psychosocial interventions for demented older persons (Folsom, 1968; Hanley, McGuire, & Boyd, 1981; Linden, 1958; Panella et al., 1984), as opposed to supportive, insight-oriented, or other forms of "talking" therapy on an individual basis. As has been mentioned, psychotropic medication is the most commonly cited and recommended treatment for Alzheimer's patients (Hollister, 1985), along with behavioral management techniques (Carstensen & Edelstein, 1987). The problem with all of these interventions is that they may deny the AD patient a sense of personal responsibility (Hollister, 1985) if they place the control in the hands of the health care professional and/or caregiver who designs and implements such programs. It is the author's contention, borne out of years of experience in working with Alzheimer's patients and their families, that psychological interventions for the patient can and must be developed and evaluated in order to help alleviate the burdens of worry, depression, anxiety, and bewilderment in the individual who is facing the slow and relentless disintegration of self that is Alzheimer's disease.

When such psychological interventions are described or merely advocated in published works, most authors focus on the undeniably critical stage of adapting to the news that the diagnosis is Alzheimer's (Rabins, 1981; Kerzner, 1984; Barnes & Raskind, 1984). This work is important and will be expanded upon later in this chapter. However, the emotional needs and reactions of the AD patient do not stop after some resolution or acceptance of the diagnosis has occurred. Instead, just as caregivers must deal with a never-ending series of changes brought about by the deterioration inherent in Alzheimer's disease, so too must patients assimilate and adapt to the losses that they are facing, at least until the capacity for insight, self-reflection, and integration of events is truly lost.

The remainder of this chapter will define and describe the treatment needs of Alzheimer's patients in relationship to the cognitive, emotional, and behavioral changes that accompany the disease. Specific forms of the psychological interventions will be discussed, including individual, couples, family, and group therapy, as well as a brief consideration of medications and behavioral management as adjunct measures. Finally, future directions for research and clinical work will be described.

EARLY TREATMENT NEEDS IN ALZHEIMER'S DISEASE: LOSSES AND REACTIONS

The need for psychological treatment in AD patients stems from the losses associated with the diagnosis itself, the progression of the illness, and the emotional reactions of the individual to these events. In addition, the responses of the patient's family, friends, and co-workers all may contribute at times to the need for some kind of psychosocial intervention.

Being given the diagnosis of Alzheimer's disease, however tentative it may be, is nothing short of being told one has a terminal illness, which to many may sound the death knell. In fact, with the success of recent efforts to educate the public, the disease has taken on the connotations and significance with which cancer has traditionally been associated. In response to these factors, many professionals and family members debate about whether or not to tell the patient that AD is the diagnosis, just as debates occurred in the past over the decision to inform cancer victims of the nature of their illness. Lipkowitz (1988) has noted that it is preferable to tell the AD patients what their diagnosis is, in order to prevent barriers from developing between them and their families and to enable the patient to participate in planning for the future. This approach makes sense from a psychological perspective as well, since it will prevent the individual from self-blame for the declines and deficits inherent in AD, and it will allow him or her to be a truly active participant in all phases of care, management, and adjustment. On the other hand, there may be rare instances in which the patient will be better off not hearing the actual term "Alzheimer's"; in these cases the nature and consequences of dementing illnesses in general may be explained without invoking the spectre of Alzheimer's disease. Any decision to withhold information from the patient should be a decision made by the family, not the professional. Furthermore, such deception or half-truths will likely backfire more often than not, especially now that so many people know about Alzheimer's disease (and suspect they have it) before they even enter the professional's office for evaluation.

Thus, the first phase in psychological interventions with AD patients begins with the diagnosis—one that is shared by the professional or team with the patient and family in an open forum with at least 60–90 minutes alloted for the session.

Families will not be served well by being given this devastating news in either a dry, overly detailed form, or in a rushed and time-limited format in which their questions, which may take some time to formulate, are left unanswered. Although these recommendations might seem superfluous in the advanced and sophisticated times of the present, this author has seen numerous families who have been evaluated at the best centers, only to have been given a hurried and cursory explanation of their loved one's diagnosis by a single professional or team who sat with downcast eyes. The families' impression is often that this news is harder for the team to give than for the patient to receive! In addition to providing an accepting, honest diagnostic and informative session, it is recommended that a second, follow-up session be routinely scheduled for the patient and family with the member(s) of the assessment team chosen by the patient or family. This provides an opportunity for further questions to be asked: not uncommonly, the shock or dismay felt at actually hearing the term Alzheimer's disease may temporarily preclude further rational thought. A second session, held a few weeks to a month after the diagnosis is given, is invaluable not only to the entire family, but also to the members of the professional team who are then able to determine whether further intervention is necessary at that time. It is in this follow-up session when the question "Are you *sure* it's Alzheimer's" is asked (or repeated), and the delicate business of dealing with denial vs. reality and acceptance begins. For some families these two information (follow-up) sessions may be all that is necessary for the time being as they then work alone to assimilate the information into their life plans. Further intervention may or may not be accepted but should always be offered.

PROMOTING ACCEPTANCE

The next point at which psychological interventions are so vital but often not available occurs after the diagnosis has been given and some rudimentary level of acceptance has occurred. The issues at hand will vary depending on a number of factors, including the stage of the disease and severity and nature of the deficits that have occurred thus far; the patient's personality characteristics, life-style, and pre-existing coping mechanisms; and finally, the nature of his or her interpersonal, social, and cultural milieu. There have been some published references to psychotherapy at this stage (Rabins, 1981; Aronson, 1988; Byrne, 1984, Gilewski, 1986), in which the goals are to foster a realistic acceptance of the illness, to vent or express feelings of anger, frustration, and fear, and finally, to develop means of coping with or compensating for the dysfunctions that are occurring. It is in this phase that depression is most likely to be seen in the AD patient, primarily in reaction to the declines in memory, complex problem solving abilities, and language skills that are becoming increasingly evident (Salzman & Gutfreund,

1986; Poon, 1986). The task of the mental health professional, then, is to provide an opportunity for the patient to express his or her emotions and to develop instrumental and effective coping styles in response to the illness. Consideration should be given to the use of antidepressant medications, although the anticholinergic effects of some of these drugs may exacerbate the cognitive impairment (Kerzner, 1984; Hollister, 1985; Jarvik & Trader, 1988).

Decisions about the nature and duration of psychotherapy most appropriate in this adjustment/adaptation phase of Alzheimer's disease must be flexible without being disorganized. Short-term interventions lasting from two to 15 sessions can often be helpful, and it is most useful to conceptualize the needs of the AD patient in terms of repeated, intermittent contacts that are brief in duration. The traditional view of therapy as an intensive "one shot" cure for a discrete problem is not generally applicable in Alzheimer's disease, which by its very nature is a continuous, dynamic process. This will result in the need to update coping styles and adaptations previously attained. In addition, expectations for long-term benefits of any short-term intervention plan are unrealistic. Rather, the goals should focus on ameliorating distress, emotional dysfunction, and excess disability (Brody, Kleban, Lawton, & Silverman, 1971) during each phase of the illness, utilizing appropriate treatment approaches as outlined below.

The patient's task of accepting the diagnosis of AD begins with hearing the professional team announce their conclusions, but does not end there. Reactions will include anger and denial, withdrawal, anxiety and agitation, and depressive reactions ranging from mild to profound. Helplessness, hopelessness, and suicidal ideation may also result. Therapists must follow the general principle of allowing the individual to maintain current defenses, while gradually working to replace those that are dysfunctional with more adaptive means of coping. Thus, denial and distortion of the diagnosis and its consequences initially may be necessary and adaptive responses to the news that one has Alzheimer's disease. However, the individual will generally fare better if at least partial acceptance can replace denial, along with a slow progression toward accommodation to the disease and the accompanying changes in life-style and daily functioning.

METHODS OF INTERVENTION

The modality of therapy to be employed with the AD patient should be determined on an individual basis (Solomon, 1980) using the same criteria that would be applied to any nondemented client. While the goals of therapy will certainly be shaped and limited by the severity of the individual's deficits, it has been the author's experience that insight-oriented psychotherapy can be just as viable in AD as in other problems. Cognitive-behavioral, client-centered, and supportive approaches all have been suggested for use with Alzheimer's patients (Solomon,

1980; Byrne, 1984; Beck, 1982; Akerlund & Norberg, 1986; Gilewski, 1986), although "organic" conditions have been listed as criteria of exclusion in at least one manual for cognitive therapy with older adults (Yost, Beutler, Corbishley, & Allender, 1986). This kind of exclusion criterion reflects a general belief that the demented elderly are inappropriate candidates for psychotherapy, a view that is being increasingly refuted in the literature. Thus far, the focus in this chapter has been on helping Alzheimer's patients begin to accept and adapt to the realities of their condition. Individual psychotherapy, usually short-term, has been found to be useful. Group psychotherapy for newly-diagnosed AD patients also may be a viable method of intervention, and although the author is aware of the existence of a few such groups across the country, published outcome studies are not yet available.

Couple and Family Therapy

It is obvious that the AD patients' reactions to the diagnosis do not occur in a vacuum. Instead, the social and family context in which patients function will have a major impact on the nature of their psychological, as well as instrumental, needs and concerns. As has been noted, interventions aimed at family members and caregivers of AD patients have dominated the literature (Aronson, 1988; Rabins, Mace, & Lucas, 1982), but more often than not, the patient is excluded from family sessions. Family support groups sponsored by ADRDA do not generally involve Alzheimer's victims, although there is no specific guideline that excludes them. While families and caregivers certainly need opportunities to receive help and express their feelings openly and in the absence of the afflicted individual, interventions that involve the family or married couple can be quite valuable in promoting acceptance of the diagnosis of Alzheimer's disease. The onset of AD, like any severe chronic illness, is an event that produces disequilibrium in the family system. This disruption, along with the emotional reactions to the diagnosis, should be a focus of intervention involving a couple or family. The adjustments to be made include, but are not limited to, changes in financial and household responsibilities, limitations in activities of daily living, socialization, transportation, interpersonal relationships, and sexuality.

Case Illustration

A common problem at this stage results when the patient is willing to accept his or her illness, but the spouse or another family member refuses to discuss the diagnosis or accept its validity. The following case illustrates the difficulties presented in this kind of situation.

> Mrs. G was a 72-year-old woman who came to a multidisciplinary geriatric assessment center for evaluation of changes in her cognitive functioning and feelings of depres-

sion. Mrs. G's husband of 45 years accompanied his wife to all of the appointments, and when interviewed by a variety of staff members, he repeatedly stated that all his wife needed was a "pill" to bring her back "up." A detailed assessment that included neuropsychological testing and psychiatric evaluations revealed that while Mrs. G did seem to be somewhat depressed, her history and the nature and severity of her cognitive and language deficits were strong evidence of Alzheimer's type dementia. A combination of psychotherapy and antidepressant medication was offered to Mrs. G; the trial of medication was undertaken by the psychiatrist in part because of the extreme pressure exerted by Mr. G. The medications were discontinued after Mrs. G complained of unpleasant side effects. Individual therapy of a supportive and exploratory nature was continued for a total of 12 sessions. While Mrs. G was understandably distressed and concerned about the implications of her diagnosis, she was able to accept it, and in fact had known that something was wrong for quite some time. The effectiveness of the therapeutic intervention aimed at helping her to deal with her feelings was hindered, however, by her husband's adamant and unwavering refusal to accept the idea that his wife had Alzheimer's disease. Although he attended a few joint therapy sessions, he was unwilling to enter into a longer-term process, and the sessions that were held were largely unproductive. Mr. G's denial created tension between him and his wife, and it led him to maintain expectations of her that she could not meet, such as his belief that she should still drive. In spite of the difficulties with her husband, Mrs. G was able to work through many of her initial fears and reactions and began to develop compensatory behaviors for some of her cognitive deficits. She stopped playing in two of her weekly card games but maintained a third that was less demanding, and she began to engage in alternate social activities that were enjoyable but did not highlight her deficits. The early sessions were held on a weekly basis. Later they were held every 2 months, and the final two sessions occurred at 4-week intervals. Therapy was terminated when the initial goals of acceptance and adaptation were reached, and Mrs. G's feelings of depression had subsided. Longer-term marital therapy was recommended, but because of some longstanding difficulties as well as the onset of his wife's Alzheimer's disease, Mr. G declined to participate. Mrs. G was assured that she could return for follow-up sessions or a renewed therapeutic contact if she felt the need for further assistance.

This case demonstrates the usefulness of psychotherapy in the early stages of Alzheimer's disease. First, it is an example of the co-existence of depression and dementia. In addition, the patient's reactions and subsequent treatment were complicated by a difficult relationship with her husband, who was convinced that all she needed was medication to cure her depression. While the ideal intervention would have involved the spouse in an active attempt to help both husband and wife deal with the diagnosis and begin to accommodate their expectations and life-style accordingly, individual therapy with the patient proved to be beneficial in helping her to achieve these goals for herself.

Family Therapy

A final note on types and methods of intervention in the early stages of AD concerns the extended family. In addition to the spouse, children, grandchildren, and siblings, nieces and nephews and even parents may be integral components of a family system. Their reactions, interpretations, and expectations about Alzheimer's disease all may affect the patient's ability to cope with the illness. When there are a number of children involved in decision making or caregiving, intervention may be helpful in achieving consensus and a smooth flow of communication and adaptation. It is generally most helpful to arrange large family meetings, as well as smaller sessions that involve only those family members who are most involved in the patient's daily life; frequently this will involve the spouse and an adult daughter or son. As with individual or couples-based therapy, family therapy conducted in the earlier stages of AD will focus on acceptance, understanding of the disease, and its implications for future planning and management.

INTERVENTIONS IN THE MIDDLE AND LATE STAGES OF ALZHEIMER'S DISEASE

The psychological needs of the AD patient and his or her family have been described in relation to the time of diagnosis and the early phases of the disease. Fear, depression, worry, denial, withdrawal, and hopelessness all have been described as possible reactions that may be dealt with in a variety of therapeutic settings and modalities. As the disease progresses and new deficits appear with concomitant declines in daily functioning, these same emotional reactions can recur or worsen. Mild depression may deepen into severe melancholia and despair; suicidal ideation and behaviors may appear in the patient who retains the capacity for insight as the decline progresses. It has often been assumed that this capacity for self-reflection and the awareness of deficits deteriorates rather rapidly in dementing diseases. While this may be true in some cases, many AD patients remain aware of their condition well into the disease process, even if this awareness seems clouded or absent at times. Professionals and families involved with AD must be continually sensitive to the feelings of anxiety and loss experienced by the afflicted individual, and symptoms of severe depression or other emotional reactions should be treated aggressively.

Case Illustration

The need to consider psychological interventions is illustrated by the case of an elderly couple who had apparently devised a double suicide pact.

> Mrs. K had been diagnosed as having a dementing disease, which began to progress fairly rapidly after a few years of minimal decline. At this point, her husband, who had a mild to moderately severe case of multi-infarct dementia, began talking of his

desire to have them both "go" at the same time. Detailed questioning revealed that Mr. K had apparently talked with his wife about his plan to drive both of them off of a cliff near their home, in order to end their suffering and to ensure that neither would be left alone. A number of interventions were immediately undertaken, including 24-hour supervision of the couple, restricted driving, and family therapy sessions. Ultimately, Mr. and Mrs. K moved to an assisted living environment with nursing care made available for Mrs. K, whose dementia continued to progress.

Behavioral Disturbances

In addition to the emotional reactions described previously, the middle and later stages of Alzheimer's disease are often characterized by other disturbances such as agitation, wandering, sleeplessness, paranoia, and hallucinations. The medical and behavioral management of these problems have been described elsewhere as useful and, at times, essential methods of intervention in many cases (Jarvik & Trader, 1988; Thal, 1988; Hollister, 1985; Carstensen & Edelstein, 1987). Nevertheless, it should be recognized that paranoid, agitated, or restless behaviors may reflect an underlying emotional need or concern of the Alzheimer's patient. In these cases, simply removing the behavior or reducing its severity with psychotropic medications or behaviorally-based interventions may not solve the problems, and the unmet need will likely be manifested in another form. While timely efforts to deal with the behavioral disturbances of the moderately or severely demented AD patient are desirable, it is often quite useful to take the time to explore with the patient the meaning of his or her behaviors and to attempt to identify and meet whatever emotional needs may be underlying the disruptive or disturbing actions. The level of cognitive and/or language impairment may preclude this type of active exploration, but efforts directed at understanding the individual phenomenology of a given behavior may facilitate effective interventions.

The Final Step: Institutionalization

Institutionalization is the final area in which psychological interventions in Alzheimer's disease can be useful. Although not all AD victims are placed in nursing homes, it is likely that the majority of those who reach the end stages of the disease will need full-time care (Aronson, 1988). The painful decision to institutionalize a relative can be made easier with short-term interventions designed to elicit and work through feelings of guilt, anxiety, and loss, as well as to provide accurate information regarding the choice of an appropriate nursing home. The creation of specialized Alzheimer's units in institutions across the country is an encouraging event, but families will need assistance in determining whether there is indeed anything "special" or beneficial about specific units, at least until standardized guidelines for these units have been developed and implemented.

Finally, the role of the mental health professional need not end once the AD patient has been placed in a nursing home. In the event that new disruptions or disturbances in the individual's behavior develop following institutionalization, the therapist who has worked with the patient and family may be in the best position to act as a consultant to the nursing home staff in developing methods of caring for and intervening with the Alzheimer's patient.

CONCLUSIONS AND FUTURE DIRECTIONS

This chapter has attempted to identify the needs and characteristics of the Alzheimer's patient as they relate to psychological interventions through the course of the disease. It has been demonstrated that while we have a sizeable body of literature to guide our efforts in assisting family members and other caregivers in their efforts to cope with the disease, there is less material available when it comes to psychotherapeutic interventions designed with the Alzheimer's patient as the identified recipient of services. It is hoped (and recent publications give reason to be optimistic) that future directions in the care of the AD victim will continue to extend beyond pharmacotherapy or behavioral management to include psychotherapeutic interventions that involve afflicted individuals and their families in individual as well as group sessions. More attention should be paid to the needs of the patient from the point of diagnosis through the mild and moderate stages of decline, and including the end phase, which may involve institutionalization. Research efforts and funding aimed at finding the cause and cure of Alzheimer's disease are indeed crucial, yet it is clear that until these goals are achieved, there will remain many victims of the disease who deserve our best efforts at easing their burden and that of their families.

REFERENCES

Akerlund, B. M., & Norberg, A. (1986). Group psychotherapy with demented patients. *Geriatric Nursing*, March/April, 83–84.

Aronson, M. K. (Ed.). (1988). *Understanding Alzheimer's Disease*. New York: Charles Scribner's Sons.

Barnes, R., & Raskind, M. (1984). Long-term clinical management of the dementia patient. In J. P. Abrahams & V. J. Crooks (Eds.), *Geriatric Mental Health* (pp. 75-93). Orlando, FL: Grune & Stratton, Inc.

Beck, P. (1982). Two successful interventions in nursing homes. The therapeutic effects of cognitive activity. *The Gerontologist, 22*(4)378–383.

Brody, E. M., Kleban, M. H., Lawton, M. P., & Silverman, H. A. (1971). Excess disabilities of mentally impaired aged: Impact of individualized treatment. *Gerontologist, 11*, 124–132.

Byrne, K. D. (1984). Psychotherapy with cognitively impaired older adults. Paper presented at the annual meeting of the Gerontological Society of America, San Antonio, Texas.

Carstensen, L. A., & Edelstein, B. A. (Eds.). (1987). *Handbook of Clinical Gerontology*. New York: Pergamon Press.

Folsom, J. C. (1968). Reality orientation therapy. *Journal of Geriatric Psychiatry, 1*, 291–307.

Gilewski, M. (1986). Group therapy with cognitively impaired older adults. In T. L. Brink (Ed.), *Clinical Gerontology* (pp. 281-296). New York: Haworth.

Godber, C. (1977). Planning services for the elderly demented patient [Supplement]. *Age and Aging,* 6,100–103.

Hanley, I., McGuire, R., & Boyd, W. (1981). Reality orientation and dementia: A controlled trial of two approaches. *British Journal of Psychiatry, 138*, 10–14.

Hollister, L. E. (1985). Alzheimer's disease: Is it worth treating? *Drugs, 29*(6), 483–488.

Jarvik, L. F., & Trader, D. W. (1988). Treatment of behavioral and mood changes. In M. K. Aronson (Ed.), *Understanding Alzheimer's Disease* (pp. 128-145). New York: Charles Scribner's Sons.

Kerzner, L. J. (1984). Diagnosis and treatment of Alzheimer's disease. In G. H. Stallerman (Ed.), *Advances in Internal Medicine*, vol. 29 (pp. 447-470). New York: Year Book Medical Publishers, Inc.

Linden, M. E. (1958). Group psychotherapy with institutionalized senile women. *International Journal of Group Psychotherapy, 3*, 150.

Lipkowitz, R. (1988). Services for Alzheimer patients and their families. In M. K. Aronson (Ed.), *Understanding Alzheimer's Disease* (pp. 198–226). New York: Charles Scribner's Sons.

National Institute on Aging Task Force Report. (1980). Senility reconsidered: Treatment possibilities for mental impairment in the elderly. *Journal of the American Medical Association,* 244, 259–265.

Panella, J. J., Lilliston, B. A., Brush, D., & McDowell, F. H. (1984). Day care for dementia patients: An analysis of a four-year program. *Journal of the American Geriatrics Society, 32*, 884.

Poon, L. (Ed.). (1986). *Handbook for Clinical Memory Assessment of Older Adults*. Washington, DC: American Psychological Association.

Rabins, P. V. (1981). Management of irreversible dementia. *Psychosomatics 22*(7), 591–597.

Rabins, P. V., Mace, N. L., & Lucas, M. J. (1982). The impact of dementia on the family. *Journal of the American Medical Association, 248*(3), 333–335.

Salzman, C., & Gutfreund, M. (1986). Clinical techniques and research strategies for studying depression and memory. In L. Poon (Ed.), *Handbook for Clinical Memory Assessment of Older Adults* (pp. 257-268). Washington, DC: American Psychological Association.

Sands, D., & Suzuki, T. (1983). Adult day care for Alzheimer's patients and their families. *The Gerontologist, 23*(1), 21–23.

Solomon, J. G. (1980). Treating an elderly woman with organic brain syndrome. *Psychosomantics, 21*(2), 165–166.

Thal, L. J. (1988). Treatment strategies: Present and future. In M. K. Aronson (Ed.), *Understanding Alzheimer's Disease* (pp. 50-68). New York: Charles Scribner's Sons.

Yesavage, J. A., & Karasu, T. B. (1982). Psychotherapy with elderly patients. *American Journal of Psychotherapy, 36*(1), 41–55.

Yost, E. B., Beutler, L. E., Corbishley, M. A., & Allender, J. R. (1986). *Group Cognitive Therapy*. New York: Pergamon Press.

Zarit, S. H., & Zarit, J. M. (1982). Families under stress. Interventions for caregivers of senile dementia patients. *Psychotherapy: Theory, Research, and Practice, 19*, 461–471.

Zarit, S. H., Zarit, J. M., & Reever, K. E. (1982). Memory training for severe memory loss: Effects on senile dementia patients and their families. *Gerontologist, 22*(4), 373–377.

10

Facilitation of New Learning in Alzheimer's Disease

Cameron J. Camp

To weave the magic of a thing, you see, one must find its true name out.
(LeGuin, 1975, p. 107)

In this chapter a memory intervention for individuals suffering from Alzheimer's disease will be described. Our initial research has focused on teaching such individuals to learn the names of strangers or to relearn the names of individuals who are familiar to them, such as those of staff at adult day health care centers. The chapter will begin with an anecdote about the first time we used this technique. The history of the intervention will then be described—how it initially was created in an experimental setting with college students, then was used in an experiment with people suffering from neurological disorders, and how it came to be used in its current form. A description of our most recent research involving three individuals with Alzheimer's disease will follow. A review of the potential strengths and weaknesses of the intervention and suggestions for future research will close the chapter.

A GLIMPSE OF MAGIC

In the fall of 1986 I was working in an adult day health care center with two student research assistants. We had been gathering initial data on a memory battery for everyday memory problems. We were especially interested in observing how individuals diagnosed as having Senile Dementia of the Alzheimer's Type (SDAT) would perform on the various subtests of the battery. After the testing session, the client was asked to recall the names of each of the two students in turn. She could not do so. After each recall failure, she was provided with the correct name. She was then asked to name the psychologist. Again she failed and was provided the correct name. A few seconds later, she was asked to name the psychologist, and did so. She was then asked to name each student in turn, and failed. The correct name was always supplied after each of these attempts and each subsequent recall failure. She was again asked to name each student in turn, and again failed. She was then asked to name the psychologist, and did so. Next, she was asked to name each of the students in turn. This was repeated twice (three pairs, six recall attempts). She failed on each recall attempt of a student's name. She then was asked to name the psychologist, and did so. Thus, the paradoxical result was that the seldom-presented psychologist's name was remembered best.

On the way out, a student asked the client how she had been able to remember the psychologist's name. The client responded that she did not know. When the research team was leaving the center, the psychologist asked the students how the woman was able to remember his name. The students responded that they did not know. At that point, the students asked the psychologist what he had used to let the woman learn his name. His response was "magic," and he then relayed the history of that seemingly "magical" intervention to his students.

History of the Spaced-Retrieval Memory Intervention

The history of a memory intervention called the "spaced-retrieval technique" may illustrate how research findings can migrate from laboratory to real life settings. Also, after showing the "secret" to this "magic," it is hoped that it will not appear to be a mere illusion.

Discovery

Landauer and Bjork (1978) described a name-learning technique called "spaced-retrieval," in which the names of faces were retrieved at increasingly long intervals over a fixed period of time. This testing technique was related to good long-term retention of face–name associations. In addition, a control procedure was used in which face–name associations were tested an equal number of times per testing session as in the spaced-retrieval condition. However, the amount of time between tests in the control procedure was a constant. This allowed a test of whether memory enhancement effects of the spaced-retrieval technique were a result of sheer practice (repetition) or of the addition of increasingly longer intervals between testings. Retention of information in the control procedure was worse than that in the spaced-retrieval technique, confirming that practice alone could not account for enhanced memory associated with spaced-retrieval. They concluded that retrieval practice serves to guide and enhance further recall attempts, especially if intervals between recalls are consistently expanded.

This initial study by Landauer and Bjork (1978) was a traditional lab-based type of research. They were interested in optimizing the effects of studying new information and used large numbers of college students as their research participants. Before long, however, the implications of their research for application on other populations became apparent. Alan Baddeley (1984) cited the spaced-retrieval technique as an example of "micro level" distribution of practice in learning, and stated that the technique combined early success with a gradual increase in distribution of practice. Moffat (1984), in the same volume, cited the general technique as potentially being useful as a strategy for memory therapy. He wrote,

> During training sessions involving rehearsal the aim should be to handle an immediate test of recall rather than encourage rapid repetition of the material. This is both more effective as a learning strategy, and offers an ongoing monitoring of an involvement by the patient. (p. 68)

Rabinowitz and Craik (1986) studied the effects of prior retrieval of information on the subsequent retrieval of that same information in younger and older adults. They found that prior retrieval of information benefited subsequent retrieval in both older and younger populations. Citing their own findings and those of Landauer and Bjork (1978), they wrote,

> On a practical level, however, the present results suggest that retrieval practice may be an effective mnemonic technique for elderly adults—techniques of self-testing under conditions that optimize the likelihood of initial retrieval could easily be taught in group settings. (p. 374)

Application of the Findings

Schacter, Rich, and Stampp (1985) used the spaced-retrieval technique with four clients suffering from memory disorders of varying etiologies. They reasoned that this technique might be more useful than other memory training procedures, because spaced-retrieval requires little cognitive effort (Bjork, 1979). Thus, clients would not have to generate mental images or engage in organizational strategies when trying to learn new information—tasks that can be very difficult for individuals with neurological impairments.

Schacter, Rich, and Stampp found that this technique did allow acquisition of new information. Working with an experimental paradigm similar to that of Landauer and Bjork (1978), they showed several faces (photographs) of individuals to each participant and provided the participants with other attributes about the target individuals, such as names or occupations. They found that some information about target characteristics was retained over a 12-day interval, though recall was far from perfect.

They also had attempted to train participants to spontaneously utilize the spaced-retrieval procedure. These attempts met with mixed results. Their two older participants did not show effective spontaneous initiation of spaced-retrieval as a rehearsal strategy to learn new information. Even for the clients who maintained the use of the strategy during the experiment, " . . . there was no evidence of continued use of the strategy outside the laboratory" (Glisky & Schacter, 1986, p. 56).

In general, it is difficult to get even healthy older adults to spontaneously utilize and maintain memory improvement training (Anschutz, Camp, Markley, & Kramer, 1987). However, Schacter, Rich, and Stampp did conclude that spaced retrieval might be useful for facilitating retention of specific pieces of information that are important for clients to remember.

Spaced-Retrieval and Alzheimer's Disease

Initial Study

The author first learned of the spaced-retrieval technique at the third George A. Talland Conference on Memory and Aging at New Seabury, MA, in 1985. After discovering the extant research literature on the topic and conducting some pilot work with the procedure (such as was described above in the anecdote), an initial study was designed to use the spaced-retrieval procedure with a client diagnosed as having SDAT at an adult day health care center.

Modifications of Procedures

For our purposes, we decided to modify previously used procedures based on the recommendations of Schacter, Rich, and Stampp (1985) and our own expertise working with this population. Landauer and Bjork (1978), as well as Schacter, Rich, and Stampp (1985), used multiple stimuli, with Schacter, Rich, and Stampp concluding that this may have hampered performance in their client population. We concentrated instead on forming a face–name association for one specific photograph.

Another change in procedure that we instituted involved intervals between tests. In the previously mentioned studies, intervals between tests were manipulated by showing a target and then presenting the target again after interjecting a variable number of intervening stimuli. For example, after showing a picture, either one, four, or 10 other pictures might be presented before retesting memory for the name of the target. In our study, intervals between tests were actual time segments (e.g., 15 sec, 30 sec, etc.), and these intervals were filled with conversation or game playing to prevent active rehearsal.

In our initial study the participant was presented with a photograph and told that the name of the person pictured (i.e., the target) was "Janet Simpson." The participant was then presented the picture and asked to recall the target's name in each of the next series of trials.

Initial Results

As shown in Figure 10.1, the first trial was given 5 sec after exposure to the target. This resulted in a correct recall. In a second trial 10 sec later (15 sec total time elapsed in the experiment), the participant again recalled the name of the target. The third trial was given 20 sec later (35 sec total time elapsed in the experiment), resulting in a correct response. Subsequent trials were presented at intervals of 40, 60, 90, 120 sec, etc.

Note that the initial interval was quite small (5 sec), the next interval was somewhat larger (10 sec), and interval size began to expand by an additional 30 sec once recall was successful at a 1-min interval. We had initially hoped to simply double the amount of time between intervals from one trial to the next; however, pilot testing had indicated that (at least for our first client) increasing the intervals in 30 sec increments led to fewer recall failures than doubling retention intervals.

Figure 10.1 also demonstrates our procedure for dealing with incorrect response. If a trial resulted in a "miss," the participant was presented the target on the next trial at the interval that had last demonstrated successful retention. In Figure 10.1, it is shown that the client did not recall the name of the person in the photograph after an interval of 180 sec. The client was told the name, asked to repeat it, and then tested after a 150-sec interval (the highest previous successful retention interval). When the name was recalled, the next expansion of the interval was only 15 sec (to 165 sec). After succeeding at that interval, the client was tested after 180 sec. When recall was achieved, the client was put back on the regular expansion of the schedule (30-sec increments of expansion).

Thus, we used a technique similar to shaping, in which closer and closer approximations of a desired response (long-term retention of new information) were elicited from the participant. When the amount of change was too great to be successfully elicited, we "retreated" to a previous level of success and then moved "forward" in smaller steps.

One week later, we returned. We began the session by asking the client to name the photograph. She could not. We then gave her the name, had her repeat it, and waited for 4 min (240 sec—the longest interval of successful retention from the week before). As shown in Figure 10.1., she could not recall the name over this interval. At that point, we gave her the name, had her repeat it, and then tested for recall after a 2-min (120-sec) interval. Thus, we "retreated" to a shorter interval by cutting the 4-min interval (longest retention interval from the week

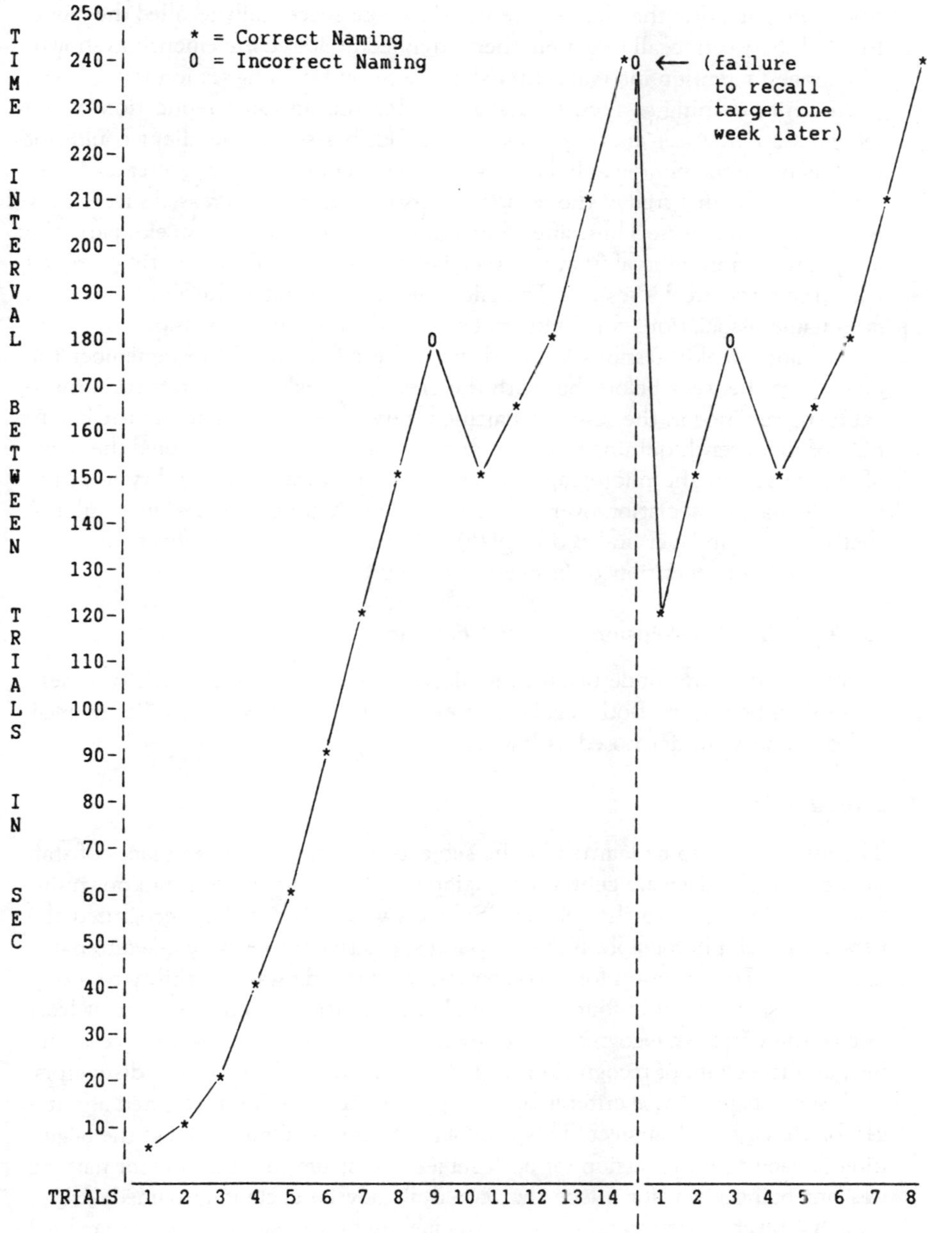

FIGURE 10.1 Recall performance as a function of trial and retention in the first two weekly training sessions.

before) in half. After the 120-sec interval, the client successfully recalled the name. Intervals between recall tests were then extended in 30-sec increments, as shown. The longest retention interval achieved in the second training session was 240 sec.

The third training session, held 1 week later, was an exact replication of the second session. After another week, at the fourth session, the client could not initially name the photograph, but was able to remember the name after a 240-sec interval on the first trial of the session. Intervals then were increased successfully in 30-sec increments. Thus, after four training sessions held 1 week apart, the longest retention interval from the week before was retained as a starting interval within the next week's session. The client also demonstrated the ability to retain face–name associations for 7-min intervals within a training session.

Two more weekly sessions followed, with the client unable to remember the name from the week before, but with the previous week's longest retention interval being retained as the session's starting interval. One week later, at the beginning of the seventh training session, the client successfully remembered the name of the person in the photograph. Thus, she demonstrated the ability to retain the face–name association over a 1-week interval. A control procedure similar to that used by Landauer and Bjork (1978) demonstrated that this effect was not a result solely of repetition of face-name testings.

Replication and Extension of Initial Findings

A second study was undertaken to replicate these initial results with two men, ages 67 and 68 years. Both regularly attended an adult day-care facility in New Orleans and were diagnosed as having SDAT.

Procedures

The associations to be learned by the subjects were the names and faces of staff members at the day care center. Photographs of four staff and four unknown distractors were shown to the subjects. Subjects were asked if they recognized the person in each photograph. If they responded positively, they were asked to name the person. The criterion for participation in the study was the ability to recognize at least three out of four of the familiar faces, the inability to name at least one of the correctly recognized faces (which then could serve as a target stimulus), and the claim of recognition made for no more than one of the distractors. Both subjects met these criteria, and a separate photograph was selected as a target for use with each subject. This same set of tests was administered at the beginning of each training session for both subjects to assure that training for naming was not being given for a face that could already be accurately named.

Each subject participated in three individual training sessions; sessions were held once a week and lasted for approximately 30 minutes. At the beginning of the first session, subjects were shown the target photograph and asked if they could name the person pictured. When the subjects could not do so, they were told the name of the person and asked to repeat it. Recall was then tested at intervals of 5 sec, then 10 sec, 20 sec, 40 sec, and 60 sec. From that point on, recall test intervals were increased in increments of 30 sec. Within all sessions, no recall failures occurred (though one participant failed to retain the initially-trained name across sessions). During the intervals between recall testing within a session, the experimenter engaged the subjects in conversation, looked at books of photographs with the subjects, or played games of checkers and cards.

Results

For the first subject, the retention interval for naming the photograph of the targeted staff member reached 3½ min by the end of the first session. On the fourth day after the session he was shown the actual staff member at the center and asked to name her, which he did. On the sixth day after the initial session, he failed to name the actual staff member. The next day, at the beginning of the second session, he correctly named the target photograph. Thus, the client was able to retain the face–name association for the photograph for 1 week, but the ability to generalize the training to the naming of the actual staff member was of a more limited duration.

At the second training session, a new target photograph was presented. In a slightly extended session, the longest testing interval reached was 5 minutes. At no time did the client mistakenly use the name of the first staff member when naming the second target photograph. Thus, the second piece of new information did not elicit intrusion errors from the original training. Generalization of training for the second target staffer showed the same pattern as the initial generalization of training.

At the start of the third and last training session, the participant correctly recognized and named the second target, but not the first (i.e., original) target that had been learned in the first week of training. Training was then reinstated for the original target item. The first retention interval for the origin target lasted 3½ min rather than 5 sec, since 3½ min represented the longest retention interval during the initial training session. Recall was successful after the 3½ min delay, with retention intervals being expanded in 30-sec increments afterward. Again, no recall failures were found within the last training session.

For the second subject, the initial training session elicited a 4-min maximum interval of retention. Generalization the following week was not obtained, nor was the subject able to name the target at the start of the second session. The first interval used in the second session was 4 min (the highest retention interval during the first training session). From this point the subject eventually reached a 6-min retention interval. The following week, generalization was found after 4 days but not after 6 days. At the third training session, the subject accurately named the target at the beginning of the session and proceeded to learn a new target, reaching a maximum retention interval of 5 min. Again, no intrusion errors from initial training were found.

Potential Problems and/or Limitations

Though we have had some encouraging initial success using the spaced-retrieval technique, there are some potential problems or limitations to its utility. It is certainly not a panacea for the memory impairments that accompany SDAT. We can only hope that it can enhance the quality of life (and care) for those suffering from a deadly and irreversible disease process. It is therefore important that we discover, acknowledge, and accept the limitations of this cognitive intervention (and other "cognitive remediations") until a true cure can be found.

How Much Information Can Be Learned?

One of the first pragmatic issues to be addressed with the use of spaced-retrieval training is: how many new pieces of information can be learned (or relearned) using this procedure? We simply do not know. It may be the case that the procedure only can be used successfully for a limited number of items. If this proves to be the case, the clinician should be quite selective in what things will be taught using the procedure.

Interference Effects

Though some new learning can be facilitated using spaced-retrieval, it is possible that the first few newly-learned items might interfere with later learning (e.g., through intrusions, perseverations, etc.). (See Chapter 5 for other examples of intrusion and/or interference errors in SDAT.) Though our initial results are encouraging, interference effects still may prove to be a limiting factor in the use of spaced-retrieval as a learning intervention.

Maintenance of Learning

At this point, we do not know how long information acquired using the spaced-retrieval procedure will be maintained. Our initial findings indicate that such learning may undergo decay and/or that retrieval of the information may become less accessible over time. This is true of new learning in college freshmen as well, though SDAT may show an acceleration of the processes found in normal populations. In any event, the amount of time necessary to train and maintain new learning using the spaced-retrieval procedure could become so large that it is not a cost-effective intervention in terms of effort expended and benefits gained.

Generalization of Learning

In our research, we have tested for the "near generalization" of training. Our participants demonstrated the ability to name actual staff members after learning to name staff photographs. However, this may be the limit of generalization. (Of course, if we had worked with the actual staff members as stimuli rather than their photographs, the issue of generalization would have been a moot point.)

The woman who was in our original study told her family that she liked to take part in our research because we were "making her smarter," but it is doubtful that the training improves general memorial ability. For training to truly generalize, participants must "learn to learn" (i.e., learn how to initialize and use the strategy across settings). This may be particularly difficult for older adults with SDAT (again, see the results of Schacter, Rich, & Stampp, 1985).

Areas for Future Research

We have only begun our investigation of the utility of the spaced-retrieval technique. A variety of topics needs to be addressed before the usefulness of this procedure can be accurately assessed. The following is meant to serve as a representative (but certainly not exhaustive) listing of future research topics in this area.

Maintaining Retention

As mentioned in the listing of limitations of the training, the ability to recall information learned through spaced-retrieval can be lost. The important question facing practitioners wishing to use the technique is: can the ability to recall new information be retained, and what is necessary to ensure relatively permanent retention of the information? Is there an optimal training schedule to ensure long-term retention (along the lines of spaced- versus massed-practice)? Would overlearning increase the ability to retain the information? What should the longest testing interval be during the training sessions? Should newly-learned items be retested on a regular basis to ensure that they are still accessible? If so, should the retesting be done daily, weekly, or monthly?

Other Types of Associations

We are engaged currently in a study using the spaced-retrieval technique to train individuals with SDAT to remember locations (e.g., where keys are kept) and other types of associations. We are interested in discovering which types of learning/memory problems can be attacked using this procedure, as well as in determining how to adapt our procedures to the demands of these new problem domains.

Multiple/Concurrent Training Schedules

Another topic to be investigated is the use of the spaced-retrieval intervention to train the retention of several new pieces of information at the same time. What might be the best way to train the retention of the names of three staff members at the same time? Will interference effects become more pronounced with the use of multiple/concurrent training schedules? Is there a maximum amount of new information that can be retained?

Stages of the Disease Effects

How is the ability to learn using the spaced-retrieval technique influenced by the stages of Alzheimer's disease? Is the technique only useful in its early stages? If information is learned using spaced-retrieval at an early stage of the disease, can it be maintained as the disease progresses?

Need to Individualize Retention Intervals During Training

Originally we had thought that we could increase recall intervals at a rate that doubled the previous interval (e.g., 1 min, 2 min, 4 min, 8 min, etc.). This did not seem to be effective with our first participant, and so we simply increased testing intervals in 30-sec increments for all of our participants. However, the optimal or highest increase in testing intervals probably varies across individuals. Our goal is to train longer and longer retention intervals. Therefore, training will be optimized by finding the greatest increase in testing intervals that can still produce high rates of successful recall for each individual.

Caregivers as Trainers

Even if the spaced-retrieval technique proves to be a highly effective means of enhancing new learning in SDAT, it will be of limited use if it remains an arcane piece of mental alchemy wielded by a small number of health professionals. Ultimately, the spaced-retrieval technique must be put into the hands of caregivers if it is to have a truly beneficial effect in dealing with memory loss associated with SDAT. The end result of research guided by questions such as those described in this section should be the delivery of a proven intervention, whose strengths and weaknesses have been well documented, into the hands of those who have the most contact with populations suffering from SDAT. A clear regimen for implementing and optimizing the effects of spaced-retrieval training must be provided if we are to fulfill our obligations as applied research scientists.

Computerization of the Training Procedure

Perhaps an optimal means of "giving away" the spaced-retrieval intervention to caregivers is through computerization of the training procedure. A computer in the home might allow the caregiver to train a person with SDAT while conducting routine activities in a familiar setting. For example, a computer program could cue the caregiver as to when to test a client. The caregiver then would simply record the success or failure of a recall trial, and the computer would then determine the next testing interval, keep a running record of the client's progress, etc. The computer could even determine the optimal amount of time to expand testing intervals for an individual client. The caregiver thus would be freed from the responsibility of acting as a timekeeper. This might be especially useful if multiple/concurrent training schedules for several items are being used. Individualizing and implementing optimal retestings to allow maintenance of new learning would also be controlled by the computer.

It might even be possible to use "meta-training" with clients who have SDAT, such as teaching them to remember to go to the computer whenever they hear a signal. At that point, the computer might present stimuli for testing, direct the client as to how to enter a response, and likewise take over the responsibility of the testing session. Thus the computer would take over the responsibility of self-testing so that the client with SDAT would not be burdened with having to remember to use the spaced-retrieval strategy.

The technology to implement these suggestions is currently available. However, before engaging in a large-scale computerization effort, the benefits gained from the use of spaced-retrieval must be demonstrably large enough to warrant the expenditure of time, effort, and cost involved in such a project. In addition, as mentioned before, the optimal way to achieve such benefits must be known in order to maximize the use of computer technology.

*The Development of a Small-*n *Experimental Paradigm*

Finally, the use of spaced-retrieval with this special population might allow the creation of a small-*n* experimental paradigm for the study of forgetting, where the *n* represents not only subjects but also experimental stimuli. The ability to study memory decay/enhancement functions for specific pieces of information in this population may lead to an increased understanding of how memory functions in normative populations.

SUMMARY

Research has been initiated using the spaced-retrieval training technique as an intervention with clients suffering from SDAT. The technique has proven to be an effective way of training these individuals to learn and retain face–name associations over relatively long time intervals. In addition, some evidence of near generalization of the training was found. Potential problems and limitations of the technique were discussed, along with areas for future research.

At this point, we do know that the spaced-retrieval technique has several positive aspects to recommend it as an intervention. The technique is nonthreatening and is embedded within the context of a social visit. Clients would look forward to the next time experimenters would arrive to "play checkers" or "chat," rather than viewing the training as "testing" sessions. The most striking thing about observing the procedure in operation is the ease and confidence with which individuals with (often severe) memory deficits remember names. One client, after successfully recalling a name after a 210-sec interval, told the experimenters, "Don't worry. I won't forget." Another client once named a photograph "Sherlock Holmes," laughed at the surprised look on the face of the experimenters, and then produced the correct name. In some instances, the task appeared almost too easy. Knowing the memory deficits of the clients involved, their performance sometimes appeared to be the work of a special type of "magic."

> But what a wizard spends his life at is finding out the names of things, and finding out how to find out the names of things.
>
> LeGuin, 1975, pp. 107–108)

ACKNOWLEDGMENTS

The author would like to thank Helen Chawkin, Gyongyvere Andrews, Leslie McKitrick, Nola Felker, Paula Cimino, and Clint Moore for their assistance. Sarah Moody-Thomas and Tom Elder offered valuable suggestions. The author also thanks Linda Greenwald, Directress, and the clients of the Kenner Adult Day Health Care Center.

Comments, inquiries, and especially reports of results when attempting to use the spaced-retrieval technique, should be sent to: Cameron J. Camp, Ph.D.; Department of Psychology, University of New Orleans, New Orleans, LA, 70148.

REFERENCES

Anschutz, L., Camp, C. J., Markley, R. P., & Kramer, J. J. (1987). Remembering mnemonics: A three-year follow-up on the effects of mnemonic training in elderly adults. *Experimental Aging Research, 13*, 141–143.

Baddeley, A. D. (1984). Memory theory and memory therapy. In B. A. Wilson & N. Moffat (Eds.), *Clinical Management of Memory Problems* (pp. 5-27). Rockville, MD: Aspen.

Bjork, R. A. (1979). Retrieval practice. Paper presented to the Conference on Developmental and Experimental Approaches to Memory, Ann Arbor, MI, October, 1979.

Glisky, E. L., & Schacter, D. L. (1986). Remediation of organic memory disorders: Current status and future prospects. *Journal of Head Trauma Rehabilitation, 1*, 54–63.

Landauer, T. K., & Bjork, R. A. (1978). Optimum rehearsal patterns and name learning. In K. M. Gruneberg, P. E. Morris, & R. N. Sykes (Eds.), *Practical Aspects of Memory*. New York: Academic Press.

LeGuin, U. K. (1975). *The Tombs of Atuan*. New York: Bantam Books.

Moffat, N. (1984). Strategies of memory therapy. In B. A. Wilson & N. Moffat (Eds.), *Clinical Management of Memory Problems* (pp. 63–87). Rockville, MD: Aspen.

Rabinowitz, J. C., & Craik, F. I. M. (1986). Prior retrieval effects in young and old adults. *Journal of Gerontology, 41*(3): 368–375.

Schacter, D. L., Rich, S. A., & Stampp, M. S. (1985). Remediation of memory disorders: Experimental evaluation of the spaced-retrieval technique. *Journal of Clinical and Experimental Neuropsychology, 7*(1):79–96.

11

Caring and Alzheimer's Disease: The Nursing Perspective

Kathleen Coen Buckwalter

Nursing care of the patient with Alzheimer's disease (AD) takes place in a variety of community-based and institutional settings. It is multifaceted, complex, and challenging. Therefore this chapter can only highlight a few of the many important roles nurses play, such as the management of behavioral problems, environmental manipulation, and evaluation of research related to professional nursing activities. One area not covered, but which remains a significant nursing function, is management of caregiver stress. However, this topic is addressed elsewhere in Chapters 9 and 12.

To date, the bulk of AD research has been focused on biomedical approaches designed to discover the cause of the disorder. Nurses tend to be concerned more with the behavioral, cognitive, and psychosocial impairments that result from brain changes in AD, rather than its etiology. This concern is tempered by understanding of the progressively deteriorating course of the illness. Despite the enormity of the care burdens associated with AD, very little study or federal monies have been directed toward improving the situation confronted by the more than 2.5 million older persons currently afflicted with AD and their families (Buckwalter, 1986). Many nurses argue that what is also needed, in addition to biomedical research, is an applied services research focus. This focus would stimulate the development of research-validated clinical and services approaches to address the immediate needs of AD patients and their families. In this effort nurses would be pivotal members of multidisciplinary research and care teams. Thus the development and implementation of appropriate, effective, and safe nursing services for AD patients and their families is a critical challenge to the nursing profession (Buckwalter, Abraham, & Neundorfer, 1988).

Of the multiple treatment roles in AD, diagnosis, staging, and prognosis are more within the domain of psychiatrists, neurologists, and psychologists. Management of AD patients and their caregivers is within nursing's domain. Nurses have developed and are testing conceptual models for planning and evaluating nursing care of the AD patient (Hall & Buckwalter, 1987; Maas, Buckwalter, & Russell, 1986). This conceptual approach is based largely on symptom presentation, which in AD can be affected by a variety of factors. These include areas of the brain affected; size of the lesions; premorbid personality including coping skills, intelligence and motivation, cultural, and ethnic affiliations; and external resources. The latter category includes elements such as demands by others, the environment, and economic resources.

CONCEPTUAL BASIS FOR CARE

From the nursing perspective, then, care planning for the AD patient is based on the four-fold patterning losses commonly associated with AD: cognitive, affective, conative, and progressively lowered stress threshold (Hall & Buckwalter, 1987). Cognitive losses include problems with short-term memory, time sense, abstraction ability, decision making ability, perceptual changes, impairments in problem solving, and judgment. Affective losses include social withdrawal, diminished inhibitions, pseudo-hallucinations and other psychotic symptoms, personality changes, avoidance of complex stimuli, agnosia and increasing self absorption. Conative or planning losses include the inability to carry out voluntary or goal-directed activities, confusion leading to frustration with voluntary tasks, apraxia, and inappropriate task performance in a variety of spheres.

The fourth area of losses, developed by Hall (Hall & Buckwalter, 1987) is called *progressively lowered stress threshold* and includes symptoms such as increased anxiety, night wakening, catastrophic behaviors, "sundown syndrome," purposeful wandering, confusion and agitation, combative behavior, and diminished reserve characteristic of the AD patient whose stress thresholds have been exceeded. Hall and Buckwalter (1987) have identified certain assumptions that underlie this nursing perspective:

1. The client exists in a 24-hour continuum.
2. The confused or agitated client is not comfortable and has the right to be comfortable.

3. All behavior is rooted and has meaning, therefore all catastrophic behavior has a cause.
4. All humans need some control over their person and environment.
5. All humans need some unconditional positive regard.

The identification of factors that heighten stress and potentiate dysfunctional behaviors in AD is an essential nursing role. These factors include fatigue; change of environment; caregiver routine; multiple competing stimuli; demands to achieve beyond abilities; and physical stressors such as illness, medications, and comfort. Hall, Kirschling, and Todd (1986) postulated that most nursing units are characterized by unending spaces and stimuli that can be overwhelming to the AD client with cognitive, affective, and conative losses, and a diminished stress threshold. Low or controlled stimulus care units have been proposed as one approach to the management of behavioral problems commonly associated with AD. These units include chairs that invite the demented patient to rest for short periods (twice daily), eating groups limited to three to four residents in their own room rather than a congregate setting, decreased disturbing stimuli such as mirrors and artwork, and decreased aural stimuli such as public address systems, telephones, and TV sets. Nurses also identify and treat the causes of excess disability in the AD population. Excess disability has been defined by Dawson et al. (1986) as a reversible deficit that is more disabling than the primary disability, existing when the magnitude of the disturbance in functioning is greater than might be accounted for by basic physical illness or cerebral physiology.

THERAPEUTIC ADAPTATIONS

Attention to multiple safety factors in both the home and institutional settings is another critical nursing concern. Therapeutic adaptations may be made in either setting to simplify the environment. These adaptations include, for example, increasing the lighting in hallways, raising the toilet seat, providing bathtub transfer rails, enhancing access to telephones, using plastic bedsheets, removal of scatter rugs and cords that might precipitate falls, preventing access to poisons, locking cupboard doors, getting rid of unused appliances, securing doorlocks, and putting an identification bracelet on the demented patient. Nightlights help orient AD patients during episodes of nighttime awakening, color contrasting helps patients to distinguish areas such as toilet seats, and use of signs and symbols rather than words helps AD patients to identify important areas such as toilet or dayroom. Painting tap faucets bright red to indicate "hot," making sure that potentially hazardous areas such as the stove are fixed so that they cannot be manipulated by the demented individual, smoke alarms, and non-skid strips in the bathroom are other essential safety features. Nurses often work closely with occupational and physical therapists to implement therapeutic and safety adaptations.

CARE PLANNING

Care planning is an important nursing function, and many care planning principles emanate from the nursing perspective described in this paper. These include reducing environmental stressors such as intake of caffeine, monitoring and diminishing misleading stimuli such as television sets, modifying the environment to decrease unending spaces and unneeded noise, and reducing the number of extra people in large groups with whom the demented person comes in contact. Also, compensation for planning and cognitive losses should be a part of the nurse's care planning effort. This might include providing a calm and consistent routine, eliminating changes in personnel or in the environment whenever possible, keeping patient choices to those that they can handle, not trying to reason, argue, or confront the demented client, not expecting or asking the client to try harder to learn to do something, not trying to teach them new routines that may frustrate or agitate them, and decreasing expectations related to recovery of lost skills.

A third focus of care planning concerns the provision of unconditional positive regard (Rogers, 1951). Some ways in which nurses provide unconditional positive regard include addressing the client by their first name, using one-to-one communication techniques, using touch as a sensation to reassure the patients, allowing the AD client to use whatever preserved social skills they may have, using reminiscence and validation approaches rather than forcing reality orientation, eliminating the number of negative responses from the environment, and using distraction rather than confrontation as a nursing approach.

A fourth important area for nurses to consider in care planning for AD patients allows for lowered stress threshold and diminished reserves in this population. This includes the implementation of "time out" periods twice daily, usually mid-morning and mid-afternoon, and alternating high stimulus activities with more restful ones when negative reactions do occur. The nurse intervenes to decrease stimuli and reevaluate the nature of the stressors, particularly physical factors such as pain, a full bladder, or adverse side effects from medications. In all these care planning efforts, careful documentation is necessary to determine potential cause-and-effect relationships.

Finally, the nursing role includes care of the AD client's family through education, such as teaching caregivers to understand the symptoms commonly associated with AD and the care plan that has been developed specifically for the AD patient. Planning for respite, visitor training, referral to support groups, and for legal and financial counseling, provision of day care, and in-home support are all included under this important aspect of care planning. The family is an essential ally for nurses in that all care planning needs to recognize the environment the patient came from. Attention to family needs is an important part of nursing care, and discharge planning must not neglect these important elements of care planning if and when the AD client moves to another level of care. Overall, the nursing objective of care is to maximize the level of safe functioning and quality of life for both AD clients and their caregivers.

BEHAVIORAL MANAGEMENT

Nurses deal with many behavioral problems associated with Alzheimer's disease. Foremost in nurses' caregiving efforts is the consideration of safety for the AD client as well as other residents and staff in institutional settings. To this end, disruptive behaviors are monitored with an attempt made to prevent their recurrence. The nurse notes when AD clients are unable to participate in care and treatment activities. When they become disturbing to other clients, intervention must occur.

Nurses should pay attention to problems not only for the demented client but also for the lucid client, particularly in those settings where AD patients are integrated with nondemented patients (Maxwell, Bader, & Watson, 1972). For the lucid client, these concerns include invasion of privacy, damage or loss of personal property, decreased socialization, interrupted sleep patterns, and fear of physical harm by the agitated AD patient. For the demented client, use of tranquilizing medications may cause decreased mobility, loss of appetite, and dependency in activities of daily living. They may be excluded from traditionally planned activities, which subsequently results in decreased socialization. They may be overwhelmed by negative restrictive feedback from their caregivers and other residents in the facility. This in turn may increase their fear and agitation as well as negative family responses that may precipitate the use of both chemical and physical restraints.

In dealing with these complex problems, the nurse or caregiver (or educator of other caregivers such as family members) strives to meet several goals. These include assisting the AD client by acting in a prosthetic manner, supporting losses, preventing stress-related behaviors to promote emotional comfort, and, as noted previously, providing the client with unconditional positive regard. To meet these goals, nurses need to have an understanding both of normal and pathological behaviors associated with aging. They must conduct holistic assessments and be able to interpret the assessments of other members of the multidisciplinary team. Only in this way can nurses identify and interpret the meaning of behaviors. Thus, care can be truly individualized and focused on remaining strengths and abilities rather than client limitations. Often the nursing role resembles a balancing act, trying to balance patient and environmental demands against diminishing internal and external resources. The enormous care burdens associated with providing quality of care to AD patients suggest that nurse administrators must look at different staffing patterns on units that house a high percentage of AD patients. For example, provision of increased time for Activities of Daily Living (ADLs), increased staff-to-patient ratios, the provision of support groups for staff needs, as well as tangible and intrinsic rewards for caregivers should be considered.

Therapeutic communication is yet another nursing function, and guidelines for nurse/patient communication in dementia have been set forth by Bartol (1979).

In general, style of speech is important, including speaking slowly, clearly, increasing volume, and decreasing tone. When questions are asked, a response should be waited for, and only one question should be asked or one command given at a time. If a request or question is repeated, it should be repeated in a similar manner. Humor is another element that can be used effectively in therapeutic communication. Nonverbal communication strategies employed by nurses include overemphasis and exaggeration of facial expressions, standing directly in front of the AD patient, always maintaining eye contact, moving slowly, and not abruptly confronting the demented client from behind. In general, increasing the complexity of stimuli and the number of trials or repetitions does not always facilitate communication. It is *how* things are said (the effect) that is more important than *what* is said (the content).

Management of untoward or catastrophic behaviors is one of the most significant nursing functions. Examples of catastrophic behaviors include "sundowning syndrome," pacing, withdrawal from activities, night wakening, noisy behaviors, purposeful wandering, fearfulness, confusion, combativeness, and agitation and frustration. Nurses have developed protocols to manage these catastrophic responses. These protocols cover both the immediate and secondary actions taken by nurses. For example, immediate measures designed to protect the patient and decrease dysfunctional behaviors may include placing the AD patient in a quiet environment, eliminating all unnecessary stimuli (especially the television), checking for and eliminating potential stressors such as a full bladder, pain, restraints, or catheters. If restraint is necessary, it should be done in the least restrictive manner and only when the client presents a hazard to themselves or others (for example, when the client is combative or persists in dangerous behaviors). Similarly, tranquilizers should be administered cautiously and conservatively, and only in response to dangerous behaviors.

When responding to catastrophic behaviors, nurses should remain calm and reassuring to patients, confirming their sense of safety and security. If at all possible nurses should ask family members or other caregivers to assist them with the untoward response. Secondary measures are designed to minimize recurrent dysfunctional episodes and are based on identification and elimination of potentially confusing environmental objects. These measures include increasing the number of daily rest periods, the use of soothing music, confronting the patients in terms of reorientation only when it does not agitate them, and efforts to minimize the number of staff who interact with the AD client. It may also be necessary for the nurse to limit or restrict large groups of family visitors to prevent recurrence of negative episodes.

Nighttime episodes are another area where nurses manage AD behaviors. In general, the AD client who awakens at night should be toileted and fed and then returned to bed. If they continue to remain awake they should be taken to the nurses' station and allowed to remain awake rather than sedated. It may be helpful to have the lights on in the room starting at sunset. Fall precautions should always be observed. Finally, in contrast to commonly held beliefs, increasing the number and length of daytime rest periods may serve to decrease nighttime episodes of awakening.

NURSING RESEARCH

Yet another important nursing role is to systematically evaluate nursing and environmental interventions on the cognitive and functional performance levels of AD patients, family attitudes toward care, staff morale and attrition, and cost effectiveness (Maas, Buckwalter, & Russell, 1986). Analysis of data from these nursing studies will allow researchers to compare various nursing environments for AD patients. This research is valuable for Alzheimer's residents, their families, and managers and policy makers of long-term care institutions concerned with the effective use of resources. Considerable costs are involved in the construction and staffing of special care units. However, the potential costs and threats to quality of care associated with care of Alzheimer's residents on traditional units make it imperative to evaluate the effectiveness of environmentally modified special care units. With the increasing number of persons expected to develop Alzheimer's disease, nurses, managers of long-term care facilities, and policy makers are faced with the difficult prospect of determining the most effective means of caring for these residents. Because there have been no comprehensive studies of special care units, there is still an absence of empirical support for the many proposed advantages (Peppard, 1985; Rabins, 1986). Few studies have used systematic measurement techniques or measures with established reliability and validity. Given the growing number of elderly persons in the United States and the expected growth in the number of nursing home residents with Alzheimer's disease, it is important for nurses to establish the value of these special treatment units for AD residents.

SUMMARY

Providing quality care for AD patients and their families is an ongoing challenge to nurses. Persons with AD display a number of behaviors, such as wandering and falling, that are difficult to manage and that are commonly treated with chemical or physical restraints. Thus nurses are challenged to develop, implement, and test less restrictive strategies for behavioral management, such as environmental modifications. Multiple, complex, and competing stimuli can contribute to the confusion, agitation, and disorientation experienced by AD patients. Special care units with environmental modifications based on the concept of progressively lowered stress thresholds in the AD patient have been suggested as one strategy to promote the safety and welfare of demented residents. These units are an attempt to reduce or control the amount of sensory stimulation in order to prevent catastrophic behaviors in AD patients and to maximize their functioning.

ACKNOWLEDGMENTS

The help of Joan Crowe in manuscript preparation and Geri Hall for care planning and conceptual contributions related to progressively lowered stress threshold is gratefully appreciated.

REFERENCES

Bartol, M. A. (1979). Nonverbal communication in patients with Alzheimer's disease. *Journal of Gerontological Nursing* 5(4),21–31.

Buckwalter, K. C. (1986). Testimony before Senate Subcommittee on Aging, July.

Buckwalter, K. C., Abraham, I. L., Neundorfer, M. (1988). Preface. *Nursing Clinics of North America* vol. 23 (pp. xi-xiii). Philadelphia: W. B. Saunders Co.

Dawson, P., Kline, K., Wiancko, D. C., & Wells, D. (1986). Preventing excess disability in patients with Alzheimer's disease. *Geriatric Nursing,* 7(6),298–330.

Hall, G. R., & Buckwalter, K. C. (1987). Progressively lowered stress threshold: A conceptual model for care of adults with Alzheimer's disease. *Archives of Psychiatric Nursing,* 1(6),399–406.

Hall, G. R., Kirschling, V. M., & Todd, S. (1986). Sheltered freedom: an Alzheimer's unit in an ICF. *Geriatric Nursing,* 7(3):132–136.

Maas, M., Buckwalter, K. C., & Russell, D. (1988). Nursing evaluation of a special Alzheimer's unit: Phase I baseline data. *Applied Nursing Research,* 9(1),41.

Maxwell, R., Bader, J., & Watson, W. (1972). Territory and self in a geriatric setting. *Gerontologist, 12*,413–417.

Peppard, N. (1985). Alzheimer special-care nursing home units. *Nursing Homes, 34*(5),25–28.

Rabins, P. (1986). Establishing Alzheimer's disease units in nursing homes: Pros and cons. *Hospital and Community Psychiatry, 37*(2),120–121.

Rogers, C. (1951). *Client centered therapy*. New York: Houghton Mifflin.

12

Caring and Alzheimer's Disease: A Social Worker's Perspective

Lisa P. Gwyther

"Best care" awaits more rigorous evidence of how much amelioration is possible for which patients with which levels of family support at which points in the family care process. However, it seems timely to challenge some assumptions and look more critically at what we offer in the name of help.

Gentle humor is a great antidote for professionals who risk taking themselves and their methods too seriously. For example, just before my 40th birthday, a close friend dragged me kicking and screaming to my first aerobics class. I was determined not to join any mass movement toward health, but she won me over by buying me a T-shirt to fit my mood; it read "Pushing 40 is exercise enough." My thesis for this chapter is much the same: Living with AD or a close relative with AD is hard enough. We would do well to lighten up on our expectations of patients, families, and professionals. In caring for AD patients and families, our greatest mistakes come in expecting too much, expecting too little, or expecting things that aren't relevant to quality of care.

For example, when I worked in an Ohio nursing home, I learned how insensitive traditional reality orientation drills could be for adults who retained little short-term memory. These patients still had exquisitely intact adult feelings of shame, embarrassment, and fear. Later Lily Tomlin in her one-woman show reminded me that "Reality is a major source of stress for those still in touch with it." We know we have to do better, but we have gone through some ridiculous stages in trying to achieve more. For example, we now have a tendency to label all social interventions "therapy," package this basic humanity in reimburseable units, and schedule it between 1:00 and 2:00 P.M. on an activity calendar. Now there are labels like humor therapy, pet therapy, touching therapy, music, art, or horticulture therapy, and perceptual therapy. We don't stop to think that people with and without AD have enjoyed humor, hugging, pets, plants, music, and the arts long before we *treated* them with it. Most of us, whether or not we're demented, would prefer these activities or experiences as spontaneous moments in life or in a care milieu. We can't use these activities to treat diseases, since any method is only "therapeutic" in its effects on individuals. Furthermore, it's risky to borrow the confidence and status of medications and curative procedures and apply them to low-tech, but highly skilled care.

A 1977 poem by Elise Maclay sums it up best. She calls it *Insights*:

> They
> Psychiatrists
> Psychologists
> The experts
> Keep reinventing the wheel
> I just read where
> Studies show
> Gazing at water
> Brooks, rivers, the sea
> Is tranquilizing
> Next thing you know
> They'll discover that crowds
> Make people nervous.
> The longer I live
> The more it seems to me
> Life is a gigantic Easter egg hunt
> We go running around like crazy
> Hunting for brilliant truths
> Hidden in plain sight

While we all have our favorite innovations and outcomes we believe are do-able using our version of truth, we can't go wrong innovating as long as we acknowledge that no single setting, strategy, therapy, or profession provides total relief for such a heterogeneous population. While there are no panaceas or all-knowing saintly care providers, there are lots of pearls. Let's begin with what we think we know about family caregiving and the health care team.

Because dementing illnesses are such equal opportunity diseases, they affect a range of persons and families who have widely divergent views of what constitutes good care. I'll never forget a lady in a nursing home in Ohio who was bemoaning the poor care she had received from her attending physician during her hospitalization. With a classic Archie Bunkerism of her era, she announced, "I was in that hospital for 10 whole days and not once did he call in one other doctor for consolation." Many families laugh at the idea of the health care team: "What team," they say, "other than our family's 20 mule team?" Yet, the team is almost sacred to geriatric practice. I used to believe that we had health care teams because older people have multiple problems. It is probably more likely that we have teams because no single discipline wants to feel as overwhelmed as the primary family caregiver does.

Families want generalists—one trusted professional dependable over time as a jack-of-all-trades. Families want that person to be expert and knowledgeable, not a "specialist" who defines his area just narrowly enough to exclude their presenting problem. Dr. Seuss's latest book, *You're Only Old Once*, warns of the dangers of that type of geriatric specialization. Families want what one family medicine marketing poster describes this way: "Don't you ever wish you had a doctor who specialized in you?" People don't want professionals who specialize in AD; they want people who specialize in them.

With or without teams, families want active treatment for their relatives and themselves. Active treatment implies medical, nursing, and social services. They want something done, not just a $1,500 work-up, a pronouncement that "you don't need to bring her back here," and referral to custodial care or a social worker. AD patients get sick, and what scares their family caregivers most is not knowing a new symptom of the dementia from a concurrent acute or reversible illness or a medication reaction. Family caregivers look to the health care professional to validate their concerns and the worthiness of their relative, to acknowledge their loss, and to recognize with the family that often the choices open for care are equally unappealing. Families ask for reassurance, back-up, and well-earned recognition for the invaluable role they play in long-term care. They also look to the professional for information to clear up misconceptions. Even more important, they want help to translate or interpret what's known about dementia to their everyday experiences (why their mother can't shop or cook or why their father insists he already bathed and he's going to drive).

Families also want professionals to be the bad guys—to make the tough decisions, but without the family losing control over their relative's life. Finally, families want more service and reimbursement options, not professional cheerleading or financial incentives to care.

Unfortunately, there are still some professionals who overly romanticize or pathologize the family caregiver as a neurotic martyr or an angry saint waiting for the liberation that only long-term psychotherapy can offer. It's more helpful to see the family facing AD as having a problem, not being the problem. There are few perfect saints or born martyrs; most families care from a sense of family solidarity or values. They can provide more effective care to the extent they have a common enemy—a disease, not each other. They appreciate flexible, tolerant professionals who remind them that there is not total predictability in the responses of persons whose brains are impaired by dementing illness. In spite of the best care or the best environment, progressive dementia gets worse.

It's dealing with the irrational, unpredictable elements of dementing illness that brings most families to seek professional help. Although a specific diagnosis like AD implies bona fide brain damage, the major noticeable manifestations of the disorder are changes in behavior, personality, mood, and function. It is these changes that drive families to seek help. To the extent these changes are dignified as disease symptoms and not labeled as character flaws, manipulation, weakness of will, or laziness, the family is better able to respond appropriately.

It's helpful to illustrate common themes with vignettes or composites that set the stage for discussion. The following scenario suggests avenues for social work support of families facing tough transitions in care. Helping families is probably one of the most effective ways to improve quality of care and quality of life for both patients and their caregivers. Supportive counseling is a bona fide therapeutic modality that is appropriate for many families of AD patients.

SCENE: SOCIAL WORKER ANSWERS HER PHONE AT AN AGENCY

It's the irate middle-aged married daughter of an 82-year-old woman with AD. The social worker spent all the past week selling this lady's mother to a wary nursing home admissions director with a preference for easier care patients. Now the daughter screams, "You were absolutely wrong about Golden Acres being the best place for my mom. She's been there 5 whole days, and they have been the 5 worst days of our lives. I'm feeling more guilty and out of control than I was when I was running between her house and ours. To top it off, that pompous administrator had the nerve to suggest that she needs more care than they are equipped to provide. How do they think I did it all these years? For that kind of money, you would think they could manage one little old lady. He says Mother has been wandering off and trying to call a cab—that's a real joke—there are no cabs way out there. She has all the visitors believing I'm the Devil Incarnate, and she really doesn't need to be there. She says they don't invite her to meals, and since I stole all her money, she can't afford to eat out. She says she can't use her private bath because there's always a crazy old lady in there staring at her. The nurse says she screams when they restrain her at night, and her roommate's husband is complaining because she steals her roommate's stuff, and yesterday she even climbed in bed with her. They say Mother slapped and cursed out a nursing assistant who was helping with her bath—I know better, however—my mother doesn't know

> any four-letter words. Whenever I arrive, Mother is always pacing the public living room shouting, 'I didn't do it. I don't belong in jail. Please honey, I'll pay you if you give me a lift to my mama's house. That woman put me here so my real mama can't find me.' So Ms. Smart Social Worker, you got any other bright ideas??

Notice the common themes in this vignette. Families report that placement in the nursing home is the hardest decision of the whole illness, but it is often the only viable alternative for adult children facing many competing demands. In our studies at Duke University, the most stressed and at-risk times for caregivers were those immediately preceding and after placement of a relative. There is no initial relief from a family's emotional responsibility, regardless of where the patient lives. Often stress levels aren't reduced until the patient dies, and adjustment takes longer than 5 days. Placement often means the family gives up control, but not responsibility.

The placement decision is a lonely one for families, particularly if it is interpreted as abandonment or rejection by the patient or other family members. It's helpful for a family to reassure themselves that the doctor or social worker made them do it. Statements like, "Your mother needs 24-hour care that most families aren't equipped to provide," can be very helpful. Professionals must be willing to assume responsibility for these recommendations, without unduly raising expectations about the success of the placement.

It is hard for laypersons to believe that health care institutions like nursing homes or even hospitals can't protect one little lady from her poor judgment or the wrath of her more intact peers. Unfortunately, as long as hospitals and nursing homes try to be all things to all people, AD patients will experience some misunderstanding or embarrassment.

AD patients can't report their care accurately, they can't remember meals, or advocate for themselves. Some families make adaptive pacts with staff: we'll only believe half of what we hear about you if you will do the same.

AD patients new to a facility face an environment in which nothing makes sense or looks familiar. Wandering and pacing may be a search for something familiar, a search for stimulation, or a way to relieve excess energy inherent in points of dementing illness. Long-term memory is the last to go, and our most primitive symbol of nurturing and security is "mother." It may be easier to remember mother than a spouse of 50 years or your children.

AD patients retain vestiges of well practiced rote behavior; this lady's social autopilot allows her to call a cab or try to pay people. All of these are attempts to retain self-esteem or an image of herself as competent and effective.

The crazy lady in the bathroom is a mirror sign. Some patients don't recognize themselves in mirrors. They may view the image as a comforting companion or a frightening spy, and their fear or pleasure with the image in the mirror should determine the professional response.

Physical restraints in a bed or gerichair increase agitation and screaming, both of which are serious problems in group living. It's scary to see a stranger in your room, and each time she sees her roommate, it's a new experience.

Loss of a sense of time, judgment, or reason means she never knows where her next meal is coming from. Five minutes seems like 5 hours, or vice versa. She may stuff food or silver in her bra or grab her roommate's stale banana for a rainy day.

Most staff injuries with AD patients occur around providing personal care. It is hard for a patient whose variable function permits her to remember that one doesn't undress in front of strangers to follow an unrecognizable aide to an unfamiliar institutional bathroom. Some patients believe it's raining in the shower room, and they refuse to be pushed in the rain. The patient may find it hard to position her body in space to get into a tub. Her uncharacteristic cursing is a symptom of her loss of impulse control: she feels attacked and instinctively fights back or defends herself.

Feelings of being punished for unintended crimes commonly lead AD patients to believe they are in jail, abandoned, or cut off from important security symbols like "mama." She sees old sick people around her, and her last memory is that she is young and has someplace and somebody looking for her. She may fear she is not living up to expectations.

What Can a Social Worker Do When Faced With This Angry Daughter?

The daughter should be encouraged to stay close to her mother at the beginning to help orient her and the staff to each other. Well-meaning offers of respite should be appreciated but ignored. Boot-camp approaches to nursing home adjustment don't work with AD patients. While staff may be less exhausted and more creative, they will depend on the family to orient them to previous comforting routines. The patient should be dressed and out of her room, close to reassuring, consistent staff most of the day.

The patient needs an individual identity within the facility. She needs a meaningful role, one that fits her image of herself and provides a vehicle to get to know and establish some parity with potentially supportive residents and staff. Familiar objects may help her find her room and may make her daughter feel better in visiting her mother when surrounded by her familiar things. Old wedding pictures, war pictures, or pictures with parents are always appreciated and provide a good stimulus for discussions with visitors.

AD patients can give and receive real support to each other, but their relationships must be guided, directed, and nurtured by staff and visitors. The daughter can be encouraged to take her mother around visiting with other residents and families. AD patients also benefit from a flexible but broad range of structured programs throughout the day and evening. Family should be encouraged to go *with* the patient to programs to encourage and guide participation. Activities should be purposeful and meaningful; religious holiday celebrations or beauty shop appointments are better than bingo for most AD patients. Activities enrich and create immediate pleasure by building on strengths or retained function. We can encourage people to laugh and have fun by laughing at ourselves. We don't need "joke therapy." We can create meaningful reasons to socialize just by arranging chairs around a card table or coffee klatch. We can provide stimulating environments for patients to just sit and fantasize or reminisce. We can offer patients the dignity of just observing and not participating until they choose. Activity programs don't just keep people busy. They keep patients involved in a reassuring way that compensates or fills in the blanks in a confusing world.

The daughter and staff should be encouraged to quietly and discreetly replace what the patient takes from her roommate without accusations or rational or moral questions about why she took it. Any explanations to the mother of why she is where she is should not "rub her nose in her disability" nor should it take away her hope. The explanation should preserve her self-esteem, lessen her fear of abandonment, and increase her sense of security. "I'll always know where to find you," or "You'll be here until they get to the bottom of your memory problem," are often kinder than "This is Golden Acres Nursing Home and this is your home now."

Distraction works well if the daughter is having difficulty getting away from her visits. One woman told her mother she was going to throw another load in the washer, and her mother didn't seem to notice her daughter didn't return for a week. The daughter should be encouraged to call, visit, or write regularly, to soothe her mother in whatever ways she finds comforting and helpful in keeping her mother connected to significant family. Walks, rides, listening to music, watching VCR family tapes, sharing favorite snacks, watching children play, or visiting with others may all improve the quality of their time together.

In summary, good care includes a variety of direct and indirect strategies, all of which promote both patient and family security without necessarily changing either's behavior. It allows patients and their families to celebrate their remaining or fluctuating capacities while treating any excess disabilities that compromise function. We can substitute or compensate for lost patient abilities or impulse control. Structured routines protect patients from embarrassment and assure more successful and pleasant moments while letting the program and environment work *for* the patient. "Helpers," regardless of discipline or professional level, should adjust to the patient, rather than expecting a compromised patient to adjust to our reality. Days are carefully balanced to include time for rest, stimulation, reminiscence, and reverie, but especially to continue meaningful work or roles within either the community or family setting. Distraction, diversion, and heading off behavioral outbursts is more successful than threatening, cajoling, reasoning, explaining, or sulking. Building in opportunities for the patient to give and to feel loved and valued models appropriate responses for other helpers, friends, or family members.

Good care is family centered, allowing family caregivers sufficient breaks and recognition to restore their perspective. Staff and families who care do better if they develop tolerance for ambiguity or confusion. A sense of humor is an antidote for the pain of loss, and a strong belief or religious faith offers an acceptable rationale for why such bad things happen to good people. Caregivers quickly acknowledge the value of old-fashioned ingenuity and cherished dependable friends. Furthermore, they learn that time alone changes not only one's perspective but also the focus or the problems one faces. Most important, successful caregivers are hopeful that together, professionals and families can make a difference and learn something that will prove invaluable for those who follow.

A quote from Elizabeth Mandlen in a 1985 Baltimore ADRDA newsletter expresses her feelings and realizations on visiting the nursing home. It inspires us to recognize what we can do in caring for AD patients:

> "Will you take me home?"
> I cannot take you home.
> But I can comfort you when the floor
> shimmers like a sunlit lake.
> I can wait while you layer, like memories
> tissue precisely on tissue
> And remember *for* you who you are
> and what you have done.
> I can give you order and refuge
> in the strange land you inhabit now
> I can love you as you are,
> ....
> But my hand
> cannot remold (such a fragile piece as you)
> No, I wish, but I cannot take you home.

And finally, my friend and colleague, Kathleen Siegle, wrote a poem about her children's response to her mother-in-law's coming to live with them:

> One of my grandmas
> Gives me presents
> On my birthday, or hugs
> Just because
>
> One of my grandmas
> Can't remember me
> or my birthdays
> So I give *her* hugs
> Just because

REFERENCES

Mandlen, E. (1985). *Baltimore ADRDA newsletter.*

Maclay, E. (1977). Insights. *Green Winters*. New York, NY: Readers Digest Press, p. 112.

Seuss, Dr. (1986). *You're only old once*. New York: Random House.

Siegle, K. (1987). *The Caregiver* 7(3):5.

13

Health Care Delivery for Dementia: Meeting the Need

Robert L. Kane

The treatment of Alzheimer's disease should not be viewed as a separate category of long-term care, although some issues obviously need to be addressed quite separately, and there are policy issues with regard to how one manages Alzheimer's patients better in the context of long-term care. The challenge facing the United States is developing a rational and compassionate system for long-term care as a whole and that, in turn, will be an environment in which the fate of Alzheimer's patients will be greatly improved.

ALTERNATIVES TO INSTITUTIONS

We are coming to recognize the error of our past ways and are re-examining some of the ideas that we have held dear for the past couple of decades. There is a growing appreciation of the need to distinguish between the site of care and the type of care. We have adopted imprecise habits of defining types of care by the way they are delivered, but fashions change with learning. Care that once was considered to require many days in the hospital can now be delivered at home or in an ambulatory setting. Indeed, terms like home care don't mean much anymore, because almost anything can be delivered at home.

The changing spectrum has meant we need new terms to fill in the gaps. In addition to hospital and long-term care, we now have an intermediate phase called "post acute care" or "aftercare." Care is increasingly viewed as a series of transitions. With our growing capacity for new kinds of technology, not simply machines but information technology, we are able to deliver many forms of care in the community that previously we used to believe could be delivered only in institutions, in both the acute care sector and the long-term care sector.

We have also come to appreciate the dangers of the "alternatives mentality" (Kane & Kane, 1987). Most of the programs launched a decade ago to test community-based care basically sought to show that community care saved money by keeping people out of institutions. However, because most of the people in the community, even the vulnerables, never went into institutions, they had a very narrow margin to work against in order to show that their care was cheaper.

One area of consensus in long-term care, whether talking to providers or consumers or their families, is that everybody wants to stay in the community as long as possible. Rather than pursuing community care as a goal in itself, we addressed the inappropriate paradigm of the alternative. Not only did we waste a lot of time and money, we created some perverse incentives. Keeping people out of institutions is good for some people and not so good for others. Institutional care may be the right answer for certain sets of the population and the wrong answer for others. The goal is to match treatments and therapies better than in the past.

A disabling by-product of this alternatives mentality is the propensity to shift attention away from the institutions just when we need more efforts to improve them. There are going to be people who need institutional care, although the institutions may look quite different from those we have today. We need to focus creative energy on finding ways to make institutions better places, hence to demand higher standards of quality.

FUNCTION

The common language of long-term care is functioning. The functional approach becomes the final common pathway of long-term care. Long-term care is essentially defined as the care of the dependent portions of the population. A nonproductive distinction is made between the so-called medical and social models, when both are sorely needed in concert.

Efforts to broaden physicians' views by encouraging them to think about patients in terms of functioning may have created some confusion. Functioning has several components. A crucial first step in enhancing functioning is to make the correct diagnosis. There is nothing laudable about treating somebody compassionately for a problem they don't have. Remedying the remediable is the first task necessary in any kind of a functional approach, but it is not sufficient. We need to look beyond that to recognize that the next component in functioning has to do with environment. Environment certainly includes the physical environment. Certain kinds of environments enhance functioning, while others make it worse. For example, the architecture for the treatment of Alzheimer's disease is diametrically opposed to that for treating physical frailties. The former requires large spaces with ultimate confinement, but as few obstructions as possible and long distances to allow people to wander around. The architecture for treating the physical frail requires immediate access to care with travel times as short as possible. Thus, if one were starting to design the most appropriate places to treat different kinds of impaired elderly, the architectural situations would probably be very different. Similarly, patients with congestive failure should not have to climb stairs. Likewise, falls can be prevented by eliminating loose rugs and improving lighting.

But the physical environment is only part of the problem. There is another environment too often ignored: namely, the social environment. What we expect of people has a great deal to do with how well they function. A special problem of social environment can be traced to risk aversion. No place is as risk averse as the hospital. Many of the procedures used by institutions to protect the patient may obstruct functioning. Risk aversion, however, is not limited to hospitals. Families are terribly risk averse. It is very hard for families, particularly with Alzheimer's patients, to trust a cognitively impaired person to live on their own and take the risk of getting into some kind of untoward event, such as leaving the stove on or starting a fire. Very often families make very protective plans for relatives that restrict their environments dramatically and infantilize them without carefully considering the relative risks and benefits of the act.

Another negative influence on the social environment comes from the quest for efficiency. It seems more efficient to do things for people than to help those people do things for themselves. Anyone who has ever tried to raise teenagers knows that. It takes much more manpower, for example, if nursing staff work with patients to help them dress and feed themselves than if the nursing staff does it for the patients. Under pressures to cut costs and minimize time spent per activity, institutions will do the thing that gets the job done fastest.

That kind of short-term mentality, which focuses on the short-run payoff, is the exact antithesis of what is needed in long-term care. Everything we know about long-term care says that the only way to succeed is to invest our efforts up front in the expectation that over time we will recoup those investments by improved functioning and better outcomes, which should potentially lead to fewer complications and down-the-road savings.

The third component of function has to do with motivation. Two paradigms are germane. One derives from the work of psychologists who experimentally demonstrated behavior they called the "innocent victim syndrome." Using studies on college students they showed very dramatically that the group that thought it could control or shock an anonymous victim was much more positive toward this person than was the group that felt impotent to help. The generalizable psychological paradigm derived from this work says simply that when people feel impotent to help other people, they become hostile toward those people (Lerner & Simmons, 1966; Lerner & Lichtman, 1968). The translation into the area of geriatrics and Alzheimer's care is obvious; if we can provide people with tools that at least give them the sense of something they can do to manage the problem, they will approach such patients more positively. Even making the worst of all assumptions, that it is all placebo, one can expect great benefits in terms of changing the attitudes of caregivers toward patients. Given the great potential for meaningful change from better information, the future seems quite optimistic.

The second observation with regard to motivation draws on a review of the work using randomized trials of geriatric assessments (Kane, 1988). The half dozen or so randomized trials of various forms of geriatric assessments generally have a positive effect, despite different people doing the assessments and doing different kinds of assessments on different kinds of people. Interventions vary from extensive multidisciplinary efforts to home visits by a public health nurse (a health visitor in England or a social worker in Denmark) once a month or once every 6 months to see how the patient is getting along. In either case, there are positive benefits. This observation suggests that much of the assessment's value may lie in empowering people to believe that they can make a difference with these people that can improve them. That belief conveys a sense of motivation to the patient: the expectation that more is possible rather than the negative self-fulfilling prophecy of hopelessness. Encouragement can make an enormous difference in enhancing function.

When we talk about functioning as the end result we need to recognize it as the end result of three very important processes: an adequate professional evaluation to remedy the remediable; the development of an environment—physical, psychological and social—to enhance that individual's capacity to function; and finally, a spirit of motivation and an expectation that improvement or maintenance is possible, that the patient is simply not on an inevitable downward course. This package represents a special challenge with a disease like Alzheimer's disease where part of the diagnosis hinges on seeing a gradual downward deterioration. It sounds like an oxymoron.

CLIENT PREFERENCES

Another inadequately addressed topic is the issue of client preferences. Americans are the victims of our own freedom. Because of our love of the Constitution, we have managed to create a very strange kind of environment. We are trapped by our sense of social justice and what we expect of our 85-year-old population. For example, federal law prohibits discrimination on the basis of race or religion.

As a consequence, and in contrast to most other countries in the Western world, we give people at the end of their lives very little choice about where they are going to spend those last years.

At one point in this country, we came close to what could have been the ultimate paradox: we almost invested more in people dying than in people living. As a consequence of the hospice movement, we were prepared to give people tremendous amounts of freedom and choice once we declared them terminally ill. But if we simply declared them chronically ill, they had to go into government-approved facilities that could not discriminate on the basis of any of these things.

We sentence nursing home residents to living situations few of us would accept. In a society where very few of us would tolerate one night in a hotel where we had to share a room with a stranger, we see nothing wrong with sending a relative to spend the next 3 years living with a series of strangers in nursing home accommodations. It is interesting that Canadians see nothing wrong with allowing people to express very clear preferences about cultural and ethnic mix. They tolerate facilities that are very clearly segregated, not only under religious auspices but also under ethnic auspices so the people can associate with people with whom they are comfortable (Kane & Kane, 1985). We have a great deal of difficulty with that in this country.

Another area where we seem to fly in the face of client preference is the question of what may be called "the mixers and the splitters": should severely cognitively impaired be managed separately from the physically frail? The arguments are familiar. They address beliefs that indeed cognitively impaired people may or may not in fact do better in the presence of other people who can stimulate them or who can act as buffers to protect them by more articulately expressing the preferences of the cognitively impaired. But this integration comes at the cost of quality of life concerns for the cognitively intact people who have to live with them. A consistent complaint from nursing home residents is invasion of their physical or social privacy by people who are demented and simply uninhibited in their behavior. The quality of life for the cognitively intact is often mortgaged in an effort to improve the quality of life for the cognitively impaired.

QUALITY ASSURANCE

Quality assurance poses difficulties with regard to long-term care, and perhaps specifically with regard to dementia (Kane & Kane, 1988). We have several basic problems with quality assurance. One major deficiency is that not many people do it, although we spend an awful lot of time with quality assessment (IOM, 1986). Americans are obsessed with measuring things. We count everything. But the challenge of quality assurance is to act on the information, at least to eliminate the providers who are well below an acceptable range of performance.

Our problem as a country, as a society, is that we don't have the will or the mechanism to do much about it! It is very hard to pull a physician's license even in the face of flagrantly poor performance. A few years ago, the heads of a Texas nursing home were brought to trial for first-degree murder for repeated examples of bad quality care; they didn't get convicted or even have their licenses removed! (Long, 1987). All across the country maximally substandard homes have simply not been closed or have been given over to new management, which is very difficult to accomplish politically and logistically. In an area of scarce nursing home beds, there is always the problem of what to do with the people that you evict from those homes. The consequence is a bizarre paradox in which we pour money into bad homes in the hope of rehabilitating them. This action creates a rather perverse set of incentives; then we wonder why we don't have stronger rules.

We need a different kind of incentive system, one that goes beyond litigation, and probably beyond fines. In what is essentially a proprietary industry we should tie the payment system into some measures of quality. We can pay people for better care. To do this we need to develop a better system of accountability by changing the very basic information technology that we use daily to record information for giving care. We should not have two separate systems of records in nursing homes, one for the inspectors and one for the caregivers. We need to use that precious caregiving time to collect information that makes meaningful differences in patient care. We ought to be measuring the importance of care not on the basis of whether one meets standards of professional orthodoxy but on the basis of whether it makes a difference in the outcomes of patients. We can develop meaningful measures of outcome in long-term care.

We must become more innovative. There are steps to take now to change the system. First, we should link payment to quality. This does not imply case-mix reimbursement, which is essentially a throwback. It didn't work in the hospitals, and it is not likely to succeed in long-term care. Case-mix reimbursement essentially pays more as the patient becomes more sick or disabled. It provides exactly the perverse incentive that we want to avoid.

In contrast, we want to emphasize the outcome rather than the process. We don't know enough about the process in long-term care. We don't know what makes a difference. Rather, a variety of actors can have very positive results if they are done in the right kind of context with the right kinds of people. We want to reward good outcomes. Simply relying on good outcomes gives credit to the kinds of patients admitted. We want to reward outcomes on the basis of a comparison that adjusts for the differences in patients, that is, to compare the observed outcomes to the expected outcomes.

We have the basis to develop statistical norms of what might be expected for different types of these patients (Kane, Bell, Riegler, Wilson, & Keeler, 1983a). We can measure those outcomes in appropriate domains for long-term care. Those domains are commonly accepted as addressing physiological functioning, activities of daily living, pain and discomfort, psychological functioning, cognitive functioning, social functioning, and patient satisfaction (Kane, Bell, Riegler, Wilson, & Kane, 1983b).

Multiple measures present another problem. The ultimate question is whether the patient is comparatively better or worse. That requires a single score derived by adding up the components. To sum the components, you have to be able to weight the different domains. Weighting the different domains means assigning values to each domain, and those values ought to be generated from measures of preference. This raises a basic question that our society is just beginning to explore: "Whose values do we use?" Do we rely on the value preferences of policy makers? Patients? Caregivers? It is encouraging to discover from early study exploring this issue that there may not be great differences among the values held by these different constituencies (Kane, Bell, & Riegler, 1986).

Focusing on outcomes shifts the whole nature of the discussion about long-term care. We stop worrying about whether they should wear a white or a blue coat. Instead we address what we want from the care system. What are its goals? We then have the capacity to send a clear market signal. We are willing to put our money where our mouth is by rewarding outcomes realistically adjusted for expectations. We want to talk about what is really important.

Such a step can lead to productive dialogue. New stimulus is created to search for better ways of achieving those outcomes. Because attention is shifted to what is accomplished instead of how and where it is done, we begin to look at whether or not it is better to put people in institutions or treat them in the community, or to look at a whole variety of different kinds of mixtures of ways to do that.

TECHNOLOGIES FOR CAREGIVING

At the same time, we can begin to think about how new kinds of technologies can be tapped. The pressing question of the next decade with regard to long-term care is going to be caregiving. We are facing a major caregiver shortage, even beyond the nursing shortage. The people who give long-term care come from two basic pools. One is families. Family is a euphemism for women. Most of the informal caregivers in the United States are women. As women enter the labor force, nothing has changed. We still turn to women to provide that informal care. There is no evidence of significant countervailing increases in male caregiving. But women are pursuing a whole set of other activities and simply do not have the resources to donate their time the way they used to.

The other major source of caregivers, also women, relies on the lowest strata of our society. Throughout the Western world, the people who provide most of the care in long-term institutions and in homes as paid caregivers tend to come from the lowest social class (Kane & Kane, 1976). Often they are immigrants, and in some countries they are actually imported to give that care. They tend not to speak the language. They tend to have a very poor education. Many are functionally illiterate. We have not done very much to really try and support them, to augment them, or to make them effective in their caregiving.

The more creatively we give care, the more we begin to move out of institutions and into the home, the more difficult it is going to be to monitor those aides on the firing line. We can use information technology to solve that problem. Techniques are available to monitor the performance of aides, to help them with decision making, to provide reminders of things they ought to be doing, and to give them cues and reinforcers to guide their behaviors. We can, for example, today use a laser reader, about the size of a credit card, to read bar codes. Supermarkets use the same kind of device to read product bar codes. Imagine what can be done simply by giving every caregiver an ID badge with a bar code identifier and putting a bar code identifier on each patient's bracelet instead of just their name. Because you can build a clock into the microchip of the bar code reader, it can tell you how much time any caregiver spends with any patient. For home care you can monitor when they arrived, when they left, and what they accomplished. By putting bar codes on all the medications and programming the microchip so that giving the wrong medication to the wrong patient or giving it at the wrong time will cause unpleasant noises, you can prevent medication errors and get an unfudgeable medication record that can only be created in real time.

You can build, as we have begun to do in Minnesota, a behavioral modification system for treating incontinence by essentially maintaining toileting schedules using bar code readers as reminders and recorders. This technology essentially offers a means to make functionally illiterate people accurate record keepers. Moreover, you can use information to improve management. You can summarize care activities and inform nursing supervisors about what is going on in their units, often for the first time. You can relate patient progress to worker performance.

We are on the verge of exciting breakthroughs in terms of technology. Lap-top computers can be programmed to do or to record assessments. You can build into the assessment structure subtle changes that reinforce desired behaviors. For example, why not make asking about preferences a basic part of assessing each activity area? Such programs provide consistent information and eliminate the enormous redundancy that we get today when everybody asks the same questions. Basically, the progress can either control access by setting up identifier codes so that people can only enter information into various sections of the assessment, or you can flash the results up on the screen and say, "We've already got that information." You can change it if it is wrong, but you do not have to ask those questions again. Such an approach can reduce assessment time by 50 to 60%. It produces better information in less time, and can be printed out in many different ways, depending on who wants it and what it is for. You can use algorithms to translate problems into care plans. You can set up prompting systems keyed to problems that will tell caregivers when to make certain kinds of observations and build in a feedback system that, when the entered data fall out of expected ranges, will tell them what step to take next. This represents a major change in the way we give care.

You can link people in their homes through telephone lines into two-way interactive television sets that will allow them to enter physiological and psychological data and to query, as the worried are prone to do, as much as they want without ever having to use anybody's time. The programs can even assess the urgency of the problem and suggest when physician attention is immediate. You can put information reminders in for those patients or their families to keep them on their medication schedules. All of this is possible with current technology without spending a lot of money. These types of technological support will permit significant change in the long-term care system, such as innovative combinations of housing and care.

You can use tracking systems that will allow you unobtrusively to track people who wander. You can set up magnetic fields around doorways and essentially monitor where people are in buildings or even track them outside. There is a whole range of things that we can do with very simple technology that can reduce some of this caregiving load as we begin to face this new manpower crisis (OTA, 1987).

POLICY ISSUES

We need to think about some basic planning issues on the macro scale with regard to long-term care. A major issue of the moment is private long-term care insurance. Administrative practice too readily confuses solving a problem with making it someone else's responsibility. Thus the facile answer of how to solve the growing public cost of care is to make somebody else pay for it. Unfortunately, our society has been brainwashed into believing that those kinds of non-answers are answers. We have grown up believing that there are two sets of books: private paybooks and public paybooks, and that moving things from the public ledger to the private ledger accomplishes something. In truth, you have accomplished nothing except to inflate the total cost of care. As a society we must confront the fact that the only way to control the cost of care in this country is to put an end to the patchwork financing of health care.

How do we do that? The first task is to establish the appropriate role of public and private financing. For a variety of reasons we must look toward greater public financing. The real question is the level of government that we want to look to for that public financing. Rather than continuing to look to the federal government where we have looked up to now, we must shift attention to the state and the local levels where more and more of this will have to be delivered.

When we talk about insurance we are basically talking about three kinds of activity. Insurance protects against relatively rare events that happen with a reasonable degree of unforeseenness. If you could predict who was going to get something you would hardly want to insure those people. The strategy of insurance is pooling the risk. To pool the risk widely, a large group of people will buy the policy at a very low rate in order to make it affordable, knowing that a certain number of them, by the laws of statistics, will cash in in the future.

One problem with most private long-term care insurance has been convincing people to buy it. The only people who seem to think they are really likely to need long-term care are quite old. By that time their probability of needing it is high enough to preclude significant risk pooling. Instead you are concentrating the risk in a small number of high-risk people. The difficulty of marketing long-term care insurance has prompted attention to including it as a fringe benefit for some workers. But a concentration on this market will lead to cheaper products that exclude the high-risk elderly. This is a situation analogous to the 1960s situation with health insurance, the inciting force for Medicare.

There are basically two reasons to buy long-term care insurance. One is to buy a different kind of care than is available without long-term care insurance. The fallback position to privately paid long-term care is Medicaid. Thus one strategy to encourage private long-term care insurance is to make Medicaid so unattractive that people will be frightened into buying it privately. Making Medicaid so inhumane that anybody who could afford to buy something else would rush out to get it seems like a pretty pathetic kind of scenario to use as the basis for setting national policy.

The second reason to buy long-term care insurance is to prevent the stigma of falling back on what is essentially a welfare program. This second reason has two components. People don't want to be thought of as welfare cases, although in our society being on welfare has become much less of a stigma than it was a generation ago—some might view it as almost a natural concomitant of aging. The other reason to avoid Medicaid is because it is enforced penury. You have to divest yourself of all your assets. Thus long-term care insurance has less to do with care than with asset protection.

Do we want to make national policy based on protecting assets and to shift our discussions away from a program that is designed to provide a humane set of care for individuals at a price that everybody can afford? You can have both. Developing a universal base for the insurance that truly pools the risk provides a universal set of benefits that avoids a two-class system and still protects people's assets. Not only is it feasible, it is affordable. Universal coverage for insurance is even compatible with mechanisms for private administration. Most of the care of the Canadian long-term care system is given by private organizations. Most of them are nonprofit, although some of them are proprietary (Kane & Kane, 1985). It is possible to have public financing with private administration.

Other models have been proposed that call for some form of mixed financing in which you have voluntary contributions from individuals, perhaps on some kind of sliding scale basis, or from private corporations as part of an employee benefit package. Others have proposed a role for government in which it subsidizes purchase of private insurance or provides some kind of a stop-loss function in which the government will guarantee all risk above a certain amount.

We have not exhausted the creative options for seeking partnerships between public and private mechanisms. Nor is it clear how many will work in practice. At the same time, at least a half dozen states are considering proposals to pursue some form of private–public approach.

Greater involvement of states in delivering this kind of care begins to look increasingly attractive. We may not have the national will to pursue the panacea to solve this crisis by some kind of national effort. America may be too large and heterogeneous a country to be able to contend with all the various constituency groups. The state may be a more appropriate target to develop this type of care. International experience supports this level of scale. Most of the countries of the Western world with long-term care programs are essentially the size of our states. Although all of Canada has a population equivalent to the size of California, the Canadian system operates at the provincial level. One of the most successful provinces in terms of mounting a long-term care program is Manitoba, with a population of only about a million people. Thus a state is not too small a unit to be able to do this in economical units of scale. It is economically and administratively feasible. Even at the state level you probably would want provisions for more local control.

A state-based program will create new problems. Current funding arrangements create large incentives for states to use Medicare over Medicaid because the former is fully federal and the latter is a shared cost. States now expend great energy trading off state dollars against federal dollars. The most feasible solution will likely come from negotiating some kind of a block grant program to states that are willing to take on this program, in which the federal government would provide a lump sum payment that could then be put toward some kind of a merged system covering both acute and long-term care.

A state system would mean greater variation around the country—one of the things we tried to avoid in 1965 by developing a single standard of care under Medicare but compromised under Medicaid by leaving to the states a fair amount of latitude to vary things. Nonetheless, we could establish a reasonable national package of basic standards. It may be realistic in a country as large, populous, and geographically diverse as the United States to set up different priorities in parts of the country. Certainly it is probably more politically feasible to begin to organize at the state level, to create appropriate units of scale among constituency groups, and to think about developing the appropriate geopolitically designated units to operate these kinds of systems on what would probably be the county level.

There are different ways to run such programs. Some people argue for competition where different firms battle against each other for market shares. A preferable approach uses geopolitical kinds of utility models, very much like the public utility models we have for power and telephones, which would then hold the organization responsible for a defined population. One great fear about a competitive situation is that the firms would compete in terms of marketing their product and not in delivering services. If, then, different kinds of people are enrolled with the different firms, great efforts will be required to compare the two populations to hold their caregivers accountable. By contrast, if a firm is accountable for a defined population, one is much more likely to find comparable groups.

In either case, the level of accountability is a population, composed of enrollees or residents of an area. The test of performance is the status of the whole group, both those who use the services and those who do not. This approach looks at the whole denominator of the population at risk rather than simply looking at the numerator of the people using services.

SERVICES

To sum up, we can put to rest suggesting some shibboleths. We can at least enunciate the parameters of what we want in a long-term care system.

- We want to change the nature of eligibility. It is time to move away from a system that defines eligibility on the basis of the ability to pay and to shift toward a more universal set of standards tied into some measure of function.
- We can affirm that the family has been and will continue to be a vital, fundamental, and central source of long-term care in this country. In all of the countries in the Western world where long-term care has been covered under various forms of universal medical coverage, the family continues to provide the bulk of that care. Formal services will not displace informal care. We want a flexible plan of care that recognizes the use of informal care but does not preclude formal care because of it.
- We need to provide flexible packages of care in which a care plan responds to the needs and the abilities of both the client and the family, rather than rigid dispensing of fixed aliquots of care in a very structured and autocratic manner.
- We need to debunk the fear of the "woodwork phenomenon" that if we were to broaden eligibility for care, people would be coming out of the woodwork demanding great amounts of free care. The experience gained from social programs in many parts of the world indicates that it does not happen. Control is achieved by a system of care coordination or case management. Care coordinators need to have an independent status that allows them to purchase care from the providers, but they should not be the providers. Few care coordinators will be sufficiently altruistic to do what is best for the patient if they are also working for the company that is likely to provide part of the care. It is a little bit like sending the wolves to tend the sheep.
- We want a system that will hold those care coordinators accountable, in both fiscal and quality terms, for the kinds of services that they are authorizing

or purchasing by some kind of a geopolitical responsibility monitoring how well they are utilizing the available resources.

These are not pipe dreams but are all components of a system of care that is feasible today. They are part of the system of care that is currently in operation in eight out of the 10 provinces in Canada and could be replicated with some modifications in this country if we had what the Canadians have, namely, a national will. The Canadians have determined that it is important to offer long-term care to all the citizens in their society. In contrast the United States is known as "The Land of the Demonstration Project." No country in the world has conducted so many social experiments and has so few social programs to show for it. It is high time we begin to change that.

REFERENCES

Institute of Medicine Committee on Regulation of Nursing Homes. (1986). *Improving the Quality of Care in Nursing Homes*. Washington, DC: National Academy Press.

Kane, R. A., & Kane, R. L. (1987). *Long-Term Care: Principles, Programs, and Policies*. New York: Springer Publishing Company.

Kane, R. A., & Kane, R. L. (1988). Long-term care: Variations on a quality assurance theme. *Inquiry, 25*(1),132-144.

Kane, R. L. (1988). Beyond caring: The challenge to geriatrics. *Journal of the American Geriatrics Society* 36,467–472.

Kane, R. L., & Kane, R. A. (1976). *Long-Term Care in Six Countries: Implications for the United States*. Washington, DC: GPO, DHEW Publ. No. (NIH) 76-1207.

Kane, R. L., Bell, R., Riegler, S., Wilson, A., & Keeler, E. (1983a). Predicting the outcomes of nursing-home patients. *Gerontologist* 23(2),200–206.

Kane, R. L., Bell, R., Riegler, S., Wilson, A., & Kane, R. A. (1983b). Assessing the outcomes of nursing-home patients. *Journal of Gerontology* 38, 385–393.

Kane, R. L., & Kane, R. A. (1985). *A Will and A Way: What Americans Can Learn About Long-Term Care From Canada*. New York: Columbia University Press.

Kane, R. L., Bell, R. M., Riegler, S. Z.. (1986). Value preferences for nursing-home outcomes. *Gerontologist* 26:303–308.

Lerner, M. J., & Simmons, C. H. (1966). Observer's reaction to the "innocent victim": Compassion or rejection. *Journal of Personality and Social Psychology* 4:203–210.

Lerner, M. J., & Lichtman, P. R. (1968). Effects of perceived norms on attitudes and altruistic behavior toward a dependent other. *Journal of Personality and Social Psychology* 9;226–232.

Long, S. (1987) *Death Without Dignity*. Texas Monthly Press. Austin, TX.

Office of Technology Assessment, U.S. Congress. (1987). *Losing a million minds. Confronting the tragedy of Alzheimer's disease and other dementias*. OTA-BA-323, Washington, DC: U.S. Government Printing Office, April.

Index